Technological Advances in Dentistry and Oral Surgery

Guest Editors

HARRY DYM, DDS
ORRETT E. OGLE, DDS

DENTAL CLINICS OF NORTH AMERICA

www.dental.theclinics.com

July 2011 • Volume 55 • Number 3

SAUNDERS an imprint of ELSEVIER, Inc.

W.B. SAUNDERS COMPANY
A Division of Elsevier Inc.

1600 John F. Kennedy Boulevard • Suite 1800 • Philadelphia, Pennsylvania 19103-2899

http://www.dental.theclinics.com

DENTAL CLINICS OF NORTH AMERICA Volume 55, Number 3
July 2011 ISSN 0011-8532, ISBN-978-1-4557-1094-2

Editor: Donald Mumford; D.Mumford@elsevier.com

Dental Clinics of North America (ISSN 0011-8532) is published quarterly by Elsevier Inc., 360 Park Avenue South, New York, NY 10010-1710. Months of issue are January, April, July, and October. Business and Editorial Offices: 1600 John F. Kennedy Boulevard, Suite 1800, Philadelphia, PA 19103-2899. Periodicals postage paid at New York, NY and additional mailing offices. Subscription prices are $240.00 per year (domestic individuals), $420.00 per year (domestic institutions), $113.00 per year (domestic students/residents), $287.00 per year (Canadian individuals), $529.00 per year (Canadian institutions), $347.00 per year (international individuals), $529.00 per year (international institutions), and $170.00 per year (international and Canadian students/residents). International air speed delivery is included in all *Clinics* subscription prices. All prices are subject to change without notice. **POSTMASTER:** Send address changes to *Dental Clinics of North America*, Elsevier Health Sciences Division, Subscription Customer Service, 3251 Riverport Lane, Maryland Heights, MO 63043. **Customer Service (orders, claims, online, change of address): Elsevier Health Sciences Division, Subscription Customer Service, 3251 Riverport Lane, Maryland Heights, MO 63043. Tel: 1-800-654-2452 (U.S. and Canada). Fax: 314-447-8029. E-mail: journalscustomerservice-usa@elsevier.com (for print support); journalsonlinesupport-usa@elsevier.com (for online support).**

Reprints. For copies of 100 or more, of articles in this publication, please contact the Commercial Reprints Department, Elsevier Inc., 360 Park Avenue South, New York, NY 10010-1710. Tel.: 212-633-3812; Fax: 212-462-1935; E-mail: reprints@elsevier.com.

The Dental Clinics of North America is covered in *MEDLINE/PubMed (Index Medicus), Current Contents/Clinical Medicine, ISI/BIOMED* and *Clinahl.*

Contributors

GUEST EDITORS

HARRY DYM, DDS
Chairman of Department of Dentistry/Oral and Maxillofacial Surgery, The Brooklyn
Hospital Center, Brooklyn; Clinical Professor, Oral and Maxillofacial Surgery, Columbia
University, College of Dental Medicine, New York; Attending, Oral and Maxillofacial
Surgery, Woodhull Medical and Mental Health Center; Attending, Oral and Maxillofacial
Surgery, New York Harbor Healthcare System, The Brooklyn VA Campus, Brooklyn,
New York

ORRETT E. OGLE, DDS
Chief; Program Director, Oral and Maxillofacial Surgery, Department of Dentistry,
Woodhull Medical and Mental Health Center, Brooklyn, New York

AUTHORS

JED M. BEST, DDS, MS
Clinical Associate Professor of Dentistry, Columbia University, Division of Pediatric
Dentistry, College of Dental Medicine; Private Practice, New York, New York

ANDREA M. BONNICK, DDS
Assistant Professor and Chair, Department of Oral and Maxillofacial Surgery, Howard
University Hospital, College of Dentistry; Director, Oral and Maxillofacial Surgery Program;
Howard University Hospital, College of Dentistry, Washington, DC

GARY DAVIDOWITZ, DDS
Assistant Clinical Professor, International Advanced Aesthetic Dentistry Program; Faculty,
Department of Cariology and Comprehensive Care, New York University College of
Dentistry, New York, New York

HARRY DYM, DDS
Chairman of Department of Dentistry/Oral and Maxillofacial Surgery, The Brooklyn
Hospital Center, Brooklyn; Clinical Professor, Oral and Maxillofacial Surgery, Columbia
University, College of Dental Medicine, New York; Attending, Oral and Maxillofacial
Surgery, Woodhull Medical and Mental Health Center; Attending, Oral and Maxillofacial
Surgery, New York Harbor Healthcare System, The Brooklyn VA Campus, Brooklyn,
New York

SCOTT D. GANZ, DMD
Assistant Clinical Professor, Department of Restorative Dentistry, University
of Medicine and Dentistry, New Jersey, New Jersey Dental School, Newark;
Maxillofacial Prosthodontist, Private Practice, Fort Lee, New Jersey

ROGER GRANNUM, DDS
Former Resident, Private Practice of Oral and Maxillofacial Surgery; Department
of Dentistry, Woodhull Medical and Mental Health Center, Brooklyn, New York

JAMES GREEN, DMD
Senior Resident, Oral and Maxillofacial Surgery, The Brooklyn Hospital Center, Brooklyn, New York

DAVID HUANG, DDS
OMFS Resident, Department of Dentistry/Oral Maxillofacial Surgery, The Brooklyn Hospital Center, Brooklyn, New York

AMANDIP KAMOH, DDS
Chief Resident, Oral and Maxillofacial Surgery, Woodhull Medical and Mental Health Center, Brooklyn, New York

ALAN KLEIMAN, DMD
Departments of Oral and Maxillofacial Surgery and Community Health, New Jersey Dental School, University of Medicine and Dentistry of New Jersey, Newark; Private Practice, Moorestown, New Jersey

PHILIP G. KOTICK, DDS
Faculty, Department of Cariology and Comprehensive Care; Assistant Clinical Professor, International Comprehensive Dentistry Program, New York University College of Dentistry, New York, New York; Fellow International Congress of Oral Implantology

GHAZAL MAHJOUBI, DMD
Resident, Oral and Maxillofacial Surgery, Department of Dentistry, Woodhull Medical and Mental Health Center, Brooklyn, New York

RORY E. MORTMAN, DDS
Co-Chairman, Endodontic Section, Atlantic Coast Dental Research Clinic, Lake Worth; Private Practice, West Palm Beach, Florida

MARK NALBANDIAN, DDS
Assistant Professor, Department of Orthodontics, Howard University College of Dentistry, Washington, DC

ORRETT E. OGLE, DDS
Chief; Program Director, Oral and Maxillofacial Surgery, Department of Dentistry, Woodhull Medical and Mental Health Center, Brooklyn, New York

ANABELLA OQUENDO, DDS
Instructor, Department of Cariology and Comprehensive Care; Advanced Program for International Dentists in Interdisciplinary Dentistry, New York University College of Dentistry, New York, New York

ORVILLE PALMER, MD, MPH, FRCSC
Chief, Division of Otolaryngology, Head and Neck Surgery, Department of Surgery, Harlem Hospital Center, New York, New York

JOSEPH PIERSE, DMD, MA
Resident, Department of Dentistry, Oral and Maxillofacial Surgery, The Brooklyn Hospital Center, Brooklyn, New York

GLENN K. ROCHLEN, DDS
Clinical Assistant Professor, Department of Cariology and Comprehensive Care, New York University College of Dentistry, New York, New York

FRANCES E. SAM, DDS
Assistant Professor, Department of Oral and Maxillofacial Surgery, Howard University College of Dentistry, Washington, DC

JOSH SHAGAM, BS (Biomedical Photographic Communications)
Visiting Lecturer, Department of Biomedical Photographic Communications, Rochester Institute of Technology, Rochester, New York

MARIANNE S. SIEWE, DDS, MS
Assistant Professor, Department of Orthodontics, Howard University College of Dentistry, Washington, DC

AVICHAI STERN, DDS
Attending, Department of Dentistry and Oral and Maxillofacial Surgery, The Brooklyn Hospital Center, Brooklyn, New York

JASON SWANTEK, DDS
Chief Resident, Oral and Maxillofacial Surgery, Woodhull Medical and Mental Health Center, Brooklyn, New York

RICHARD D. TRUSHKOWSKY, DDS
Associate Clinical Professor, Department of Cariology and Comprehensive Care; Associate Program Director, Advanced Program for International Dentists in Aesthetic Dentistry; Program Director, Advanced Program for International Dentists in Interdisciplinary Dentistry, New York University College of Dentistry, New York, New York

RAM M. VADERHOBLI, DDS, MS
Clinical X Assistant Professor; Assistant Program Director, AEGD Residency Program, Department of Preventive and Restorative Dentistry, University of California San Francisco, San Francisco, California

ADAM WEISS, DDS
Senior Resident, Departments of Dentistry and Oral and Maxillofacial Surgery, The Brooklyn Hospital Center, Brooklyn, New York

JOSHUA WOLF, DDS
Resident, Department of Oral and Maxillofacial Surgery, The Brooklyn Hospital Center, Brooklyn, New York

MARK S. WOLFF, DDS, PhD
Professor and Chair, Department of Cariology and Comprehensive Care, New York University College of Dentistry, New York, New York

EDMUND WUN, DDS
OMFS Chief Resident, Department of Dentistry/Oral Maxillofacial Surgery, The Brooklyn Hospital Center, Brooklyn, New York

RICHARD K. YOON, DDS
Associate Professor of Clinical Dentistry and Program Director, Residency in Pediatric Dentistry, Division of Pediatric Dentistry, Columbia University, College of Dental Medicine, New York, New York

Contents

optical occurrence tomography are 2 new imaging technologies that can assist the practitioner in the diagnosis of pulpal disease. The self-adjusting file and the Apexum device can be used for instrumentation and bulk debridement of an apical lesion, respectively. Neodymium:yttrium-aluminum-garnet laser, erbium:chromium:yttrium-scandium-gallium-garnet laser, EndoActivator, EndoVac, and light-activated disinfection may assist the practitioner in cleaning the root canal system. Computed tomography-guided surgery shows promise in making endodontic surgery easier, as does mineral trioxide aggregate cement for regenerative endodontic procedures.

Local pain management is the most critical aspect of patient care in dentistry. The improvements in agents and techniques for local anesthesia are probably the most significant advances that have occurred in dental science. This article provides an update on the most recently introduced local anesthetic agents along with new technologies used to deliver local anesthetics. Safety devices are also discussed, along with an innovative method for reducing the annoying numbness of the lip and tongue following local anesthesia.

There have been several exciting technological advances in extraction techniques and outpatient oral surgery within the last decade. A variety of new instruments and techniques are revolutionizing the fields of oral and maxillofacial surgery and dentistry. This article reviews the newer innovations in dentistry including the powered periotome, piezosurgery, the Physics Forceps, laser therapy, orthodontic techniques, and use of polyurethane foam.

Computed tomography (CT) and cone-beam CT (CBCT) technology allows three-dimensional evaluation of each patient's individual anatomy. This article highlights the presurgical planning phase of dental implant procedures that benefit from lower dose CBCT technology so that educated treatment decisions can be accurately determined. Clinicians should gain an understanding of how each view can be individually significant, with unique levels of detail helping to provide a comprehensive overview of the patient's anatomic presentation. This article outlines the benefits of using CBCT technology for dental implant applications for increased accuracy and avoidance of potential surgical and restorative complications.

There are approximately 21,000 new cases of oral cancer every year. Although the oral cavity is relatively accessible to examination, malignant

processes tend to present late with poor prognosis. To improve tumor outcome, early detection and treatment is essential. This article reviews the
realms of oral cancer and its causes, as well as early detection methods
and screening technologies that may be used. Currently available screening tools may help in visualizing an existing lesion or its borders, but they
add little in discriminating between a premalignant, malignant, or inflammatory process.

The role of computers in dental practice has dramatically changed over the
past 30 years. We have witnessed the progression from administrative roles
to complete integration leading to chartless offices. As the dental community gradually adopts this contemporary development, the move to electronic health records is imminent because of upcoming changes in the
health care system. The past, present, and future of dental office computer
systems is explored in this article. An understanding of the benefits and current challenges of contemporary dental practice software is also reviewed.

Computer-aided design (CAD) and computer-aided manufacturing (CAM)
have become an increasingly popular part of dentistry over the past 25
years. The technology, which is used in both the dental laboratory and
the dental office, can be applied to inlays, onlays, veneers, crowns, fixed
partial dentures, implant abutments, and even full-mouth reconstruction.
This article discusses the history of CAD/CAM in dentistry and gives an
overview of how it works. It also provides information on the advantages
and disadvantages, describes the main products available, discusses
how to incorporate the new technology into your practice, and addresses
future applications.

New technological advances have helped the orthodontic profession
progress in traditional and surgical methods of treatment. The profession
has seen transitions from traditional braces to self-ligating brackets, lingual braces, removable aligners, and more advanced technology, which
have helped to address concerns that include but are not limited to better
diagnostics, anchorage control, length of treatment, and esthetics. An increase in the number of adult patients seeking orthodontic treatment and
the need for a timely efficient care will continue to drive technology and the
use of cone beam computed tomography, miniscrews, piezocision, distraction osteogenesis, and bioengineering.

Advances in technology are changing the ways that patients experience
dental treatment. Technology helps to decrease treatment time and makes

the treatment more comfortable for the patient. One technological advance is the use of lasers in dentistry. Lasers are providing more efficient, more comfortable, and more predictable outcomes for patients. Lasers are used in all aspects of dentistry, including operative, periodontal, endodontic, orthodontic, and oral and maxillofacial surgery. Lasers are used for soft and hard tissue procedures in the treatment of pathologic conditions and for esthetic procedures. This article discusses how lasers work and their application in the various specialties within dentistry.

Dentinal hypersensitivity is exemplified by brief, sharp, well-localized pain in response to thermal, evaporative, tactile, osmotic, or chemical stimuli that cannot be ascribed to any other form of dental defect or pathology. Pulpal pain is usually more prolonged, dull, aching, and poorly localized and lasts longer than the applied stimulus. Up to 30% of adults have dentinal hypersensitivity at some time. Current techniques for treatment may be only transient in nature and results are not always predictable. Two methods of treatment of dentin hypersensitivity are tubular occlusion and blockage of nerve activity. A differential diagnosis needs to be accomplished before any treatment.

In light of preoperative and postoperative mortality and morbidity, continued advancement in pain and anxiety management would benefit millions. Although significant strides have been made in the past few decades, it is imperative that research and development continue. This article discusses types of pain and anxiety, the relationship between pain and anxiety, the physiology of pain and anxiety, and current trends in pain and anxiety management.

The use of materials to rehabilitate tooth structures is constantly changing. Over the past decade, newer material processing techniques and technologies have significantly improved the dependability and predictability of dental material for clinicians. The greatest obstacle, however, is in choosing the right combination for continued success. Finding predictable approaches for successful restorative procedures has been the goal of clinical and material scientists. This article provides a broad perspective on the advances made in various classes of dental restorative materials in terms of their functionality with respect to pit and fissure sealants, glass ionomers, and dental composites.

Digital photography is a constantly evolving medium that can be used in dentistry for a number of applications including documentation and patient education. In the past 5 years, it has become standard professional practice for photographers to shoot in raw format, organize and edit in Adobe Photoshop Lightroom, and archive files using portable hard drives and offsite storage. Concurrently, cameras have increased resolution, improved antidust technology, and added versatile flash accessories for macro imaging. Adopting professional photographic practices and taking advantage of technological developments in a dental practice can be an invaluable tool in education and documentation.

The technologic advances in temporomandibular joint arthroscopy and arthrocentesis have given oral surgeons a treatment for patients who have not responded to conservative and pharmacologic treatment without the surgical risks and long-term recovery of open joint surgery.

FORTHCOMING ISSUES

RECENT ISSUES

THE CLINICS ARE NOW AVAILABLE ONLINE!

Access your subscription at:
www.theclinics.com

Preface

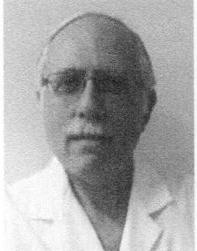 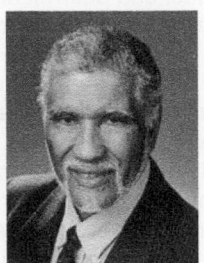

Harry Dym, DDS   Orrett E. Ogle, DDS
Guest Editors

"Progress is impossible without change and those who cannot change their minds cannot change anything"
—*George Bernard Shaw*

I attended dental school over thirty-five years ago, and like all other dental schools during that time period, we were mired in the past. Copper band impression techniques, zinc phosphate cements, and other traditional well-entrenched historical techniques and procedures were the order of the day and our prosthetic and operative instructors would shoot down any suggestions of even trying anything new and different. Academic clinical leadership was almost always led by older individuals who were suckled on the words of Dr G.V. Black, who thought that any deviations from our time-honored traditions were almost heretical in nature.

I agree with the author Tom Clancy, who wrote, "the human condition today is better than it's ever been and technology is one of the reasons for that."

Dentistry, like medicine, has seen a monumental growth in technology these past few decades and our profession and our patients are much better off as a result. Our patients have embraced technology in their business and personal use and expect no less from the dental profession. Those general dentists and dental specialists who incorporate new technological advances in their daily clinical practice will experience renewed enthusiasm, better clinical outcomes, and enhanced patient satisfaction.

This text includes much of the new technologies, which may already have been incorporated by many practitioners into their practice, and was not meant to be all inclusive. We hope the reader finds this issue useful and informative and that it stimulates many to pursue these technological advancements in their clinical practice.

We are certain that in the next decade will bring newer technologies such as chairside DNA salivary diagnoses of systemic diseases, robotic-guided oral surgery and dentistry, stem cell regenerative procedures, etc, that will further change the clinical practice of dentistry and oral surgery.

The editors are also keenly aware that many technological advances are viewed as controversial and that there will be those who fear it, talk against it, and even mock it; failure is not fatal but a failure to change one's views or procedures might be.

Dent Clin N Am 55 (2011) xiii–xiv
doi:10.1016/j.cden.2011.04.001
0011-8532/11/$ – see front matter

Harry Dym would like to take this opportunity to thank the following people:

1. Peter M. Sherman, DDS—mentor, colleague, and dear friend for over thirty-one years. A true leader and visionary in dentistry and oral maxillofacial surgery education for over four decades.
2. Orrett Ogle, DDS—my co-editor, who is also a cherished colleague and dear friend that I first met when I was a resident and he was an attending in my Oral and Maxillofacial Surgery residency program, thirty years ago. He is a true human-itarian and a teacher dedicated to resident education and humane patient care. It has been a privilege for me to have worked with him again in this endeavor.
3. Earl Clarkson, DDS—a colleague and friend for over thirty years—who leads by quiet example and is a role model for our oral and maxillofacial surgery residents and dental students.
4. Richard Becker, MD—Chief Executive Officer and President of The Brooklyn Hospital Center, who continues to lead the fight for quality patient care in a time of financial constraints.
5. Paul Albertson—Chief Operating Officer of The Brooklyn Hospital Center, for his ongoing friendship and commitment to total patient care.
6. J. Carlos Naudon and The Board of Trustees at The Brooklyn Hospital Center, for their strong commitment to Dentistry and Oral and Maxillofacial Surgery and their dedication and sacrifice on behalf of the communities we serve.
7. Ms Jennifer Nimako, Mrs Gloria Stallings, and Mr Felipe DeJesus, for their ongoing administrative/office management support.
8. George Harris and The Lucius N. Littauer Foundation, for their continued support to our residency educational programs and to the community patients we serve.
9. Donald Mumford—Editor for the *Dental Clinics of North America*, for his guidance.
10. Benson Yeh, MD—Vice President of Academic Affairs at The Brooklyn Hospital Center, for his dedication and enthusiasm for graduate medical/dental education.
11. My attending staff, Dr Ricardo Boyce, Dr Michael Chan, Dr Avichai Stern, who helped ease my clinical burden and allowed me the time to pursue my academic interests.
12. My wife, Freidy, and my family, for their continued support of all my endeavors.
13. My residents, who continue to teach me on a daily basis.

Finally, my sincerest thanks to all our authors, who have all done an outstanding job in elucidating the new technological advancements in the field of dentistry and oral surgery/medicine.

Harry Dym, DDS
Department of Dentistry/Oral and Maxillofacial Surgery
The Brooklyn Hospital Center
121 DeKalb Avenue
Brooklyn, NY 11201, USA

Orrett E. Ogle, DDS
Oral and Maxillofacial Surgery, Department of Dentistry
Woodhull Medical and Mental Health Center
760 Broadway
Brooklyn, NY 11206, USA

E-mail addresses:
hdymdds@yahoo.com (H. Dym)
Orrett.Ogle@WoodhullHC.NYCHHC.org (O.E. Ogle)

Advances in Pediatric Dentistry

Richard K. Yoon, DDS[a],*, Jed M. Best, DDS, MS[a,b]

KEYWORDS

- Caries detection diagnostic imaging tools • Early interventions
- Primary prevention • Caries-risk assessments
- Dental materials • Pediatric procedures

The use of new technology is shifting the practice of dentistry. New imaging devices, restorative procedures, and the application of the Internet and powerful electronic devices are examples of advances that have made a foremost impact on dentistry. Even though pediatric dentists may not have as many new tools of treatments compared with dentistry colleagues, their practices have nonetheless been improved significantly in recent years by advancements. Newer-generation imaging devices have allowed us to view details of the dental anatomy that heretofore were not visible to us before. This article summarizes the current state of pediatric dentistry.

CARIES DETECTION DIAGNOSTIC/IMAGING TOOLS

Early detection is crucial in the management of dental caries. When detected at an early stage at which the enamel surface has not collapsed, the incipient lesion can be treated with preventative therapies that can retard and eventually arrest the progression of early lesions and preserve the enamel tooth structure, function, and aesthetics.

Traditionally, a subjective method of visual inspection has been used as the most ubiquitous caries detection method. Key features, such as color and texture, are assessed. The assessment indicates some information on the severity of the caries process but falls short of true quantification. In addition to its limited detection threshold, the ability of this assessment to detect early, noncavitated lesions is poor.[1]

To meet the challenges in dentistry, there is a tremendous need for a range of caries detection and quantification systems to augment the practitioner's diagnostic pathway.[2] A range of relatively new detection systems, including diagnodent laser device (KaVo, Biberach, Germany), digital imaging fiber-optic transillumination (DIFOTI, KaVo Dental, Lake Zurich, IL, USA), and quantitative light-induced fluorescence (QLF, QLF-clin, Inspektor Research Systems BV, Amsterdam, Netherlands),

---

The authors have nothing to disclose.
a Division of Pediatric Dentistry, Columbia University, College of Dental Medicine, 722 West 168th Street, New York, NY 10032, USA
b Private Practice, 180 West End Avenue, New York, NY 10023, USA
* Corresponding author. CDM–Pediatrics, 722 West 168th Street, Room 8, New York, NY 10032.
E-mail address: rky1@columbia.edu

Dent Clin N Am 55 (2011) 419–432
doi:10.1016/j.cden.2011.02.004
0011-8532/11/$ – see front matter © 2011 Elsevier Inc. All rights reserved.

are considered as possible supplemental techniques for detecting incipient carious lesions.

Diagnodent Laser Device

Many studies have demonstrated that the diagnodent device is a valuable addition to the clinical examination and appropriate also for longitudinal monitoring of the occlusal and smooth surface caries process because of its objective readings.[3–5]

The device emits fluorescence after application of pulsed red light with a wavelength of 655 nm, and the fluorescence emitted from the tooth is translated into a numerical scale from 0 to 99.[6] When irradiated by light of a given wavelength, the tooth surface fluoresces.[7] The laser light is absorbed by organic and inorganic substances present in the dental tissues and also by metabolites from oral bacteria. It is these metabolites that result in the red fluorescence of carious dentin.[8] There is a baseline fluorescence level for sound enamel and a different fluorescence level after the caries process has initiated. It has been shown that deeper and hence more demineralized lesions have a higher fluorescence reading at the surface of the tooth. Nonetheless, whether this increased reading corresponds to an increased bacterial load within the lesion has yet to be demonstrated.[3]

DIFOTI

Different diagnostic tools, including digital bitewing radiographs, fiber-optic transillumination (FOTI), and DIFOTI, are used for a more accurate and reliable diagnosis for interproximal carious lesions. The basic principle behind transillumination is that demineralized areas of enamel or dentin scatter light more than sound areas of enamel and dentin.[9]

The system of FOTI is made of a high intensity light and a gray scale camera that can be fitted with 1 of 2 heads; one for smooth surfaces and one for occlusal surfaces. Images can then be displayed on a computer monitor and be archived for later examination. However, quantification of the images is not possible, and hence the analysis is to be undertaken in conjunction with a visual examination by the clinician who has to decide subjectively based on the appearance of scattering. Because there are no continuous data outputted, longitudinal monitoring is not possible. Therefore, some degree of training is recommended to be competent at this level of FOTI use.[10]

Digital imaging is a more recent development combining FOTI with a charge-coupled digital intraoral camera.[10] This technology involves light, a charge-coupled device camera, and a computer-controlled image acquisition. Digital imaging's advantages over traditional radiography include the absence of ionizing radiation, the lack of a need for film, real-time diagnosis, and higher sensitivity in detection of early lesions that are not apparent in radiography.[10]

QLF

QLF is a visible light system that offers an opportunity for early detection of caries and also its longitudinal monitoring. With 2 forms of fluorescent detection, green and red, QLF can determine if a lesion is active or not and can document the progression of any given lesion. Here, the visible light has a wavelength of 370 nm, which is in the blue region of the spectrum. The resultant autofluorescence of human enamel is then detected by filtering out the excitation light using a bandpass filter at a wavelength greater than 540 nm via a small intraoral camera, which produces an image of only green and red channels because blue light has been filtered out. The color of the enamel is green and the demineralization of enamel results in a reduction of this autofluorescence. The loss can then be quantified with proprietary software.[11,12]

Live images are displayed via a computer, and the accompanying software enables the patient's details to be entered and the individual images of the teeth of interest to be captured and stored. The captured images can be analyzed to quantitatively assess demineralization. The images can be stored and transmitted for referral purposes if needed. The images could also be used as patient motivators as well. This device is one of the most promising technologies in the caries detection presently despite the fact that further research is required to demonstrate its ability to correctly monitor lesion changes over time.[2]

Optical Coherence Tomography

There are several other techniques for detecting caries using optical methods. Systems such as optical coherence tomography (OCT) and near-infrared imaging OCT are in their infancy but may prove useful in the future.[13] There is significant work involved in developing these systems into clinically and commercially acceptable applications, and so, it may be some time until these new methodologies can be properly assessed in clinical trials.

EARLY INTERVENTIONS TO PREVENT DISEASES PROGRESSION

Although dental disease is preventable, its effect ranges from a minor inconvenience requiring restorative treatment to discomfort and loss of function. The role of bacterial plaque in caries causation is clear, yet strategies at eliminating specific microorganisms have proven to be difficult. The benefits of the use of topical antimicrobials and the use of topical fluorides in a wide array of formulations and methods of delivery are accepted by the pediatric scientific and practicing community. Remineralization strategies other than fluoride as well as the use of high-concentration fluoride preparations intended to slow the dental caries process are addressed.

Antiseptics

A topical antiseptic prevents or arrests the growth or action of microorganisms when applied to living tissues. Antiseptics have a considerably broader spectrum of activity than antibiotics. Unlike antibiotics, antiseptics have multiple intracellular targets that reduce the likelihood of resistance development. However, antiseptics application should be limited to infected wounds, skin, and mucosa.[14] There are studies on the utility of antiseptic agents to slow progression of caries in older self-compliant patients.[15,16] Some clinicians are advocates of combining antimicrobials and topical fluorides to provide more comprehensive protection against the caries progression process in young children.[17]

Chlorhexidine Digluconate

Chlorhexidine (CHX) rinses are biguanide antimicrobials with broad-spectrum antimicrobial properties that have been used as a first defense in treating dental caries.[18] At present, several CHX rinses are available commercially that differ in formulation, and the regimen of use is United States Food and Drug Administration (FDA) approved for gingivitis control. The 0.12% and 0.2% commercial formulations when rinsed according to the respective manufacturer's instructions produced similar large and prolonged reductions in salivary bacterial counts.[19] At present, no formulation has the FDA approval for caries control in children.[20] Besides the antiplaque and antigingivitis activities, the formulation is also effective in the prevention of infectious complications of oral origin.[21]

Research on the effectiveness of a CHX varnish coating has shown mixed results. A systematic review of 14 publications of controlled clinical trials concluded that there was a moderate caries-reducing effect when the varnish was applied every 3 months.[22] At present, the evidence is inconclusive regarding CHX varnishes and CHX-containing vehicles; no products for children are available in the United States.[20] Although CHX is being considered as the gold standard for antiplaque and antigingivitis agents, it is noted that the side effects of CHX include staining of teeth and poor taste.[23]

Povidone-Iodine

Iodine has been used for more than 150 years in mucosal antisepsis, therapies for skin infections and burns, and wound management. As povidone-iodine (PI) was introduced in the 1960s, it was possible to use this highly efficient microbicide for bacterial, fungal, and viral infections.[24]

Intraorally, short durations of PI contact with various periodontopathic bacteria are effective in in vitro killing and exhibit marked anticytomegaloviral activity.[25,26] PI is water soluble and hence does not irritate healthy oral mucosa. PI does not show adverse side effects, such as discoloration of teeth and tongue and change in taste sensation as noted with CHX.[23] Small-scale studies of PI utility in young children, some with established active early childhood caries, demonstrate promising data.[27-30] Contraindications are patients with iodine hypersensitivity and thyroid pathosis, as well as pregnant and nursing women for protection of the infant[30]; however, more studies need to be followed.

Topical Fluorides

Professionally applied topical fluorides are used restrictively in dental offices and may be supplied in solutions, gels, varnishes, foams, or prophylactic pastes. Fluoride can be applied using different methods: 1100-ppm fluoride dentifrice, 5000-ppm fluoride gels and foams, 223-ppm fluoride rinse, and 23,000-ppm fluoride varnish. Fluoride's basic mode of action, which is well established, is to enhance remineralization and simultaneously inhibit demineralization.[31] Fluoride ions are incorporated into remineralizing enamel/dentin, changing carbonated apatite to a fluorapatitelike form that is more acid tolerant and makes the hard tissues more acid resistant. Further, fluoride inhibits bacterial intracellular enzymes.

Fluoride varnish

Sodium fluoride varnishes are being used for caries arrest in children, and data suggest that these using this varnish is more effective that older technologies.[32,33] Varnishes are safe for at-risk infants and toddlers and provide an easy-to-use fluoride vehicle for young children. Although varnishes are being adopted in public health dental-medical settings, its use in private dental settings lags.[20]

Silver diamine fluoride

Historically, silver has been used in water purification, wound care, bone prostheses, reconstructive orthopedic surgery, cardiac devices, catheters, and surgical appliances. Advancing biotechnology has enabled incorporation of ionizable silver into fabrics for clinical use to reduce the risk of nosocomial infections and for personal hygiene.[34]

Silver diamine fluorides (SDFs) can be used to halt the cariogenic process and further prevent new caries with silver salt–stimulated sclerotic or calcified dentin formation,[35] silver nitrate's potent germicidal effect,[36-38] and fluoride's ability to reduce decay.[33] The antimicrobial action of silver compounds is proportional to the bioactive silver ion released and the availability of the ion to interact with bacterial or fungal cell membranes.[34] The specific interest in SDF centers around its presumed attributes[39]: control of pain and infection, ease and simplicity of use (paint on), affordability of material, minimal requirement for personnel time and training, and noninvasiveness. The side effects of SDF include teeth staining and unpleasant poor taste.

A 38% (44,800-ppm fluoride ions) SDF solution is commonly used to arrest caries in primary teeth, especially of those children who are young and less cooperative. In these cases, SDF allows definitive restoration to be performed when these children grow older and become more receptive to dental procedures.[34,40] Research has demonstrated the value of SDF to both arrest and prevent caries recurrence. Current evidence suggests that SDF is 2 times as effective as sodium fluoride varnish[41,42]; however, further research is needed to learn how the compound works.

Calcium phosphate fluoride

There are developing, interesting, and novel remineralizing agents, such as casein phosphopeptide–amorphous calcium phosphate, formulated as professionally applied pastes and toothpastes. Two studies have demonstrated increased incorporation of fluoride ions into the enamel subsurface to promote remineralization of incipient lesions.[43,44] More studies on early control of dental caries in young children are needed. These remineralizing agents may complement and increase the established clinical effectiveness of topical fluorides.

Xylitol

Xylitol is a naturally occurring alcohol sugar that is not metabolized by *Streptococcus mutans* (mutans streptococci [MS]). Xylitol inhibits the attachment of the biofilm and interferes with intracellular metabolism.[45] Xylitol is available in many forms: gum, lozenges, mints, sprays, rinses, pastes, and a baking substitute for sugar or other sweeteners.[45] Studies indicate that a dose of 6 g to 10 g per day significantly reduces levels of MS.[46] Patients should also be cautioned that xylitol can create gastrointestinal distress at high levels of consumption.[47] The American Academy of Pediatric Dentistry (AAPD) supports the use of xylitol chewing gum as a caries inhibitor but recommends further research.[47] Two key studies demonstrated that when mothers of very young children chewed high-content xylitol gum, their children had delayed colonization and lower levels of MS and reduced caries experience.[48,49]

Sealants

Among school-aged children, most dental caries has been detected on pit and fissure surfaces of their first and second molars. Occlusal sealants were introduced in the 1960s for protecting pits and fissures from dental caries.[50] At present, there are 2 main types of sealant materials available: resin-based sealants and glass ionomer cements.[51] The resin-based sealants are divided into generations according to their mechanism for polymerization or their content. The development of sealants has progressed from first-generation sealants (no longer available) to second- and third-generation sealants, which are autopolymerized and visible light activated, and finally to fourth-generation sealants containing fluoride. The effectiveness of resin-based sealants has been shown,[52] and the effectiveness depends on the longevity of sealant coverage.[53] The second main type of sealant material is glass ionomer cements that were introduced in 1974.[54] The results of studies using glass ionomer sealants have thus far been conflicting. The main disadvantage of glass ionomer sealant has been inadequate retention. Nevertheless, it has been suggested that glass ionomer sealants, through their fluoride release, can prevent the development of caries even after the visible loss of sealant material.[55]

RISK ASSESSMENTS

There is a range of risk assessments accessible today to determine the risk status of young children for dental caries: (1) tools that determine risk level based primarily on a set of factors on a child patient's history and (2) tools that use technology by assessing outcome measures as determinants of a child patient's risk for dental caries.

The AAPD Caries-Risk Assessment Tool

A clinician can assess a risk and provide a risk score by which to manage the disease in a specialized way based on the individual patient from examining the historical, environmental, and behavioral factors that relate to the initiation and progression of caries. For children, the AAPD developed an evidence-based screening tool called the caries-risk assessment tool (CAT) that identifies the risk of caries.[56,57] However, hypersensitivity toward and overdetection of high-risk individuals may occur because of mixed population factors, which may lead to overtreatment if not placed into the context of an overall accurate diagnosis.[58]

QLF

The QLF may be a useful risk assessment tool because of its ability to detect caries at a very early stage via light transmission to evoke fluorescence and its ability to monitor the progression of a carious lesion. Fluoresced tooth data from an image of the tooth surface are retrieved, and demineralization is calculated. The software provides detailed analysis of the tooth surface and can overlap scans over previous scans to identify the effects of early interventions over time and may be useful to generate individualized caries management plans for the child patient.[58]

TRENDS IN PEDIATRIC PROCEDURES AND DENTAL MATERIALS

Maintaining the integrity and health of the oral tissues is the major objective of pulpal treatment. It is desirable to maintain pulp vitality wherever possible. Pulp autolysis can be stabilized and maintained by different conservative treatments, or the pulp can be entirely eliminated. Current research in understanding cellular changes during tissue repair offers the opportunity to assess the biologic validity of various pulp treatments.[59] The aim of vital pulp therapy is to treat reversible pulpal injuries in primary teeth, maintaining pulp vitality and function.[60] In addition to these, in primary teeth, it is important to preserve the tooth until its natural exfoliation time, thus preserving arch integrity.[59] Vital pulp therapy includes 2 therapeutic approaches: indirect pulp treatment (IPT) in cases of deep dentinal cavities or pulpotomy in cases of a carious pulp exposure.[60]

IPT

Consequently, IPT can be an acceptable procedure for primary teeth with reversible pulp inflammation, provided that the diagnosis is based on a careful history taking and an accurate clinical and radiographic examination and if the restoration is free of marginal leakage.[59] This type of vital pulp therapy aims to treat reversible pulpal injury in cases in which dentin and pulp are affected by caries because the dental pulp possesses the ability to form tertiary dentin as part of the repair in the dentin-pulp organ.[61]

Fuks[62] presents that whenever the dentin-pulp system is affected by caries, 3 physiopathologic conditions may be observed at the dentin-pulp border as shown in **Fig. 1**. In mild carious injuries as in noncavitated enamel caries or slowly progressing dentinal caries, the odontoblasts responsible for matrix secretion is stimulated to form a tertiary

	Type	Response	Tubular Structure	Treatment
1	Mild	Reactionary	Continuous	IPT
2	Advanced	Reparative	Reduced Permeability	IPT
3	Advanced	Reparative	Not continuous	Pulpotomy

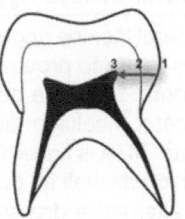

Fig. 1. Dentin response to caries. (1) In noncavitated enamel caries or slowly progressing dentinal caries, the odontoblasts responsible for matrix secretion are stimulated to form a tertiary or reactionary dentin matrix beneath the injury. (2) Advanced carious injuries without pulp exposure, odontoblasts may be damaged subjacent to the affected dentin. If suitable conditions exist within the dentin-pulp complex, odontoblastlike cells might differentiate and form tubular tertiary dentin or reparative dentin. (3) Pulp exposure caused by caries shows a narrow potential for healing as a result of bacterial infection and compromises the defense reaction.

or reactionary dentin matrix beneath the injury. Reactionary dentin shows many similarities to the primary dentin matrix and can effectively oppose exogenous destructive stimuli to protect the pulp.[63]

With advanced carious injuries without pulp exposure, odontoblasts may be damaged subjacent to the affected dentin.[62,63] If suitable conditions exist within the dentin-pulp complex, odontoblastlike cells might differentiate and form tubular tertiary dentin or reparative dentin.[61,64] Under clinical conditions, the matrix formed at the pulp-dentin interface often comprises reactionary dentin or reparative dentin formation and it is impossible to distinguish these processes at the in vivo level. Pulp exposure caused by caries shows a very narrow potential for healing as a result of bacterial infection and compromises the defense reaction.[65]

Ricketts and colleagues[66] conclude that, "in deep lesions, partial caries removal is preferable to complete caries removal to reduce the risk of carious exposure." Four articles have reported the success of this practice in primary teeth.[67–70] On the basis of the biologic changes previously described by Fuks[62] and the growing evidence of IPT success in the primary dentition, IPT may be the most suitable treatment of symptom-free primary teeth with deep caries, provided that the tooth is restored with a leakage-free restoration.

TRENDS IN PEDIATRIC DRESSING MATERIALS

Formocresol has been the most popular pulp dressing material for pulpotomized primary molars for many years, but, for reasons, the use of formocresol is decreasing considerably worldwide.

Ferric Sulfate

More recently, ferric sulfate has been subjected to long-term prospective randomized clinical trials with appropriate inferential statistical analysis and demonstrated equivalency to the formocresol pulpotomy and a wider margin of safety.[71–73] Ferric sulfate produces a local but reversible inflammatory response in oral soft tissues without toxic or harmful effects.[74] In pediatric dentistry, ferric sulfate is widely used in pulpotomy procedures of primary teeth.

Mineral Trioxide Aggregate

Mineral trioxide aggregate (MTA) promises to be one of the most versatile dental materials that also prove to promote healing of pulp wounds in the coronal or apical part of a tooth. MTA is a powder composed of tricalcium silicate, bismuth oxide, dicalcium silicate, tricalcium aluminate, tetracalcium aluminoferrite, and calcium sulfate dehydrate. MTA is known for its physical properties and its ability to stimulate tissue regeneration as well as good pulp response.[75] In pediatric dentistry, MTA can be used as an alternative dressing material for pulpotomy of primary molars with the features of stimulating cytokine release from bone cells, inducing hard tissue formation, having a dentinogenic effect on the pulp, having antimicrobial properties, and maintaining pulp integrity after pulp capping and pulpotomy without cytotoxic effect.[76–79]

TRENDS IN PEDIATRIC RESTORATIVE MATERIALS

Although stainless steel crowns, composites, and compomers remain the major restorative materials in pediatric dentistry, an important advancement in materials

---

Box 1
Current tools and technology available

Caries detection diagnostic tools

  Diagnodent

  DIFOTI

  QLF

Early interventions to slow and arrest disease progression

  Antiseptics

  CHX digluconate

  PI

  Topical fluorides

  • Fluoride varnish

  • SDF

  • Calcium phosphate fluoride

  Xylitol

  Sealants

Risk assessment tools

  CAT (AAPD), history data based

  QLF, technology data based

Procedures

  IPTs

Dressing materials

  Ferric sulfate

  MTA

Restorative materials

  RMGIs

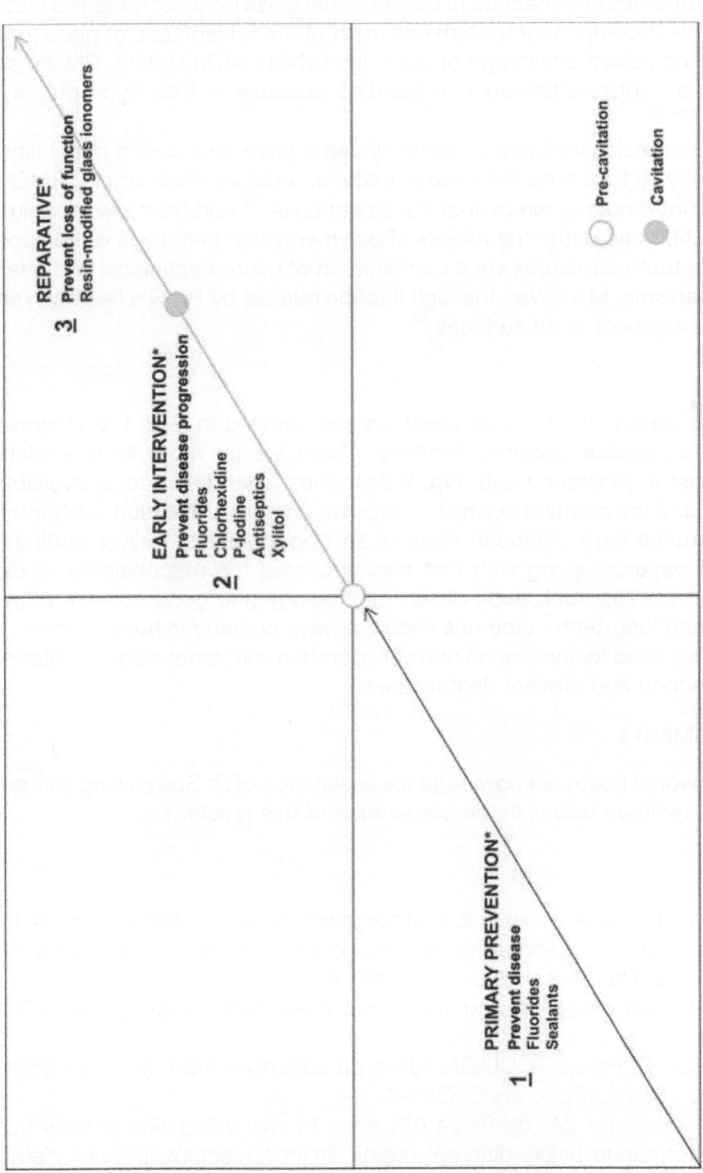

Fig. 2. Moments (*asterisk*) of intervention in the caries disease process. (1) Topical fluorides and occlusal sealants are useful in the prevention of disease. (2) Topical fluorides and other remineralization techniques are useful in prevention of disease progression. (3) Restorative materials such as RMGIs, composites, amalgams and stainless steel crowns are useful in prevention of loss of function.

was the development of resin-modified glass ionomer (RMGI) materials. Originally introduced as liners and bases requiring spatulation, the newer versions are provided in an encapsulated paste/liquid system.

RMGIs

RMGIs have properties intermediate to conventional glass ionomer materials and resin composites. This 2-component system has most of the advantages of glass ionomer materials with the added advantage of water insolubility while setting. RMGIs exhibit a high degree of moisture tolerance in bonding because of their hydrophilicity and water content.[80–82]

In addition, the resins included in some systems have dual curing capability, and hence, the ability to light cure the excess material reduces chair time.[83] RMGIs are self-adhesive, not requiring removal of the smear layer,[83] and their low modulus and ionomeric reaction can buffer the effects of polymerization shrinkage of composites. RMGIs bond to tooth structures via a combination of micromechanical and chemical bonding mechanisms. Moreover, the high fluoride release by RMGIs has been shown to help protect adjacent tooth surfaces.[84]

SUMMARY

With numerous advances at our disposal, as summarized in **Box 1**, it is indeed an exciting time to practice pediatric dentistry. There are far more tools available at present than just a generation ago. **Fig. 2** describes when those tools available are most effective and the moment in which to provide primary prevention, early intervention, and reparative care. Although there is an opportunity to deliver cutting-edge dental care to patients, along with that choice comes the responsibility to closely monitor outcomes. The application of new technology and good science to assess effectiveness and long-term outcomes should always go hand in hand. Further, there continues to be a need for innovation and collaboration with other scientific disciplines to fully comprehend and prevent dental caries.

ACKNOWLEDGMENTS

The authors would like to acknowledge the assistance of Dr Sue Hwang (at the time, a postdoctoral resident fellow) in the preparation of this article.

REFERENCES

1. Maupome G, Pretty IA. A closer look at diagnosis in clinical dental practice. Part 4. Effectiveness of nonradiographic diagnostic procedures and devices in dental practice. J Can Dent Assoc 2004;70(7):470–4.
2. Pretty IA. Caries detection and diagnosis: novel technology. J Dent 2006;24: 727–39.
3. Lussi A, Hibst R, Paulus R. DIAGNOdent: an optical method for caries detection. J Dent Res 2004;83(Spec Iss C):C80–3.
4. Diniz MB, Rodrigues JA, de Paula AB, et al. In vivo evaluation of laser fluorescence performance using different cut-off limits for occlusal caries detection. Lasers Med Sci 2009;24:295–300.
5. Rodrigues JA, Diniz MB, Josgrilberg EB, et al. In vitro comparison of laser fluorescence performance with visual examination for detection of occlusal caries in permanent and primary molars. Lasers Med Sci 2009;24:501–6.
6. Hibst R, Paulus R, Lussi A. Detection of occlusal caries by laser fluorescence: basic and clinical investigations. Med Laser Appl 2001;16:205–13.

7. Stübel H. Die fluoreszenz tierischer gewebe im ultravioletten licht. Pflugers Arch 1911;142:1–14 [in German].
8. Buchalla W, Attin T, Niedmann Y, et al. Porphyrins are the cause of red fluorescence of carious dentine: verified by gradient reversed-phase HPLC [abstract]. Caries Res 2008;42:223.
9. Pretty IA, Maupome G. A closer look at diagnosis in clinical dental practice, part 5: emerging technologies for caries detection and diagnosis. J Can Dent Assoc 2004; 70(8):540, 540a–540i.
10. Schneiderman A, Elbaum M, Shultz T, et al. Assessment of dental caries with digital imaging fiber-optic transillumination (DIFOTI): in vitro study. Caries Res 1997;31(2):103–10.
11. Bader JD, Shugars DA, Bonito AJ. Systematic reviews of selected dental caries diagnostic and management methods. J Dent Educ 2001;65:960–8.
12. Ando M, Hall AF, Eckert GJ, et al. Relative ability of laser fluorescence techniques to quantitate early mineral loss in vitro. Caries Res 1997;31(2): 125–31.
13. Ngaotheppitak P, Darling CL, Fried D. Measurement of the severity of natural smooth surface (interproximal) caries lesions with polarization sensitive optical coherence tomography. Lasers Surg Med 2005;37(1):78–88.
14. Slots J. Selection of antimicrobial agents in periodontal therapy. J Periodontal Res 2002;37:389–98.
15. Kohler B, Anderson I. Influence of caries-preventive measures in mothers on cariogenic bacteria and caries experience in their children. Arch Oral Biol 1994;39:907–11.
16. Zikert I, Emilson CG, Krasse B. Effect of caries preventive measures in children highly infected with the bacterium Streptococcus mutans. Arch Oral Biol 1982; 27:861–8.
17. Featherstone JD. Delivery challenges for fluoride, chlorhexidine and xylitol. BMC Oral Health 2006;15(6 Suppl 1):S8.
18. Anderson MH. A review of the efficacy of chlorhexidine on dental caries and the caries infection. J Calif Dent Assoc 2003;31(3):211–4.
19. Addy M, Jenkins S, Newcombe R. The effect of some chlorhexidine-containing mouthrinses on salivary bacterial counts. J Clin Periodontol 1991;18:90–3.
20. Milgrom P, Zero DT, Tanzer JM. An examination of the advances in science and technology of prevention of tooth decay in young children since the Surgeon General's Report on Oral Health. Acad Pediatr 2009;9:404–9.
21. Caso A, Hung LK, Beirne OR. Prevention of alveolar osteitis with chlorhexidine: a meta-analytic review. Oral Surg Oral Med Oral Pathol Oral Radiol Endod 2005;99:155–9.
22. Zhang Q, van Palenstein Helderman WH, van't Hof MA, et al. Chlorhexidine varnish for preventing dental caries in children, adolescents and young adults: a systematic review. Eur J Oral Sci 2006;114:449–55.
23. Löe H. Oral hygiene in the prevention of caries and periodontal disease. Int Dent J 2000;50:129–39.
24. Higashitsutsumi M, Kamoi K, Miyata H, et al. Bactericidal effects of povidone-iodine solution to oral pathogenic bacteria in vitro. Postgrad Med J 1993;69: S10–4.
25. Numazaki K, Asanuma H. Inhibitory effect of povidone-iodine for the antigen expression of human cytomegalovirus. In Vivo 1999;13:239–41.
26. Linder N, Davidovitch N, Reichman B, et al. Topical iodine-containing antiseptics and subclinical hypothyroidism in preterm infants. J Pediatr 1998;133:309–10.

27. Tinanoff N, O'Sullivan DM. Early childhood caries: overview and recent findings. Pediatr Dent 1997;19:12–6.
28. Zahn L, Featherstone JDB, Gansky SA, et al. Antibacterial treatment needed for severe early childhood caries. J Public Health Dent 2006;66:174–9.
29. Amin MS, Harrison RL, Benton TS, et al. Effect of povidone-iodine on Streptococcus mutans in children with extensive dental caries. Pediatr Dent 2004;26:5–10.
30. Lopez L, Berkowitz RJ, Spiekerman C, et al. Topical antimicrobial therapy in the prevention of early childhood caries: a follow-up report. Pediatr Dent 2004;24: 204–6.
31. Featherstone JD. The science and practice of caries prevention. J Am Dent Assoc 2000;131(7):887–99.
32. National Institutes of Health (US). Diagnosis and management of dental caries throughout life. NIH Consens Statement 2001;18:1–23.
33. Marinho VCC, Higgins JPT, Logan S, et al. Fluoride varnishes for preventing dental caries in children and adolescents. Cochrane Database Syst Rev 2002;1: CD002279. Available at: http://doi.wiley.com/10.1002/14651858.CD002279. Accessed August 13, 2010.
34. Lansdown AB. Silver in health care: antimicrobial effects and safety in use. Curr Probl Dermatol 2006;33:17–34.
35. Stebbins EA. What value has argenti nitras as a therapeutic agent in dentistry? Int Dent J 1891;12:661–70.
36. Miller WD. Preventive effect of silver nitrate. Dent Cosmos 1905;47:901–13.
37. Howe PR. A method of sterilizing and at the same time impregnating with a metal affected dentinal tissue. Dent Cosmos 1917;59:891–904.
38. Klein H, Knutson JW. Studies on dental caries XIII: effects of ammoniac silver nitrate on caries in the first permanent molars. J Am Dent Assoc 1942;29:420–7.
39. Bedi R, Sardo-Infirri J. Oral health care in disadvantaged communities. London: FDI World; 1999.
40. Chu CH, Lo EC. Promoting caries arrest in children with silver diamine fluoride: a review. Oral Health Prev Dent 2008;6(4):315–21.
41. Chu CH, Lo ECM, Lin HC. Effectiveness of silver diamine fluoride and sodium fluoride varnish in arresting dentin caries in Chinese pre-school children. J Dent Res 2002;81:767–70.
42. Llodra JC, Rodriguez A, Ferrer B, et al. Efficacy of silver diamine fluoride for caries reduction in primary teeth and first permanent molars of school children: 36-month clinical trial. J Dent Res 2005;84:721–4.
43. Reynolds EC, Cai F, Shen P, et al. Retention in plaque and remineralization of enamel lesions by various forms of calcium in a mouthrinse or sugar-free chewing gum. J Dent Res 2003;82:206–11.
44. Reynolds EC, Cai F, Cochrane NJ, et al. Fluoride and casein phosphor-peptide-amorphous calcium phosphate. J Dent Res 2008;87:344–8.
45. Anderson M. Chlorhexidine and xylitol gum in caries prevention. Spec Care Dentist 2003;23(5):173–6.
46. Milgrom P, Ly KA, Roberts MC, et al. Mutans streptococci dose response to xylitol chewing gum. J Dent Res 2006;85(2):177–81.
47. American Academy of Pediatric Dentistry. Policy on the use of xylitol in caries prevention. 2006. Available at: http://www.aapd.org/media/Policies_Guidelines/ P_Xylitol.pdf. Accessed August 13, 2010.
48. Soderling E, Isokangas P, Pienihakkinen K, et al. Influence of maternal xylitol consumption on mother-child transmission of mutans streptococci: 6-year follow-up. Caries Res 2001;35:173–7.

49. Isokangas P, Soderling E, Pienihakkinene K, et al. Occurrence of dental decay in children after maternal consumption of xylitol chewing gum, a follow-up from 0 to 5 years of age. J Dent Res 2000;79:1885–9.
50. Brown LJ, Selwitz RH. The impact of recent changes in the epidemiology of dental caries on guidelines for the use of dental sealants. J Public Health Dent 1995;55(Spec No 5):274–91.
51. Nicholson JW. Polyacid-modified composite resins ("compomers") and their use in clinical dentistry. Dent Mater 2007;23(5):615–22.
52. Mejàre I, Lingström P, Petersson LG, et al. Caries-preventive effect of fissure sealants: a systematic review. Acta Odontol Scand 2003;61(6):321–30.
53. Ripa LW. Sealants revisited: an update of the effectiveness of pit and-fissure sealants. Caries Res 1993;27(1):77–82.
54. McLean JW, Wilson AD. Fissure sealing and filling with an adhesive glass-ionomer cement. Br Dent J 1974;136(7):269–76.
55. Seppä L, Forss H. Resistance of occlusal fissures to demineralization after loss of glass ionomer sealants in vitro. Pediatr Dent 1991;13(1):39–42.
56. American Academy of Pediatric Dentistry. Policy on the use of a caries-risk assessment tool (CAT) for infants, children, and adolescents. Council on Clinical Affairs. 2002. Available at: http://www.aapd.org/pdf/policycariesriskassessmenttool.pdf. Accessed August 14, 2010.
57. Hale KJ, American Academy of Pediatrics Section on Pediatric Dentistry. Oral health risk assessment timing and establishment of the dental home. Pediatrics 2003;111:1113–6.
58. Berg J. The marketplace for new caries management products: dental caries detection and caries management by risk assessment. BMC Oral Health 2006; 6(1):S6.
59. Fuks AB. Current concepts in vital primary pulp therapy. Eur J Paediatr Dent 2002;3:115–20.
60. Tziafas D. The future role of a molecular approach to pulp dentinal regeneration. Caries Res 2004;38:314–20.
61. Baume LJ. The biology of pulp and dentine. In: Myers HM, editor. Monographs in oral science 1980. Basel (Switzerland): Karger; 1980. p. 67–182.
62. Fuks AB. Vital pulp therapy with new materials for primary teeth: new directions and treatment perspective. Pediatr Dent 2008;30(3):211–9.
63. BjØrndal L, Mjor IA. Pulp-dentin biology in restorative dentistry: 4-dental caries: characteristics of lesions and pulpal reactions. Quintessence Int 2001;32:717–36.
64. BjØrndal L, Darnnavan T. A light microscopic study of odontoblastic and nonodontoblastic cells involved in tertiary dentinogenesis in well-defined cavitated carious lesions. Caries Res 1999;33:50–60.
65. Bergenholz G. Factors in pulpal repair after oral exposure. Adv Dent Res 2001; 15:84.
66. Ricketts DNJ, Kidd EAM, Innes N, et al. Complete or ultraconservative removal of decayed tissue in unfilled teeth. Cochrane Database Syst Rev 2006;6:CD003808.
67. Farooq NS, Coll JA, Kuwabara A, et al. Success rates of formocresol pulpotomy and indirect pulp treatment of deep dentinal caries in primary teeth. Pediatr Dent 2000;22:278–86.
68. Falster CA, Araujo FB, Straffon LH, et al. Indirect pulp treatment: In vivo outcomes of an adhesive resin system vs calcium hydroxide for protection of the dentin-pulp complex. Pediatr Dent 2002;24:241–8.
69. Al-Zayer MA, Straffon LH, Feigal RJ, et al. Indirect pulp treatment of primary posterior teeth: a retrospective study. Pediatr Dent 2003;25:29–36.

70. Marchi JJ, de Araujo FB, Froner AM, et al. Indirect pulp capping in the primary dentition: a 4-year follow-up study. J Clin Pediatr Dent 2006;31:68–71.
71. Ibricevic H, Al-Jame Q. Ferric sulphate and formocresol in pulpotomy of primary molars: long term follow-up study. Eur J Paediatr Dent 2003;4(1):28–32.
72. Loh A, O'Hoy P, Tran X, et al. Evidence based assessment: evaluation of the formocresol versus ferric sulfate primary molar pulpotomy. Pediatr Dent 2004; 26(5):401–9.
73. Casas MJ, Kenny DJ, Johnston DH, et al. Long-term outcomes of primary molar ferric sulfate pulpotomy and root canal therapy. Pediatr Dent 2004;26(1):44–8.
74. Eidelman E, Holan G, Fuks AB. Mineral trioxide aggregate vs. formocresol in pulpotomized primary molars: a preliminary report. Pediatr Dent 2001;23(1):15–8.
75. Dentsply Endodontics. Materials safety data sheet (MSDS): ProRoot MTA (mineral trioxide aggregate) root canal repair material. Effective March 1, 2001.
76. Osorio RM, Hefti A, Vertucci FJ, et al. Cytotoxicity of endodontic materials. J Endod 1998;24:91–6.
77. Tziafas D, Pantelidou O, Alvanou A, et al. The dentinogenic effect of mineral trioxide aggregate (MTA) in short-term capping experiments. Int Endod J 2002; 35:245–54.
78. Sakar NK, Saunderi B, Moiseyevai R, et al. Interaction of mineral trioxide aggregate (MTA) with a synthetic tissue fluid. J Dent Res;81(Special issue A):A-391 [abstract no: 3155].
79. Torabinejad M, Chivian N. Clinical applications of mineral trioxide aggregate. J Endod 1999;25:197–205.
80. Mitra SB, Lee CY, Bui HT, et al. Long-term adhesion and mechanism of bonding of a paste-liquid resin modified glass-ionomer. Dent Mater 2009;25:459–66.
81. Friedl KH, Powers JM, Hiller KA. Influence of different factors on bond strength of hybrid ionomers. Oper Dent 1995;20(2):74–80.
82. Croll TP, Nicholson JW. Glass-ionomer: history and current status. Inside Dent 2008;6(8):1–2.
83. Ferrari M. Uses of glass-ionomers as bondings, linings, or bases. In: Davidson CL, Mjor IA, editors. Advances in glass ionomer cements. Carol Stream (IL): Quintessence Publishing Co. Inc; 1999. p. 137–48.
84. Mitra SB. In vitro fluoride release from a light-cured glass ionomer liner/base. J Dent Res 1991;70:75–8.

Hemostatic Agents

Orrett E. Ogle, DDS*, Jason Swantek, DDS, Amandip Kamoh, DDS

KEYWORDS

• Hemostasis • Hemostatic agents • Dental surgery

Bleeding during surgery is a serious clinical problem that can be very disconcerting to the patient and could have serious consequences. During the course of nearly all types of surgery, blood vessels will be disrupted, causing some bleeding, but in the dental setting, this is usually easily controlled. In oral surgery, pressure is commonly used to control bleeding, and this is successful in most cases. In major oral and maxillofacial surgical procedures electrocautery and suture ligatures are most commonly used to control bleeding from small and major vessels. At times, however, where generalized oozing is present and the use of pressure is not effective, and the use of electrosurgical instruments could endanger teeth or nerves, topical hemostatic agents may be needed.

During the recent military conflicts, particularly Iraq, there have been significant advances in hemostatic materials that have proved to be very effective in hemorrhage control on the battlefield. Several of these products are now being adapted for civilian use, and now there is a multibillion dollar hemostasis market with new products and solutions rapidly emerging. This article presents some of these products that are useful for oral surgery or that may become useful. Although the emphasis will be on agents that may be used within the oral cavity, the article will also describe agents that could be useful to oral and maxillofacial surgeons.

The authors hope that the reader will not be lulled into believing that hemostatic agents will become the panacea to the control of surgical hemorrhage. The most important step to always remember in bleeding control is direct pressure, and hemostatic agents should always be considered secondarily. The dentist should be familiar with the general techniques of hemorrhage control for different types of bleeding episodes—small vessels, large vessels, oozing, drug-induced, or when an underlying coagulation defect is present.

Having a general knowledge of the coagulation process will allow the clinician to better understand how the hemostatic agents work and when they should be applied. Hemostatic agents provide control of external bleeding by enhancing or accelerating the natural clotting process through various physical reactions between the agent and blood.

The authors have nothing to disclose.
Oral and Maxillofacial Surgery, Woodhull Medical & Mental Health Center, 760 Broadway, Brooklyn, NY 11206, USA
* Corresponding author.
E-mail address: Orrett.Ogle@WoodhullHC.NYCHHC.org

HEMOSTASIS

The process of hemostasis is a very complex one that involves 3 major steps: (1) vasoconstriction, (2) formation of a platelet plug, and (3) coagulation (secondary hemostasis).

The first step is an immediate constriction of damaged blood vessels caused by vasoconstrictive paracrine released by the endothelium. This results in a temporary decrease in blood flow within the injured vessel. The second step is a mechanical blockage of the defect by a plug that forms as platelets stick to the exposed collagen (platelet adhesion) and become activated, releasing cytokines (serotonin, thromboxane A2, and endothelin1) into the area around the injury. Released platelet factors (ADP, fibronectin, thrombospondin, fibrinogen and PDGF) reinforce the vasoconstriction and activate more platelets that stick to one another (platelet aggregation) to form the platelet plug. At the same time, exposed collagen and tissue factor initiate the third step, a series of reactions known as the coagulation cascade that ends in the formation of fibrin polymer. The fibrin protein fiber mesh reinforces and stabilizes the platelet plug to become a clot.

The clotting cascade (secondary hemostasis) is traditionally broken up into 2 basic pathways, the intrinsic pathway and the extrinsic pathway. The intrinsic pathway is primarily activated by collagen, which is exposed and binds factor 12 to initiate this cascade. The extrinsic pathway is stimulated by tissue factor, which is exposed by the tissue injury and through factor 7 activation initiates this pathway. These 2 pathways then converge in a common pathway where thrombin converts fibrinogen to fibrin and then the final clot.

Intrinsic Pathway (Contact Activation Pathway)

The intrinsic cascade is initiated when contact is made between blood and exposed negatively charged surfaces. Upon exposure of a negatively charged surface, prekallikrein, high molecular weight kininogen, and factors 12 and 11 initiate the intrinsic pathway. Upon contact activation, prekallikrein is converted to kallikrein, which activates factor 12 to 12a, which in turn activates factor 11 to 11a. With Ca+ present, factor 11a activates factor 9 to 9a, which cleaves factor 10 to 10a, the beginning of the common pathway. Contact activation of the intrinsic pathway can also occur on the surface of bacteria, and through the interaction with urate crystals, fatty acids, protoporphyrin, amyloid β, and homocysteine.

Extrinsic Pathway (Tissue Factor Pathway)

Factor 3 (tissue factor) is released from the tissue immediately after injury and initiates the extrinsic pathway. Factor 3 forms a complex with factor 7a, which catalyzes the activation of factor 10, which cleaves to become factor 10a.

Common Pathway

The intrinsic and extrinsic coagulation cascades converge at activated factor 10a, resulting in the conversion of prothrombin (factor 2) to thrombin (2a). Thrombin activation occurs on activated platelets. Thrombin then converts fibrinogen to fibrin monomers, activates factor 13 to 13a (transglutaminase), which then cross-link the monomers—with the aid of calcium—to form fibrin polymer and thus the clot **Fig. 1**.

HEMOSTATIC AGENTS

A hemostatic agent (antihemorrhagic) is a substance that promotes hemostasis (ie, stops bleeding). These agents act to stop bleeding either mechanically or by

Coagulation Cascade

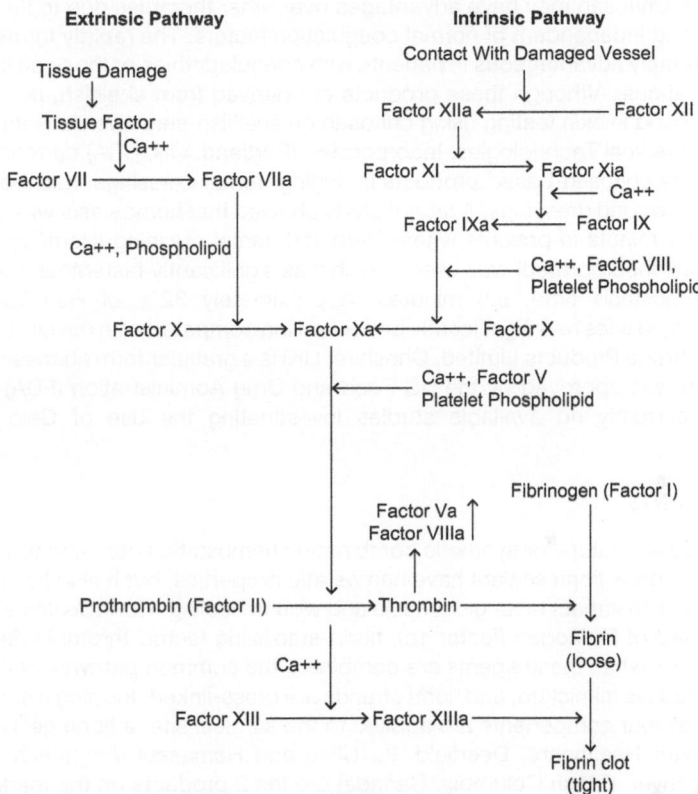

Fig 1. Coagulation cascade: intrinsic and extrinsic pathways.

augmenting the coagulation cascade. The ideal hemostatic agent should be effective, and the agent itself, along with its metabolic breakdown products, should be safe to use within the body. The locally acting hemostatic agents generally work by increasing the rate of vasoconstriction, sealing vessels/vascular channels, or by promoting platelet aggregation. Gelfoam (Pfizer Incorporated, NY, USA) and Surgicel (Ethicon Incorporated, Somerville, NJ, USA), which work proximally in the intrinsic coagulation pathway via contact activation, have been used in dentistry for many decades and remain the major hemostatic agents in oral surgery. Bone wax controls bleeding by mechanically sealing bleeding channels in cancellous bone. All three agents have been proven to be effective and safe. The authors will present other hemostatic agents that have recently been introduced.

CHITOSAN PRODUCTS

Chitosan-based products are a new generation of hemostatic medical products that have been shown to achieve early hemostasis and improve postoperative healing. Chitosan is a naturally occurring, biocompatible, electro positively charged polysaccharide that is derived from shrimp shell chitin. This charge attracts the negatively charged red blood cells, forming an extremely viscous coagulum that seals the wound and causes hemostasis. It is thought that chitosan may enhance hemostasis by inter-acting with cellular components forming a cellular lattice that entraps cells to form an artificial clot. Chitosan may have advantages over other therapies due to its ability to inhibit bleeding independent of normal coagulation factors. The rapidly formed coag-ulum is extremely advantageous in patients with coagulopathies or those on anticoag-ulant medications. Although these products are derived from shellfish, no reactions have been found in skin testing using chitosan on shellfish-sensitive patients.

HemCon Medical Technologies, Incorporated (Portland, OR, USA) currently manu-factures many chitosan-based products including dental dressings, nasal packings, and bandage wound dressings. A recent study showed that hemostasis was achieved in less than 1 minute in patients where HemCon dental dressing (HemCon Medical Technologies, Incorporated) was used, which was significantly faster than the control average hemostasis time, 9.5 minutes. Approximately 32% of HemCon dental dressing-treated sites had significantly better healing compared with the control sites.[1]

Celo (Medtrade Products Limited, Cheshire, UK) is a granular form chitosan-derived product that was approved by the US Food and Drug Administration (FDA) in 2007. There are currently no available studies investigating the use of Celo for oral procedures.

FIBRIN SEALANTS

Fibrin sealant is a natural or synthetic combination hemostatic agent and tissue adhe-sive. Not only does fibrin sealant have hemostatic properties, but it also has adhesive properties and an impact on angiogenesis and wound healing. Fibrin sealants are usu-ally comprised of fibrinogen (factor 1a), fibrin-stabilizing factor, thrombin (factor 2a), and aprotinin.[2] When these agents are combined, the common pathway of the coag-ulation cascade is mimicked, and fibrin strands are cross-linked, forming a stable fibrin clot. When all four components are applied to the surgical site, a fibrin gel is formed. Tisseel (Baxter Healthcare, Deerfield, IL, USA) and Hemaseel (Angiotech Incorpo-rated, Vancouver, British Columbia, Canada) are the 2 products on the market. Both of these products are identical with no difference in clinical use.[2] Davis and colleagues[3] conducted a study that included 71 patients who underwent various oral and maxillofacial procedures (dentoalveolar, cosmetic, and reconstructive) in which Tiseel was used. Seventy patients had successful outcomes 6 months postop-eratively with 1 recurrent oroantral fistula. Some clinicians have suggested that fibrin glue could be used in bone grafting procedures, particularly sinus lift surgery. There are currently few studies evaluating the use of fibrin sealant as a bone grafting adjunc-tive material,[4] and the available data have been inconsistent, indicating more research is needed before concrete conclusions can be made about using fibrin sealants as an adjunctive agent in bone grafting.

The only contraindication to using synthetic fibrin sealant is in patients with sensi-tivity to bovine proteins. There have been reports of tissue necrosis when fibrin sealant is used improperly. An excessively thick sealant layer may prevent revascularization at the surgical site, causing tissue necrosis.

OSTENE

For many years, bone wax was the only option to control bone bleeding. Bone wax is mainly composed of water-insoluble beeswax and is widely used for bone hemostasis in a variety of situations. It has no hemostasis quality but rather tamponades the vascular spaces within cancellous bone. There are negative issues regarding the use of bone wax in the jaws, however. Bone wax is water-insoluble and will remain at the site indefinitely, forming a physical barrier that inhibits bone healing. In defects where bone wax was applied and removed after 10 minutes, there was complete inhibition of bone regeneration.[5] Bone wax also increases infection rates by decreasing the bacterial clearance of cancellous bone and providing a nidus for infection. In a recent study evaluating the infection rates following spinal surgery, surgical site infections occurred in 6 of 42 cases (14%) when bone wax was used and 1 of 72 cases (1.4%) when it was not used.[6] Bone wax has also been shown to increase inflammation,[7] causing a foreign body giant cell reaction at the site of application due to its water insolubility and longevity.

Ostene (Ceremed, Incorporated, Los Angeles, CA, USA) is a synthetic bone hemostatic material that was first approved by the FDA in 2004 for use in cranial and spinal procedures as a bone hemostatic agent. It is a sterile mixture of water-soluble alkylene oxide copolymers that produces minimal postoperative inflammation, making it ideal for cranial and spinal surgery, where inflammation may be harmful to neural tissues. Because Ostene is water-soluble, it does not remain at the site of application and addresses all of the known negative events associated with bone wax. It dissolves in 48 hours, does not swell, and is not metabolized. The material's main polymer component inherently reduces bacterial adhesion and the incidence of infection. Wellisz and colleagues[8] showed that Ostene-treated rabbit tibial cortical defects had a significantly lower rate of osteomyelitis and positive bone cultures compared with the bone-wax treated defects.

Ostene is applied in a similar fashion as bone wax. It requires no mixing and is used straight from its sterile foil packet; it should be applied to a thickness of 1 to 2 mm. It has a putty-like consistency when warmed to body temperature by kneading it with gloved fingers. Ostene is supplied in 2.5 gram- or 3.5 gram-sized bars within sterile peel pouches with either 10 or 12 bars in a box. Although Ostene is more expensive than bone wax, its benefit compensates for the increase cost.

ACTCEL AND GELITACEL

ActCel (Coreva Health Science, LLC, Westlake Village, CA, USA) is a new topical hemostatic agent that is made from treated and sterilized cellulose and available in similar fabric meshwork as Surgicel. Once the meshwork comes into contact with blood, it expands to 3 to 4 times its original size and is almost immediately converted to a gel. Complete dissolution of the product takes place within 1 to 2 weeks. Because of its purity and the fact that it degrades rapidly into biocompatible end products (glucose, water), it does not adversely affect wound healing. It is known that when Surgicel is placed in the mandibular canal with the inferior alveolar nerve exposed there have been reports of neurotoxic effects. ActCel's mechanisms of action are multiple, enhancing the coagulation process biochemically by enhancing platelet aggregation and physically by 3-dimensional clot stabilization. ActCel has been used in third molar sites and is advertised to help prevent dry sockets. It has also been used in periodontal and orthognathic surgery.

Gelitacel (Gelita Medical B.V. Amsterdam, The Netherlands) is a fast-working, oxidized resorbable cellulose haemostatic gauze of natural origin made from highest alpha-grade selected cotton. It is not based on viscose and has state-of-the-art knitting technology for easy passage in endoscopic procedures. The special biochemical characteristics of its resorbable cellulose allows resorption as quick as 96 hours, therefore giving it decreased risk for encapsulation. Gelitacel is approved for dental surgery in Europe, is available at half the cost of Surgicel, and has better absorbing properties.

The authors were unable to find FDA approval for this product.

FLOSEAL

FloSeal Matrix Hemostatic Sealant (Fusion Medical Technologies, Mountain View, CA, USA) is a proprietary combination of 2 independent hemostasis-promoting agents. It consists of bovine-derived gelatin granules coated in human-derived thrombin that work in combination to form a stable clot at the bleeding site. When applied to a bleeding site, the gelatin granules swell by about 10% to 20% as it contacts blood, causing a seal at the bleeding site. The thrombin portion of the product activates the common pathway of the coagulation cascade and converts fibrinogen to a fibrin polymer, forming a clot around the stable matrix. It is resorbed by the body within 6 to 8 weeks, consistent with the time frame of normal wound healing. Because of the products flowability, it can adapt to irregular wounds. FloSeal can be used in all surgical procedures (other than ophthalmic) as an adjunct to hemostasis when control of bleeding by ligature or conventional procedures is ineffective or impractical. It is effective on hard and soft tissue. FloSeal matrix hemostatic sealant has been used as a first-line hemostatic agent in major oral surgical cases.

Because FloSeal is made from human plasma, it may carry a risk of transmitting infectious agents (eg, viruses) and theoretically, the Creutzfeldt-Jakob disease (CJD) agent. It should also not be used in patients with known allergies to materials of bovine origin.

QUIKCLOT

QuikClot (Z-Medica, Wallingford, CT, USA) brand products derive their primary hemostatic properties from kaolinite, a naturally occurring mineral material. When kaolin is exposed to human plasma, factors 12 and 11 are activated, thereby activating the intrinsic coagulation pathway. QuikClot is a granular hemostatic agent that effectively controls external hemorrhage by pouring it into a wound followed by a pressure dressing to achieve hemostasis. The proposed mechanism of action is that the Quick-Clot adsorbs water, concentrating clotting factors. This exothermic reaction produces significant heat that may create secondary injury.

In order to be effective, QuikClot must be applied to the source of the bleeding, the torn blood vessel itself. There is currently no dental use for this product, but the authors believe that it could eventually be modified to be used in oral surgery.

SUMMARY

Hemostasis is an integral and very important aspect of surgical practice. As a rule, most bleeding from dental surgery can be controlled by pressure. When the application of pressure does not yield satisfactory results, or where more effective hemostasis is required, hemostatic agents should be used. These agents act to stop bleeding either mechanically or by augmenting the coagulation cascade. Some of the newer agents that are available to the dental profession have been presented.

REFERENCES

1. Malmquist JP, Clemens SC, Oien HJ, et al. Hemostasis of oral surgery wounds with the hemcon dental dressing. J Oral Maxillofac Surg 2008;66:1177–83.
2. Fattahi T, Mohan M, Caldwell GT. Clinical applications of fibrin sealants. J Oral Maxillofac Surg 2004;62:218–24.
3. Davis BR, Sandor GK. Use of fibrin glue in maxillofacial surgery. J Otolaryngol 1998;27:107–12.

4. Kim WB, Kim SG, Lim SC, et al. Effect of Tisseel on bone healing with particulate dentin and plaster of Paris mixture. Oral Surg Oral Med Oral Pathol Oral Radiol Endod 2010;109(2):e34–40.
5. Ibarrola JL, Bjorenson JE, Austin BP, et al. Osseous reactions to three hemostatic agents. J Endod 1985;11(2):75–83.
6. Gibbs L, Kakis A, Weinstein P, et al. Bone wax as a risk factor for surgical-site infection following neurospinal surgery. Infect Control Hosp Epidemiol 2004;25: 346–8.
7. Allison RT. Foreign body reactions and an associated histological artifact due to bone wax. Br J Biomed Sci 1994;51:14–7.
8. Wellisz T, Yuehuei H, Wen X, et al. Infection rates and healing using bone wax and a soluble polymer material. Clin Orthop Relat Res 2008;466:481–6.

Technological Advances in Caries Diagnosis

Glenn K. Rochlen, DDS, Mark S. Wolff, DDS, PhD*

KEYWORDS

• Caries diagnosis • Radiology • Transillumination
• Laser fluorescence

"Any dentist who cannot find any cavity of decay on any tooth with the explorer and mouth glass needs a competent assistant to make his examinations for him, and not a roentgen-ray machine."
C. Edmund Kells before the American Dental Association November 10–14, 1924[1]

Finding an accurate method for detecting and diagnosing any disease has been the goal of the healing arts since the time of Socrates. In the opening quote, Dr. Kells, speaking before the American Dental Association, voiced his opinion that bitewing radiographs should not be used to identify teeth with interproximal caries. His concern focused on: who would take the radiographs (a radiodontist was emerging as a dental specialty), who would pay for the radiographs, and, more significantly, would the radiographs disclose findings of clinical importance to patient care or would they result in overtreatment? This debate took place nearly 100 years ago, yet never has the diagnostic quandary over the detection of dental caries been greater and never has the importance of appropriate detection and diagnosis been more significant. Today, European and American caries experts do not share the same criteria in diagnosing caries and use a distinctly different language than most practitioners. In clinical practice, we describe dental caries with terms such as Class I or Class II caries with a surface attached to that "diagnosis." Unfortunately, that classification tells us little about the actual surface with caries. For instance, is the caries on the mesial surface or the mesial and occlusal surface in the Class II? How deep has the carious lesion penetrated? What was the dynamic process of caries? Is the lesion active or has it become inactive? The decision of how and what to treat related to dental caries is no less confusing. Clinical research has demonstrated very different thresholds for the need for surgical caries treatment than have traditionally been practiced in the dental community. To best understand the controversy in how we diagnose dental

Department of Cariology and Comprehensive Care, New York University College of Dentistry, 345 East 24th Street, New York, NY 10010, USA
* Corresponding author.
E-mail address: mark.wolff@nyu.edu

Dent Clin N Am 55 (2011) 441–452
doi:10.1016/j.cden.2011.02.018
0011-8532/11/$ – see front matter © 2011 Elsevier Inc. All rights reserved.

dental.theclinics.com

caries, we need to understand the genesis of how the American diagnostic philosophy developed.

Miller[2] proposed a two-step process whereby mixed bacteria, when exposed to fermentable carbohydrates, produced acids. In the second step, it acted on tooth structure to dissolve the hydroxyapatite and release free calcium and phosphates. The dental examination evolved in the late 1800s and was described by Green Vardiman Black[3] in multiple writings. He defined caries as "a chemical dissolution of the calcium salts of the tooth by lactic acid, followed by the decomposition of the organic matrix..." This was consistent with Miller's observations and fits the model of a destructive disease of the teeth. Black recognized that caries needed to be recognized early if it were to be prevented, stating that "decays must be discovered early, before the etching of the enamel has made much progress, if the preparation of a cavity and placing of a restoration is to be avoided"[4] Essentially it was believed that caries could be "avoided" but there was no indication that it could be reversed. He advocated that the use of "small right and left explorers with curved tines, sharply pointed, are very effective in detecting the slightest estchings."[4] He suggested the use of firm pressure in the examination as well as a gentle pass over clean dry tooth surface. Black recommended an examination technique that started with the removal of surface deposits, using three explorers and a mouth mirror in a methodical process that would "reveal the beginnings of decay anywhere."[3] The only treatment available for dental caries, even for the slightest of enamel etching, was a restoration. Black developed a caries classification system that defined how we spoke about caries for the following century. He stated, "This classification is especially intended for use in technical procedures" and classified caries as Class I through V depending on the surfaces involved.[3] The therapeutic modalities available in 1900 were extremely limited. Black's amalgam formulation, cavity preparation, and restorations were effective and this classification system made perfect sense. There was only one bullet available: restoration; no fluoride, no modern toothpaste, and no remineralizing technologies. A simple caries classification system was perfectly effective. By the mid-twentieth century, the accumulation of plaque, subsequent production of acids within that plaque (in response to a glucose exposure), and subsequent recovery of the plaque pH to near neutrality had been demonstrated by Stephan.[5] It was demonstrated that the introduction of dietary carbohydrate, even in thin layers of plaque, resulted in significant production of acid. The extent of the pH drop and the longevity of that drop are heavily regulated by both a patient's saliva and their salivary components.[5–8] This process of acid production in the demineralization of tooth structure (enamel and dentin) and the subsequent development of caries-generated tooth cavitation is a broadly accepted model.

Today it is recognized that dental caries is a dynamic process fluctuating between demineralization and remineralization over time.[9] It is the net gain or loss of mineral over time that determines whether cavitation eventually occurs. The failure of naturally occurring and ongoing remineralization processes to keep up with the rate or severity of the demineralization challenge produces the eventual cavitation. The dynamic nature of the caries disease mandates that the recognition of the lesion be descriptive and specific enough to allow monitoring and assessment if the lesion advances over time (with advancing severity of the lesions being de facto evidence of ongoing disease activity).[10] Because caries is a dynamic process, ideally the assessment of disease activity would be made over time.[11] In clinical practice this is not practical. It is critical that the diagnosis of caries be improved to permit immediate and appropriate clinical decisions. Black's edict to treat the earliest of all lesions with surgical modalities is no longer acceptable because there are multiple treatment and prevention technologies that can reverse early carious disease. Proper and comprehensive detection is critical.

CARIES DETECTION IN THE TWENTY-FIRST CENTURY

Caries detection starts before the physical examination with a patient's medical and social history. Like any of the healing arts, listening to the patient often tells the doctor the nature of the conditions afflicting them and, more importantly, the cause. No longer is starting a patient examination with just a medical history adequate. It must be comprehensive in that it includes the patient's past dental treatment, dietary habits, and their oral health knowledge. This often discloses the cause of a patient's caries problem, as well as their risk of developing new disease. This comprehensive history is critical in developing a patient-centered care plan tailored to their actual risk.

Visual and Visual-tactile Detection

The physical detection of caries starts with a process of careful examination. The use of the sharp explorer to locate carious teeth was described by Taft[12] in his text, *A Practical Treatise to Operative Dentistry*, in 1859 and later editions 1888, but there was no mention of the use of any pressure in the examination. Radike[13] (1968) enhanced Black's original diagnostic criteria by describing areas as carious when the explorer catches with moderate to firm pressure in the pits and fissures, as well as translucency around the fissures. On the smooth surface, evidence of demineralization or white spot, even without softness, was classified as a carious lesion, even without cavitation. The determination that an area was diagnosed as carious because it was a demineralization or white spot unfortunately continued to lend credence to the need for surgical restoration of these early lesions. Though diagnosis of caries with an explorer continued to have strong acceptance in the United States through the twentieth century, European cariologists had begun to use a different criteria for the diagnosis of caries. Including the early signs of caries during diagnosis favors the tracking of the disease process that is a fluid continuum. Visual or tactile examination using an explorer with moderate pressure, as recommended by Black and Radike, has fallen into significant disfavor. Ekstrand and colleagues[14] (1987) demonstrated that use of a sharp explorer in a compressive fashion when examining the occlusal surface of teeth produced irreversible traumatic defects in the occlusal fissures that actually favored lesion progression. Further, a study of 34 dentists examining 61 teeth for occlusal caries revealed that there was no difference in diagnostic accuracy between those that used the traditional explorer and those that used visual-only examinations. The explorer did not add to the accuracy of the examination. The percentage of "clinically" correct treatment decisions was about 73% for both techniques with examinations using explorers having higher incidence of overtreatment and examinations using only visual having a higher incidence of "undertreatment."[15] Teeth classified in the undertreatment category using the visual only examination technique probably should be recommended for sealant therapy, rendering this underdiagnosis probably nonclinically significant.[16,17] The findings of overtreatment with the explorer were reported earlier by Bergman and Linden (1969).[18] In addition, their experiments indicated that the explorer could convert a white spot lesion into actual cavitation. Ekstrand and colleagues[19] (2007) demonstrated that the use of a periodontal probe lightly moved across the lesion to detect roughness improved a practitioner's ability to determine lesion activity. Roughness detected when lightly stroking the periodontal probe across the enamel in question is a sign of the current acid activity on the enamel surface. By 2001, the National Institutes of Health[20] Consensus Development

Conference on Dental Caries Diagnosis and Management Throughout Life concluded that "the use of sharp explorers in the detection of primary occlusal caries appears to add little diagnostic information to other modalities and may be detrimental" (**Fig. 1**). The use of the explorer in a compressive force mode does not add diagnostic reliability if proper visual and radiographic examinations are conducted first. In fact, the use of the explorer after visual and radiographic examination is minimally likely to locate undiagnosed lesions and rather more likely to inappropriately diagnose as carious lesions that at best should be sealed (**Fig. 2**). Avoiding damage created by explorers is important as Ismail[21] (2004) emphasized that the "disease process may reverse or stop, resulting in complete healing of the demineralized dental tissue or in preservation of minutely damaged tissue."

Radiology

Described in 1923 as "the most revolutionary aid in dental diagnosis which has come into general application during the present decade," the dental x-ray has always been used with some controversy.[22] With the introduction of early dental radiology techniques questions arose about who should administer the radiographs (a dentist or a specialized dental radiologist), then questions about their diagnostic quality[1] (problems with tooth overlap and film positioning), and, through decades of x-ray use, concerns about ionizing radiation dose and exposure have existed. Bitewing radiology has demonstrated the ability to identify caries in the approximal region earlier than by visual examination alone.[23] During the past decade, considerable discussion has been had about the quality of caries detection with the varied speed of the films available (eg, D-, E-, or F-speed film), but the one noted change is that film-based radiology is rapidly being replaced by digital capture and display. Film-based radiology has always been plagued by problems. The most noted were improper exposure time, inadequate processing quality, and poor positioning of the film. Digital radiology with generally lower radiation exposures has many of the same possible problems with the quality of the image. However, with digital radiology, postexposure manipulation of an image often enhances the image to produce results that are at least as satisfactory as film and often better.[24] As the technology has continued to improve, many manufacturers have developed image analysis software that can highlight areas of discrepancy in image density, consistent with approximal caries, thus, alerting practitioners to areas that need closer evaluation.[25] Currently in the research environment, technologies are available to monitor changes both in the density of the tooth as well as changes in the size of the lesion. This technique, subtraction radiography, requires extreme standardization of exposure, both dose and position, to optimize the accuracy of the data collected. The practicality in a private practice environment is poor.

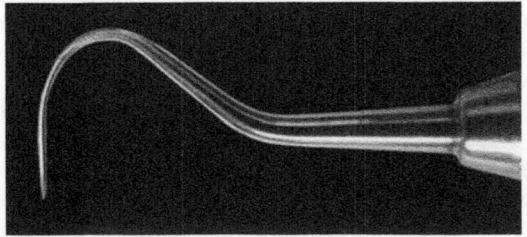

Fig. 1. The explorer tip is actually "large" with respect to the pits and fissure in the posterior teeth.

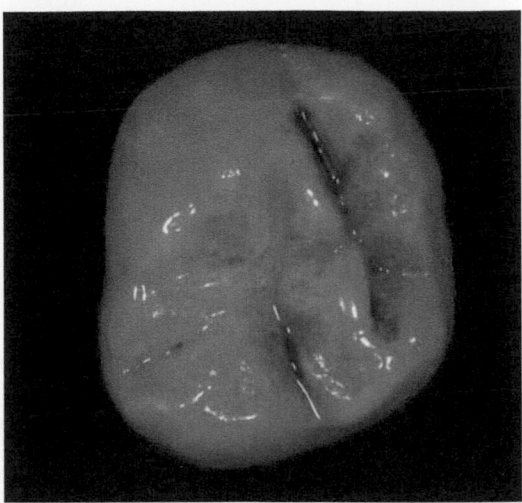

Fig. 2. The occlusal surface of a molar presents diagnostic difficulties as the result of stain and multiple irregularities in which an explorer may "stick," but there is no evidence of demineralization requiring surgical repair. Placement of a sealant based on risk assessment is the best therapeutic choice.

Within dental clinical practice, the appropriate interval for radiographic reexamination has changed over the past 50 years in recognition that ionizing radiation has the potential for side effects that may be harmful to the patient's health. The current therapeutic interval should be adjusted to the patient's caries disease risk always using as low as reasonably achievable (ALARA) exposure.

CARIES DIAGNOSIS USING LIGHT

Light has always been used in dental diagnosis. Early dental offices were designed to allow the use of daylight through windows to improve the diagnosis of dental disease. Dentists wore reflectors and early candle-powered "head-lamps" to illuminate the dental cavity with light. Today, the varied spectrums of light are used in different ways to examine for dental caries.

Transillumination

Transillumination is whole-spectrum high-intensity light narrowly focused to use light to penetrate the tooth structure and permit the identification of varied tooth density and light scattering to identify caries (similar to the variations in tooth density detected using the ionizing radiation, x-ray).[26] As the light scatters passing through the lesion, it appears darker against a light background (**Fig. 3**). It can be easily moved and compared without the negative effects of ionizing radiation allowing a three-dimensional rendering of the lesion. Fiberoptic transillumination (FOTI), when used to identify carious lesions on the occlusal surface, demonstrated its value with high correlations to both visual and histologic determinations with the greatest difficulty in both sensitivity and specificity in lesions just penetrating the dentinoenamel junction.[27] When looking at small approximal lesions, it was found that FOTI was significantly less sensitive in lesion detection than bitewing radiographs. In an era of conservative nonsurgical intervention, the clinical significance of underdetecting lesions could have a significant effect on the clinical decision.[28] When combined with other diagnostic techniques, FOTI improves both sensitivity and specificity.

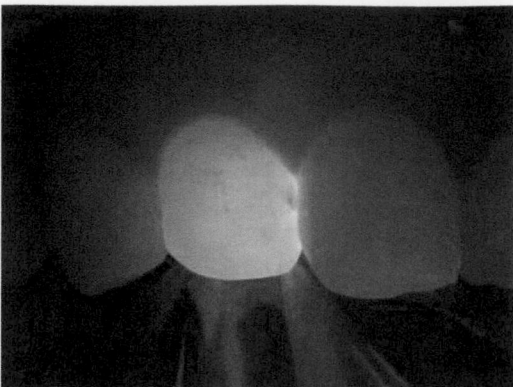

Fig. 3. FOTI reveals subtle changes in tooth density displaying early caries lesions.

Laser Fluorescence

Laser fluorescence has become a commonly used caries diagnostic aid. The principle of this device is that a monochromatic light source (655 nm wavelength) passes unhindered through a mature enamel crystal with little or no alteration. The 655 nm light has the ability to excite bacterial photoporphyrins, resulting in fluorescence. With changes in the enamel, increasing amounts of the light are scattered. Changes in fluorescence can be quantified to describe the presence and severity of the caries (**Fig. 4**).[29] Readings from the laser fluorescence can be confounded by the presence of stain in the pits and fissure and many restorative agents.[30,31] These devices have been found to have high sensitivity of detection, but have only moderate specificity when readings are used without other detection aids and techniques.[32–34] Good and proper clinical practice mandates that the practitioner have the knowledge that these devices may

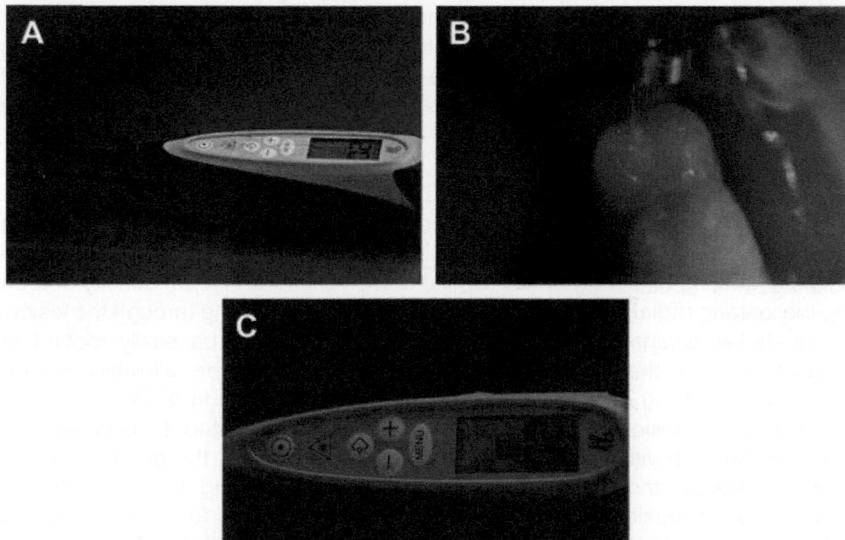

Fig. 4. (*A*) DIAGNOdent pen (KaVo America, Lake Zurich, IL, USA). (*B*) DIAGNOdent pen with the tip examining a fissure, note the device is angled to investigate the areas around the fissure. (*C*) DIAGNOdent pen Digital read-out indicating sound tooth structure.

have the potential of overdiagnosis. It is critical that the practitioner use these devices in conjunction with good visual and radiographic detection, not as a sole diagnostic.

Quantitative Light- (or Laser-) Induced Fluorescence

Quantitative light- (or laser-) induced fluorescence (QLF) is an intraoral imaging technique that uses a specific wave-length of light to cause the fluorescence of dentin. Fluorescence is the emission of light by a substance that has been exposed to or has absorbed light of a different wavelength. In dental caries, as enamel lesions progress deeper, more of the light is scattered and there is less fluorescence from dentin present.[35] The image of demineralization is seen as a dark area against a green background.[36] The image captured can be quantified for the loss of fluorescence and the surface area using digital image software. The image from a baseline measurement can be superimposed on the image from a later date, allowing the ability to track the changes in the size and volume of a lesion with a wide variety of therapeutic methods. Differences are measured in the change in fluorescence and changes in the surface area. QLF has been heavily used by the research community in multiple research projects to assess both the presence of caries on smooth surfaces[37] and to follow the natural process of remineralization.[38] Examination of teeth with QLF demonstrated an extremely high sensitivity (95.5%) for locating demineralized regions, but if used without a visual examination the sensitivity (overdiagnosis) was only 11%. Utilizing a visual examination to eliminate obvious noncarious teeth, the specificity rose to 90.9%. Obviously, QLF needs to be performed in adjunct to a visual examination. QLF can detect precavitated demineralized dentin, monitor and quantify changes in mineral content, and can be used in short-term studies to evaluate the impact of dental products on tooth health.[39] QLF units are expensive, limited to identifying caries on the surfaces of readily accessible teeth, and complicated to use, making use in private clinical practice rare.

Light-Induced Fluorescence and Light-Emitting Diode Caries Detectors

A recently released device uses the light-induced fluorescence technologies and developed a light-emitting diode (LED) technology. The diodes emit light at the 450 nm wavelength and the device focuses on the autofluorescence of the different layers of the tooth. Changes in the mineralization of the tooth can be identified in the process. The device records large areas of the tooth in one image and isolates areas of altered fluorescence. Organic deposits (as in stain), porosities, and crystalline destructuring disrupt the autofluorescence signal and may lead to incorrect assessment of the tooth surface with false-positive renderings.[40]

Another LED technology uses two LEDs (infrared 880 nm and red 660 nm) corresponding to a spectral area where differences are found between healthy and decayed areas. This technology provides a simple output in which a color indicator changes from green to red and an audible alarm that sounds more rapidly as caries is found (**Fig. 5**). Both this technology and the light-induced fluorescence have few nonindustrial-sponsored published research studies and are scientifically supported principally by abstracts presented at conferences. All the research available has been conducted by the sponsors and none has been published in major dental journals.

ELECTRICAL CONDUCTANCE MEASUREMENT

The use of electric current for caries detection dates back to 1878 when first suggested by Magitot.[41] Intact enamel surface has little conductance. As the thickness

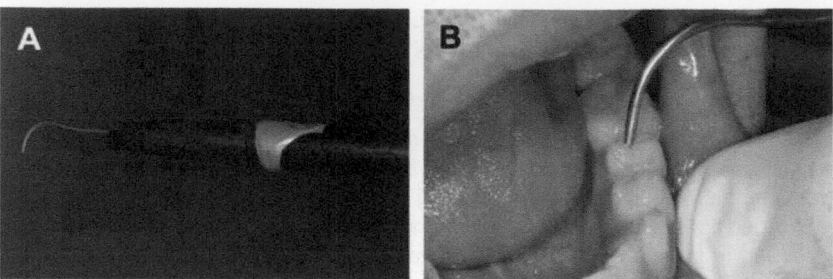

Fig. 5. (*A*) Midwest Caries I.D. (Dentsply Professional, York, PA, USA) with audible and LED displays for caries identification. (*B*) Midwest Caries I.D. fiberoptic probe in contact with dental fissure.

of dentin decreases and porosity of tooth structure increases, the resistance decreases and the electrical conductance increases.[41] The porosities in the tooth are filled with fluid from the oral environment that includes ions, resulting in decreased resistance (or impedance) and increases in conductance. Electrical conductance measurement (ECM) uses a single, fixed-frequency alternating current to measure resistance of the tooth structure. New electrical caries measurement devices use multiple frequencies (electrical impedance spectroscopy), as different substrates respond differently to the resistance test at different frequencies (**Fig. 6**).[42] As Ekstrand and colleagues[11] (1998) demonstrated, there was an excellent correlation between a comprehensive nonexplorer visual, ECM, and radiographic examination and a histologic evaluation of the teeth. After careful examination, no hidden caries or demineralization in dentin was noted in the study. Longbottom and Huysmans[42] (2004) report that ECM has higher sensitivity, but lower specificity, than clinical visual

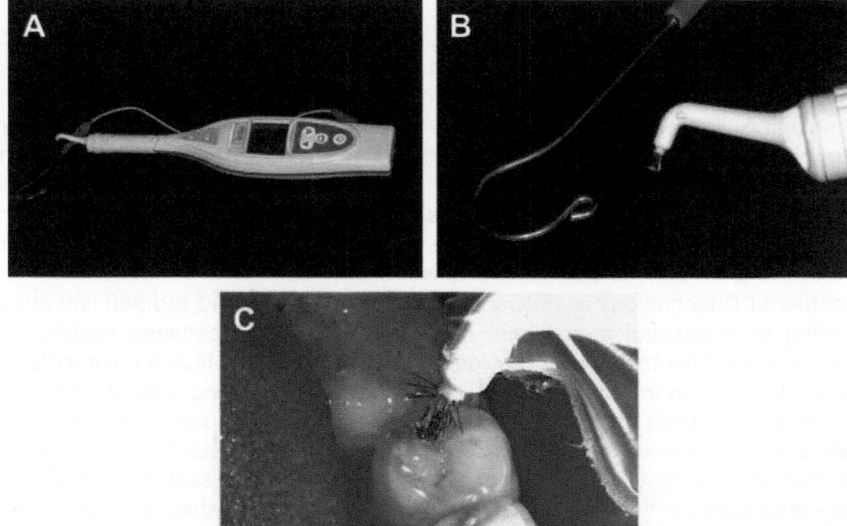

Fig. 6. (*A*) CarieScan Pro (CarieScan LLC, Charlotte, NC, USA) using electrical impedance technology provides painless clear LED indicators of the probability of caries being present. (*B*) Note the CarieScan Pro requires the placement of a lip clip to complete the electric circuit. (*C*) The CarieScan Pro sensing brush is moved over the pits and fissures of the tooth scanning for dental caries.

Table 1 ICDAS II caries severity codes	
Code	Description
0	Sound tooth surface
1	First visual change in enamel seen only after prolonged drying
2	Distinct visual change in enamel
3	Localized enamel breakdown in opaque or discolored enamel, no dentin visible
4	Dentinal shadow (not cavitated into dentin)
5	Distinct cavity with visible dentin
6	Extensive distinct cavity with visible dentin

methods, confirming the need to combine methodologies for best outcomes. With ECM, the tip of a narrow probe is placed in intimate contact with the examined tooth surface and impedance, conductivity, or resistance measurements are made relative to a tissue reference.

COMPUTER SOFTWARE
Caries Classification System: Caries Activity and Risk Assessment

Black[43] defined dental caries based on the surfaces of the teeth to be restored (eg, Class I, II, III, IV, and V). Today, in an era of nonsurgical as well as minimally invasive surgical treatments, it is necessary to carefully document the location and activity of both early and advanced carious lesions. Early lesions on the root surface may indicate a more severe disease activity in a patient than in an active demineralization of the facial surface of a tooth years after removal of an orthodontic bracket (see **Fig. 1**). The need to track the location and activity mandates the development of additional classification systems for recording caries. In 2002, a group of cariologists proposed the International Caries Detection and Assessment System (ICDAS) based on a nonexplorer visual examination.[44] The ICDAS system was revised in 2003 to what is currently referred to as ICDAS II criteria.[45] The system is a seven-category classification of dental caries based on a visual identification, both wet and dry, with no use of the sharp explorer. Originally designed for application on the occlusal surface, it is currently expanded for use on all surfaces (**Table 1**). Studies conducted to determine the accuracy of the system in predicting the penetration of caries into dentin found histologic validity of the caries classification system.[11,46] The ICDAS system, when combined with adjunctive diagnostics such as radiographs and FOTI, permits the monitoring and nonsurgical treatment of early carious lesions. When combined with the determination of lesion activity, as indicated by plaque accumulation, gingival redness, and loss of surface luster,[47] as well as patient risk based on past or present caries activity and xerostomia, an ideal treatment regimen can be determined.[48]

SUMMARY

Understanding the nature of the caries lesion detected on a tooth surface, estimation of lesion depth, the disease activity of the lesion, and the patient's general caries risk are all used in determining the nature of dental care to be delivered.

This can range from simple observation of the tooth surface to disease-specific surgical intervention.[27] Minimally invasive dentistry, or minimal-intervention dentistry as it is more frequently referred to, is a dental care concept based on an assessment of a patient's caries risk and the application of the current therapies to prevent, control, and treat the disease.[49,50] It is often referred to as treating dental caries with a biologic, therapeutic, or medical model.[51] Tyas and colleagues[51] state that this model has several tenants, including, at a minimum, (1) remineralization of early lesions; (2) reduction in cariogenic bacteria to eliminate the risk of further demineralization and cavitation; (3) minimum surgical intervention of cavitated lesions; (4) repair, rather than replacement, of defective restorations; and (5) disease control. When properly performed, an examination of the patient using a comprehensive health and social history, careful clinical examination, and an examination with appropriate technologies allows a dentist to properly assess the depth of lesion, activity of the lesion, and suggest a logical management intervention.[11] In 1921, describing the findings on a radiograph, Bennett Feldman, DDS. reminded the reader, "the radiograph is after all, only an aid to diagnosis."[52] When using diagnostic technologies, it is critical that they be used to improve the dental health of our patient not to find more work to perform. Earlier diagnosis enables the dentist to engage in a full range of nonsurgical therapies to restore dental health.

ACKNOWLEDGMENTS

Special thanks to dentists-to-be Mona Agarwal, Kenny Cheung, and Jake Fried for the preparation of the illustrations.

REFERENCES

1. Raper HR. Practical clinical preventive dentistry based upon periodic roentgenray examinations. J Am Dent Assoc 1925;112(9):1084–100.
2. Köhler W. W. D. MILLER (1853–1907), The Micro-Organisms of the Human Mouth (Unaltered Reprint of the Original Work Published in 1890 in Philadelphia). X + 390 S. 128 Abb., 3 Tafeln. Basel-München-Paris-London-New York-Sydney 1973: S. Karger, DM 56,-. Zeitschrift für allgemeine Mikrobiologie 1974;14:84. DOI:10.1002/jobm.19740140117.
3. Black GV. A work on operative dentistry in two volumes. The pathology of the hard tissues of the teeth, vol. I. Chicago: Medico-Dental Publiching Company; 1908.
4. Black AD. G.V. Black's work on operative dentistry. Pathology of the hard tissues of teeth oral diagnosis, vol. I. Chicago: Medico-Dental Publishing Company; 1936.
5. Stephan RM. Intra oral hydrogen ion concentrations associated with dental caries activity. J Dent Res 1944;23:257–66.
6. Kleinberg I. Formation and accumulation of acid on the tooth surface. J Dent Res 1970;49(6):1300–17.
7. Kleinberg I, Jenkins GN, Chatterjee R, et al. The antimony pH electrode and its role in the assessment and interpretation of dental plaque pH. J Dent Res 1982;61(10):1139–47.
8. Stephan RM. Changes in hydrogen ion concentration or tooth surfaces and in carious lesions. J Am Dent Assoc 1940;27:718–23.
9. Fejerskov O. Concepts of dental caries and their consequences for understanding the disease. Community Dent Oral Epidemiol 1997;25:5–12.
10. Featherstone J. Clinical implications: new strategy for caries prevention. In: Stooky G, editor. Early detection of dental caries. Indianapolis (IN): Indiana University; 1996. p. 287–95.
11. Ekstrand KR, Ricketts DN, Kidd EA, et al. Detection, diagnosing, monitoring and logical treatment of occlusal caries in relation to lesion activity and severity: and in vivo examination and histologic validation. Caries Res 1998;32:247–54.

12. Taft J. A practical treatise on operative dentistry. 4th edition. Philadelphia: P. Blakiston, Son and Co; 1883.
13. Radike AW. Criteria for diagnosing dental caries. Chicago: American Dental Association; 1968.
14. Ekstrand KR, Qvist V, Thylstrup A. Light microscope study of the effect of probing in occlusal surfaces. Caries Res 1987;21:368–74.
15. Lussi A. Validity of diagnostic and treatment decisions of fissure caries. Caries Res 1991;25:296–303.
16. Griffin SO, Oong E, Kohn W, et al. The effectiveness of sealants in managing caries lesions. J Dent Res 2008;87(2):169–74.
17. Beauchamp J, Caufield PW, Crall JJ, et al. Evidence-based clinical recommendations for the use of pit-and-fissure sealants: a report of the American Dental Association Council on Scientific Affairs. J Am Dent Assoc 2008;139:257–68.
18. Bergman G, Linden LA. The action of the explorer on incipient caries. Sven Tandlak Tidskr 1969;62:629–34.
19. Ekstrand KR, Martignon S, Ricketts DJ, et al. Detection and activity assessment of primary coronal caries lesions: a methodologic study. Oper Dent 2007;32(3): 225–35.
20. National Institutes of Health (U.S.). Diagnosis and management of dental caries throughout life. NIH Consens Statement 2001;18(1):1–30.
21. Ismail AI. Visual and visula-tactile detection of dental caries. J Dent Res 2004; 83(Spec Iss C):C56–66.
22. Luthringer J. The diagnostic spread in dentistry: some features of the x-ray. J Am Dent Assoc 1923;1050–7.
23. Bloemendal E, de Vet HC, Bouter LM. The value of bitewing radiographs in epidemiological caries research: a systematic review of the literature. J Dent Educ 2004;32:255–64.
24. Haak R, Wicht MJ, Noack MJ. Conventional, digital and contrast-enhanced bitewing radiographs in the decision to restore approximal lesions. Caries Res 2001; 35:193–9.
25. Gakenheimer D. The efficacy of a computerized caries detector in intraoral digital radiology. J Am Dent Assoc 2002;7(133):883–90.
26. Neuhaus K, Ellwood R, Lussi A, et al. Traditional lesion detection aids. In: Pitts N, editor. Detection, asessment, diagnosis and monitoring of caries, vol. 21. Basel (Switzerland): Karger; 2009. p. 43–51.
27. Cortes DF, Ekstrand KR, Elias-Boneta AR, et al. An in vitro comparison of the ability of fibre-optic transillumination, visual inspection and radiographs to detect occlusal caries and evaluate lesion depth. Caries Res 2000;34:443–7.
28. Vaarkamp J, ten Bosch JJ, Verdonschot EH, et al. The real performance of bitewing radiography and fiber-optic transillumination in approximal caries diagnosis. J Dent Res 2000;70:1747–51.
29. Lussi A, Francescut P. Performance of conventional and new methods for the detection of occlusal caries in deciduous teeth. Caries Res 2003;37:2–7.
30. Francescut P, Lussi A. Correlation between fissure discoloration, Diagnodent measurements, and caries depth: an in vitro study. Pediatr Dent 2003;25:559–64.
31. Lussi A, Zimmerli B, Hellwig E, et al. The influence of the condition of the adjacent tooth surface on fluorescence measurements for the detection of approximal caries. Eur J Oral Sci 2006;114:478–82.
32. Lussi A, Megert B, Longbottom C, et al. Clinical performance of a laser fluorescence device for detection of occlusal caries lesions. Eur J Oral Sci 2001;109: 14–9.

33. Iussi A, Hibst R, Paulus R. Diagnodent: an optical method for caries detection. J Dent Res 2004;83(Spec Iss C):80–3.
34. Bader J, Shugars DA. A systematic review of the performance of a laser fluorescence device for detecting caries. J Am Dent Assoc 2004;135:1413–26.
35. ten Bosch J. Light scattering and related methods in caries diagnosis. In: Stookey G, editor. Proceedings of the First Annual Indiana Conference: early detection of dental caries. Indianapolis (IN): Indiana University School of Dentistry; 1996. p. 81–90.
36. Neuhaus K, Longbottom C, Ellwood R, et al. Novel lesion detection aids. In: Pitts N, editor. Detectio, assessment, diagnosis and monitoring of caries. Basel (Switzerland): Karger; 2009. p. 52–62.
37. Kuhnisch J, Ifland S, Tranaeus S, et al. In vivo detection of non-cavitated caries lesions on occlusal surfaces by visual inspection and quantitative light-induced fluoresence. Acta Odontol Scand 2007;65:183–8.
38. Van der Veen M, Mattousch T, Boersma JG. Longitudinal development of caries lesions after orthodontic treatment followed by quantitative light-induced fluorescence. Am J Orthod Dentofacial Orthop 2007;131:294–8.
39. Stookey GK. Quantitative light fluorescence: a technology for early monitoring of the caries process. Dent Clin North Am 2005;49(4):753–70.
40. Terrer E, KoDionne A, Weisrock G, et al. A new concept in restorative dentistry: light-induced fluorescence evaluator for diagnosis and treatment. Part 1: Diagnosis and treatment initial occlusal caries. J Contemp Dent Pract 2009;10(6):1–11.
41. Angmar-Mansson B, Al-Khateeb S, Tranaeus S. Caries diagnosis. J Dent Educ 1998;62:771–9.
42. Longbottom C, Huysmans MC. Electrical measurements for use in caries clinical trials. J Dent Res 2004;83(Spec Iss C):C76–9.
43. Black GV. A work on operative dentistry: the technical procedures in filling teeth. Chicago: Medico-Dental Publishing; 1917. p. 5.
44. Pitts N. ICDAS-an international system for caries detection and assessment being developed to facilitate caries epidemiology, research and appropriate clinical management. Community Dent Oral Epidemiol 2004;21(3):193–8.
45. Topping G, Pitts NB. Clinical visual caries detection. In: Pitts N, editor. Detection, assessment, diagnosis and monitoring of caries, vol. 21. Basel (Switzerland): Karger; 2009. p. 15–41.
46. Ekstrand K, Kuzmina I, Bjorndal L, et al. Relationship between external and histological features of progressive stages in caries in the occlusal fossa. Caries Res 1995;29:243–50.
47. Nyvad B, Machiulskiene V, Baelum V. Reliability of a new caries diagnostic system differentiating between active and inactive caries lesions. Caries Res 1999;4:252–60.
48. Domejean-Orliaguet S, Gansky SA, Featherstone JD. Caries risk assessment in an educational environment. J Dent Educ 2006;70(12):1346–54.
49. McIntyre J. Minimal intervention dentistry. Ann R Australas Coll Dent Surg 1994;12:72–9.
50. Chalmers J. Minimal intervention dentistry: part 1. Strategies for addressing the new caries challenges in older patients. J Can Dent Assoc 2006;72(5):427–33.
51. Tyas M, Anusavice KJ, Frencken JE, et al. Minimal intervention dentistry- a review of FDI Commission Project 1-97. Int Dent J 2000;50:1–12.
52. Feldman B. The radiograph as a diagnostic aid. Dental Cosmos 1921;63(6):654–5.

Advanced Techniques in Bone Grafting Procedures

Harry Dym, DDS[a,b,*], Joseph Pierse, DMD, MA[b]

KEYWORDS

- Bone grafting • Bone morphogenic protein
- Bone marrow aspirate

Implant placement for the rehabilitation of edentulous spaces is now often viewed as the preferred treatment alternative; however, this technique requires an adequate bone site to allow for proper osseointegration.

Oral and maxillofacial surgeons and general dentists have been searching for the ideal hard tissue bone graft other than autogenous bone to aid in alveolar ridge augmentation or socket preservation before implant placement for years. All sorts of alloplastic materials and allografts (**Table 1**) have been used, but none are ideal, especially when the amount of bone needed to be added is significant or when the recipient site is significantly deficient (as in a 1- or 2-walled bony defect) (**Fig. 1**). Autogenous bone grafts from the hip and tibia do work well, and are considered to be the gold standard for large bony defects. However, the procedure usually requires hospitalization and general anesthesia and has serious potential postoperative complications associated with the donor site, which increase in the elderly patient population, (who are the most in need of this procedure before implant placement, making them less likely to agree to undergo such a procedure) (**Box 1**). Thus, the need for finding graft material that is osteoinductive (see **Box 1**; **Table 2**) and can help reduce the need for autogenous grafting became essential.

BMPs are members of the transforming growth factor-β superfamily that were first described by Urist[1] after observing ectopic bone formation in a rodent model from implanted devitalized cadaveric bone. This family of proteins is highly osteoinductive and contains powerful stimulants of endochondral and intramembranous bone

[a] Oral & Maxillofacial Surgery, Columbia University College of Dental Medicine, 630 West 168th Street, New York, NY 10032-3795, USA
[b] Department of Dentistry, Oral and Maxillofacial Surgery, The Brooklyn Hospital Center, 121 Dekalb Avenue, Brooklyn, NY 11201, USA
* Corresponding author. Department of Dentistry, Oral and Maxillofacial Surgery, The Brooklyn Hospital Center, 121 Dekalb Avenue, Brooklyn, NY 11201.
E-mail address: hdymdds@yahoo.com

Dent Clin N Am 55 (2011) 453–460
doi:10.1016/j.cden.2011.02.003
0011-8532/11/$ – see front matter © 2011 Elsevier Inc. All rights reserved.

dental.theclinics.com

Table 1 Bone substitute synopsis		
Graft Material	**Characteristics**	**Examples**
Allograft	A graft that is taken from a member of the same species as the host but is genetically dissimilar	Cadaver cortical/ cancellous bone, FDBA, DFDBA
Xenograft	Graft derived from a genetically Different species than the host	Bio-Oss, coralline HA, red algae
Alloplast (synthetic materials)	Fabricated graft materials	Calcium sulfate, bioactive glasses, HA, NiTi

Abbreviations: DFDBA, decalcified freeze-dried bone allograft; FBBA, freeze-dried bone allograft; HA, hydroxyapatite; NiTi, porous nickel titanium.
Data from Kao ST, Scott DD. A review of bone substitutes. Oral Maxillofac Surg Clin North Am 2007;19:514.

formation from pluripotent mesenchymal cells. Several types of BMPs were isolated and cloned using recombinant DNA technology; however, the most studied has been bone morphogenic protein-2 (rhBMP-2). BMPs act as growth and differentiation factors and chemotactic agents. BMPs stimulate angiogenesis and migration, proliferation, and differentiation of mesenchymal stem cells into cartilage and hard-forming cells in an area of bone injury.

The identification and development of bone recombinant human bone morphologic protein-2 (RhBMP) has led to the commercial availability for the first time of an osteoinductive autograft replacement (Infuse Bone Graft, Medtronic Spinal and Biologics, Memphis, TN, USA). Infuse bone graft is cleared for use in interbody spine fusion, fresh tibial fractures, and oral maxillofacial bone grafting procedures.

In March 2007, Infuse bone graft was approved by the US Food and Drug Drug Administration (FDA) as an alternative to autogenous bone graft for use in sinus augmentation and localized alveolar ridge augmentation, for defects associated with extraction sockets. Prior to FDA approval, extensive preclinical and clinical research was performed to examine the feasibility, safety, and efficacy of using Rh-BMP-2/ absorbable collagen sponge (ACS) for treating common oral maxillofacial defects. These studies were first performed in several animal species, and they were

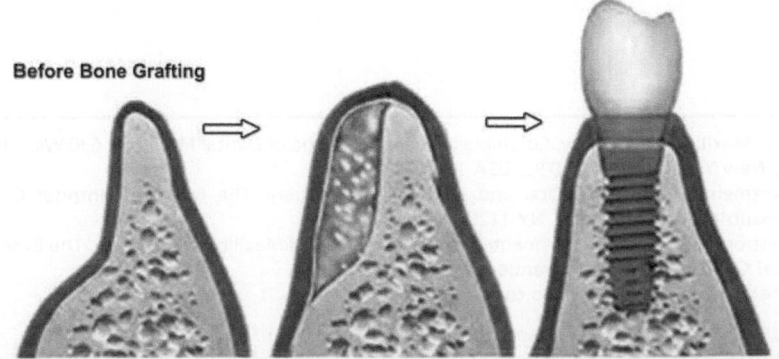

Before Bone Grafting

Fig. 1. Commonly occurring alveolar buccal atrophy in need of preimplant reconstruction.

> **Box 1**
> **Bone regenerative properties of bone graft materials**
>
> *Osteogenesis*
>
> Osteogenesis refers to living cells, such as osteoblasts, that form new bone. The success of any bone grafting procedure is dependent on having enough bone-forming or osteogenic cells in the area. Iliac Crest Bone Graft (ICBG), a type of autograft, is the only bone graft that contains enough cells to be considered osteogenic. Local bone from the primary surgical site generally contains cortical bone with much fewer cells. However, the presence of mesenchymal stem cells does not make a bone graft osteogenic. These stem cells require a signal, such as bone morphogenetic protein (BMP), to differentiate into osteoblasts.[1]
>
> *Osteoconduction*
>
> Osteoconduction refers to the ability of some materials to serve as a scaffold onto which bone cells can attach, migrate, grow, and divide. In this way, the bone healing response is conducted through the graft site, just as a vine uses a trellis for support. Osteogenic cells generally work much better when they have a matrix or scaffold for attachment. Ceramics are strictly osteoconductive scaffolds and fall in the category of autograft extender or bone void filler.
>
> *Osteoinduction*
>
> Osteoinduction refers to the capacity of normal growth factors in the body to attract, proliferate, and differentiate primitive stem cells or immature bone cells to grow and mature, forming healthy bone tissue. Most of these signals are part of a group of protein molecules called BMPs, which are found in normal bone. Highly osteoinductive bone grafts have been evaluated as an autograft alternative in certain indications.

followed by clinical investigation. The work demonstrated that Rh-BMP-2/ACS was effective in inducing viable de novo bone formation.

Two major clinical studies were performed to examine the feasibility, safety, and efficacy of using Rh-BMP-2/ACS. Boyne and colleagues[2] and Fiorellini and colleagues[3] performed randomized prospective controlled studies on the use of Rh-BMP-2/ACS in maxillary sinus augmentation procedures and in extraction site

Table 2
Bone graft material characteristics

Characteristic	Graft Material
Osteogenesis	Autograft
Osteoinduction	BMP
	DFDBA
	DBM
Osteoconduction	Bio-Oss
	Calcium phosphates
	Calcium sulfate
	Collagen
	FDBA
	Glass ionomers
	HA
	NiTi
	BMP

Abbreviations: BMP, bone morphogenetic protein; DBM, dimineralized bone matrix; DFDBA, decalcified freeze-dried bone allograft; FBBA, freesz-dried bone allograft; HA, hydroxyapatite; NiTi, porous nickel titanium.

Data from Kao ST, Scott DD. A review of bone substitutes. Oral Maxillofacial Surg Clin North Am 2007;19:514.

augmentation. Both studies demonstrated that Rh-BMP-2/ACS at 1.5 mg/cc induced significant bone formation suitable for implant placement. The bone induced by Rh-BMP-2/ACS was found to be biologically similar to native bone and capable of implant osseointegration and supporting the functional loading of a dental prosthesis.

SAFETY ASSESSMENTS

In the clinical study by Boyne and colleagues,[2] those patients in the RhBMP-2/ACS treatment group did experience a significantly greater amount of facial edema than those in the bone-grafted treatment group. This edema is thought not to be the result of surgical trauma or an allergic response but rather due to the activity of the RhBMP-2 causing an influx of fluid and cells into the treatment area related to the chemotaxis and neovascularization of the site.[4] Other than the facial edema, none of the other reported events were felt to be related to the RhBMP-2.

SURGICAL PROCEDURE

The Rh-BMP-2/ACS (Infuse) device comes packaged as a powder and liquid with an ACS (**Fig. 2**). The carrier component or ACS is derived from highly purified bovine tendon type-1 collagen and provides the matrix for the delivery of the Rh-BMP-2.

The Rh-BMP-2 comes as a powder that must first be reconstituted with dilution and then evenly expressed onto the ACS carrier (need to wait 15 minutes). Once the material is prepared, it is placed onto the maxillary sinus or the extraction site defect and closed with a tension-free soft tissue closure. In the author's experience, when augmenting a buccal wall defect, it is best to secure (using small bone screws) a 0.2 mm titanium mesh to maintain the Rh-BMP-2 in place. This titanium mesh technique is not always used and should be based on the individual surgeon's preference and past experience. One of the authors (HD) also perforates the buccal plate with a small round burr before placing Rh-BMP-2/ACS when augmenting a buccal wall defect. The titanium mesh material is available in sheets, which are easily custom fitted by the treating clinician, although prebent and contoured titanium mesh is now available from select vendors.

CASE 1

A 78-year-old woman who had a failed implant removed in the #6 position was seen by cone beam studies to have small bone fragments with no plate of bone remaining.

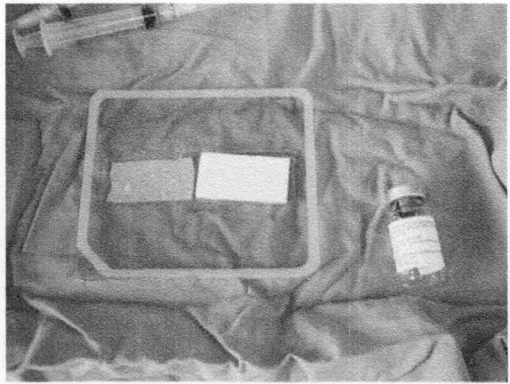

Fig. 2. Powder/liquid and absorbable collagen sponge of Infuse (Medtronic Spinal and Biologics, Memphis, TN, USA) product.

Infuse graft was placed with a titanium mesh technique. The patient returned 6 months later for implant placement. Excellent results were obtained without having to resort to using an autologous onlay graft or particulate allograft and membrane (**Fig. 3**).

CASE 2

This case involved a 72-year-old woman with a history of failed endosseous implants in the upper left maxilla. The patient had no existing alveolar bone and was in need of

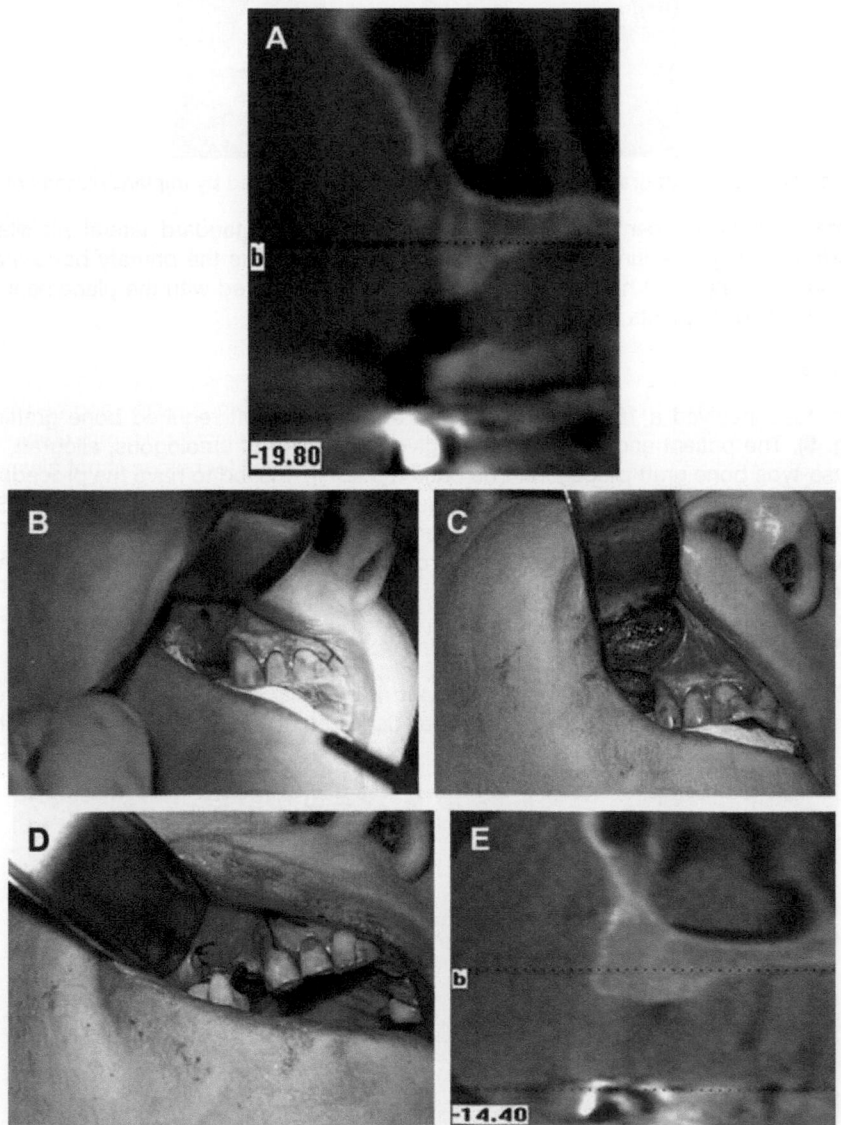

Fig. 3. (*A*) Cone beam study showing buccal wall defect in the #6 area. (*B*) Buccal alveolar defect in area of #6. (*C*) Titanium mesh secured to alveolus containing BMP-2 collagen sponge. (*D*) Primary closure obtained with buccal flap. (*E*) Buccal plate regenerated, 6 months after Infuse placement.

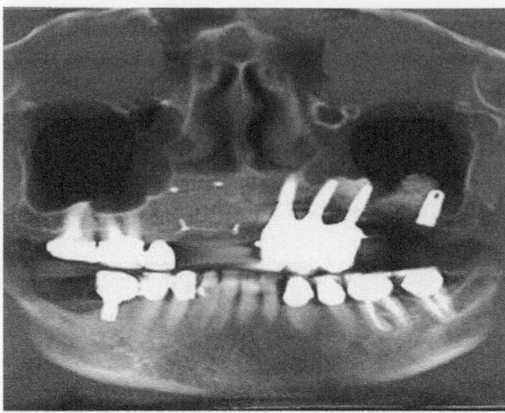

Fig. 4. Maxillary sinus grafted only with Infuse material followed by implant placement.

a major sinus augmentation. The patient underwent a standard lateral maxillary window sinus procedure, but only Infuse graft was used as the primary bone graft materials. The patient had excellent results and was restored with the placement of 4 endosseous implants (**Fig. 4**).

CASE 3

This case involved a 16-year-old boy with an alveolar cleft required bone grafting (**Fig. 5**). The patient and his family were given an option of autologous, allograft, or Infuse-type bone graft procedure. The patient's family wished to have the procedure done with Infuse graft. The standard exposure was performed and Infuse inserted. Six months later, good bone bridging was seen.

Note: this was an off-label use of the product, and the patient and his family were made aware of this before its use.

CASE 4

A 26-year-old woman with a history of right mandibular molar extractions required bone grafting to augment her mandibular-deficient alveolus in both vertical and

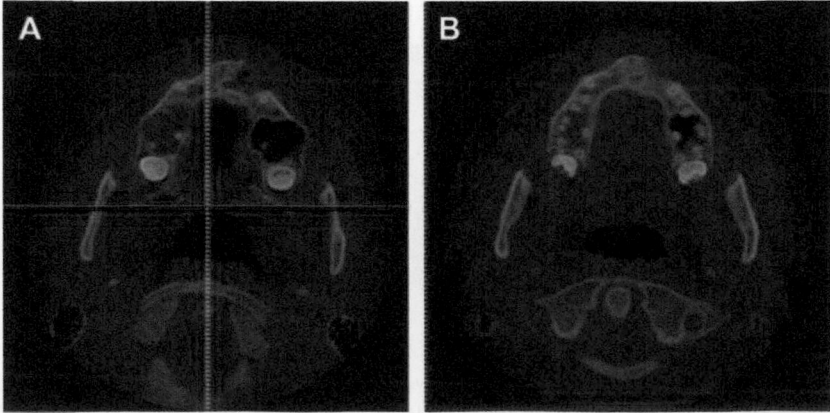

Fig. 5. (*A*) Preoperative axial cone beam view showing alveolar anterior bone cleft defect. (*B*). Six months following Infuse bone graft showing bone growth.

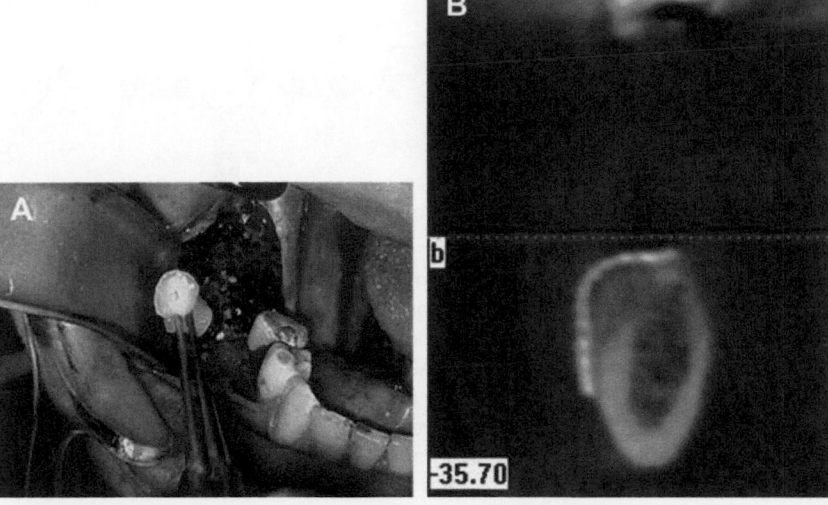

Fig. 6. (*A*) Clinical photo showing Infuse-impregnated collagen sponge about to be inserted underneath the titanium mesh material. (*B*) Six-month follow-up digital picture of atrophic posterior mandible augmented with Infuse material using mesh.

horizontal dimension. The patient underwent an Infuse bone graft procedure with the use of titanium mesh. Excellent results were obtained without the need of resorting to autologous block bone graft procedure, and implants were place into site 6 months later (**Fig. 6**).

BONE MARROW ASPIRATE CONCENTRATE

Many surgeons have used unconcentrated bone marrow aspirate (BMA) to help increase the bioactivity of bone grafted with nonautologous substitutes. Bone marrow is a rich source of autologous adult pleuropotential stem cells and growth factors that can contribute bioactive cells to the grafted site.

Hernigou and colleagues[5] determined that the efficacy of bone marrow aggregate grafting appears to be related to the number of the progenitor cells available in the graft and that the number of progenitors available in bone marrow concentrate appears to be less than optimal in the absence of concentration. A procedure that could concentrate the stem cells without diminishing their biologic potential would be critical to enhancing this procedure.

Box 2
Iliac crest bone marrow aspirate
Endothelial progenitor cells
Hematopoietic stem cells
Mesenchymal stem cells: (convert to osteoblasts in support of new bone formation)
Platelets
Lymphocytes
Granulocytes

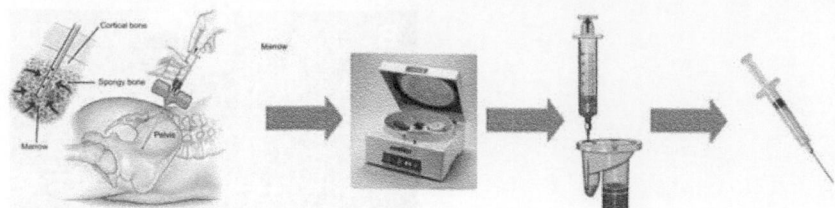

Fig. 7. Hip aspirated followed by concentration centrifuge procedure.

The best source of harvesting BMA is from the iliac crest, as it contains the full scope of regenerative cells needed for angiogenesis and bone formation (**Box 2**).

Harvest Technologies Corporation (Plymouth, MA, USA) have developed a system for the harvesting and concentrating (BMAC, bone marrow aspirate concentrate) the bone marrow aspirate while retaining their cellular viability and proliferative potential.

One of the authors (HD) has used Harvest Technology BMAC$_2$ multiple times for treating mandibular defects, using allografts as the BMAC-carrying medium. The literature includes multiple positive reports of using BMAC with xenografts, demineralized bone matrix, and allografts. The BMAC can be harvested percutaneously from the hip with the patient asleep with general anesthesia or using local anesthesia. Usually 60 mL of aspirate are required, but 30 mL can also be aspirated if the volume of BMAC required is small.

Once harvested the aspirate is injected into dual-chamber disposables and centrifuged, at which time the enucleated cells are separated and concentrated (**Fig. 7**). Most of the plasma is removed, and the cells are resuspended before augmentation; BMAC is mixed with thrombin and freeze-dried allograft particulate bone and placed into the intended site for augmentation.

SUMMARY

Technological advancement in bone grafting procedures using purified proteins or stem cells to induce osteogenesis is a significant contribution to patient care. Patients who would otherwise not have been suitable candidates for major autologous bone grafting procedures can continue to benefit from implant reconstruction, with a less debilitating bone reconstructive procedure.

REFERENCES

1. Urist MR. Bone: formation by autoinduction. Science 1965;150:893–9.
2. Boyne PJ, Lilly LC, Marx RE, et al. De novo bone induction by recombinant human morphogenetic protien-2 (rhBMP-2) in maxillary sinus floor augmentation. J Oral Maxillofac Surg 2005;63:1693–707.
3. Fiorellini JP, Howell TH, Cochran D, et al. Randomized study evaluating recombinant bone morphogenetic protein-2 for extraction socket augmentation. J Periodontol 2005;76(4):605–13.
4. Triplett RG, Nevins M, Marx RE, et al. Pivotal, parallel evaluation of recombinant human bone morphogenetic protein-2/ absorbable collagen sponge and autogenous bone graft for maxillary sinus floor augmentation. J Oral Maxillofac Surg 2009;67(9):1947–60.
5. Henrigou P, Poignard A, Beaujean F, et al. Percutaneous autologous bone marrow grafting for nonunion; influence of the number and concentration of progenitor cells. J Bone Joint Surg Am 2005;87:1430–7.

Technologic Advances in Endodontics

Rory E. Mortman, DDS[a,b],*

KEYWORDS

• Endodontics • Endodontist • Root canal • Review

According to the Merriam-Webster dictionary, technology is the practical application of knowledge especially in a particular area. It is also the specialized aspects of a particular field of endeavor.[1,2] What is modern endodontic technology? As mentioned by various endodontic Web sites, modern technology is listed as: rotary nickel titanium (NiTi) instruments, apex locators, ultrasonics, the dental operating microscope, bonded resin root canal obturation, and mineral trioxide aggregate (MTA). Although all these technologies are considered technologic advances in root canal treatment, many have been commercially available for more than 10 years. Trade journals have advertisements about new techniques and advances in endodontics. Claims such as "300% less likely to separate," "The right tool for the job," "GP free endodontics," and "Truly revolutionary" were listed. The trade journals are also filled with testimonials such as "This stuff was sent straight down from the top of Mount Olympus," and "Stress free, superior Endo, While saving time and money. You'll be a winner." So what is the difference between advertising, marketing, and proven technology? The answer is the dental literature. How does a practitioner know when to make the leap to a new, possibly, unproved technology? Is it intuition, preliminary research, case studies, or controlled studies based on outcome?

This article addresses the technologic advances in endodontics pertaining to new and emerging technology. These technologic advances are separated into 5 categories: diagnosis, instrumentation, irrigation, surgery, and MTA cement. Dentists should use caution with a new device or material that lacks definitive published research.

DIAGNOSIS

To assist in a pulpal diagnosis, tests such as biting, chewing, percussion, apical palpation, hot, cold, and an electric pulp test are used. On November 8, 1895, Wilhelm Röntgen produced and detected radiographs.[3] Otto Walkhoff, DDS MD, in Brunswick, Germany took the first dental radiograph in January 1896. Since then, dental

The author has nothing to disclose.
[a] Endodontic Section, Atlantic Coast Dental Research Clinic, 4200 South Congress Avenue, Lake Worth, FL 33461, USA
[b] Private Practice, 1501 Presidential Way, Suite 7, West Palm Beach, FL 33401, USA
* 1501 Presidential Way, Suite 7, West Palm Beach, FL 33401.
E-mail address: rmortman@aol.com

radiographs have become a fundamental part of diagnosing disease of pulpal origin. They are used to determine the presence of multiple roots, multiple canals, resorptive defects, caries, restoration defects, root fractures, the extent of root maturation, and the detection of pathosis.

Many investigators became aware of the limitations of dental radiographs. Drs Bender and Seltzer realized that lesions in cancellous bone cannot be detected roentographically, and early stages of bone disease cannot be detected by means of roentgenograms. In addition, the size of a rarefied area on the roentgenogram is not correlated with the amount of tissue destruction.[4,5] In an article by Goldman and colleagues,[6] there was agreement for the presence of pathosis in only 50% of the radiographically evaluated cases.

Two imaging technologies in endodontics are presented in this section: cone-beam computerized tomography (CBCT) and optical coherence tomography (OCT). CBCT is frequently cited in dental literature, and is a necessary radiographic adjunct for diagnosis for some endodontic cases. OCT is an emerging technology in dentistry, but well proved in ophthalmology.

CBCT

CBCT is more sensitive in detecting apical periodontitis compared with periapical radiographs (PARs).[7] It is a reliable method to detect the MB2 canal in the maxillary first molars,[8] and aids in determining the severity of root canal curvature.[9] With the assistance of a CBCT scan, La and colleagues identified independent middle mesial canals in the mandibular first molar.[10] CBCT scans are also effective for detecting vertical root fractures of different thickness.[11] A CBCT scan seems useful in the evaluation of inflammatory root resorption, and its diagnostic performance is proved to be better than that of periapical radiography.[12] Similar to PARs, a CBCT scan is not a reliable diagnostic method for differentiating radicular cysts from granulomas.[13]

The CBCT can detect an apical radiolucency that may not readily show up on a PAR because of minimal cortical plate erosion. **Fig. 1**A shows a digital PAR and **Fig. 1**B shows a CBCT scan of teeth numbers 2 and 3.

CBCT with proprietary software can reassemble a virtual tooth on a computer, showing exact root morphology. **Fig. 2**A shows tooth number 25 with periapical radiolucency. **Fig. 2**B and C, both taken with a CBCT scan, illustrate the vertical root fracture, making this tooth nonrestorable.

Fig. 3A shows tooth number 14 with periapical radiolucency over the mesiobuccal root. On the other hand, the CBCT series (see **Fig. 3**B) shows the absence of an obturated mesiolingual and distal buccal canals with a lesion surrounding the entire apex of

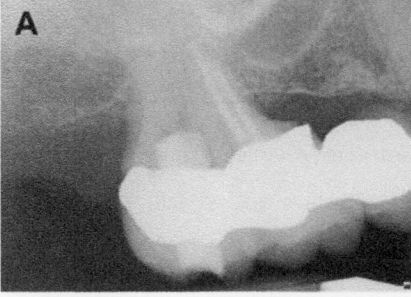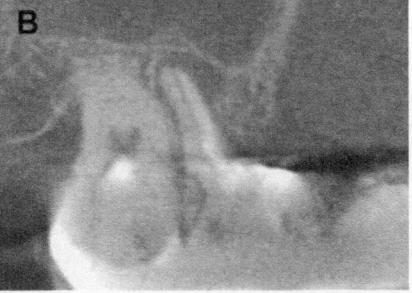

Fig. 1. (A) shows no conclusive periapical radiolucency. (B) clearly shows a periapical radiolucency surrounding the palatal canal.

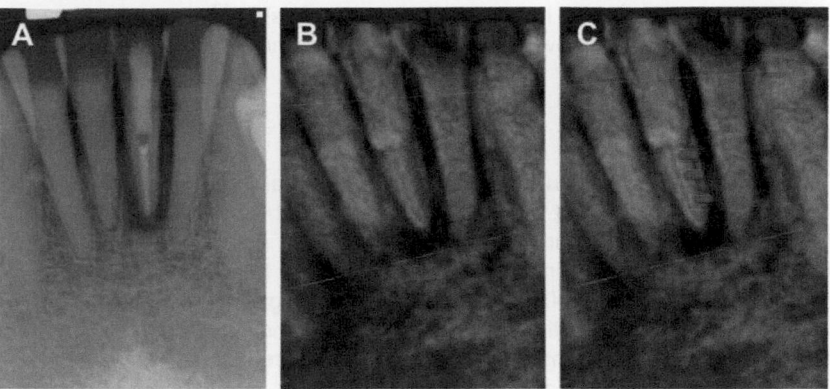

Fig. 2. (*A*) Dental digital radiograph. (*B*) CBCT image. (*C*) CBCT image with arrows pointing to the vertical fracture.

the tooth. The additional information provided by a CBCT scan is invaluable in determining the prognosis of an endodontic retreatment. A recent study on the outcome of root canal treatment in dogs determined by periapical radiography and CBCT scans, concluded that CBCT was a more accurate way to determine the presence or absence of apical lesions after root canal treatment.[14] CBCT may be the future standard to determine if periapical disease has resolved after completion of root canal treatment.

The CBCT has proved itself to be a necessary tool for endodontic diagnosis, as long as clear guidelines for endodontics are addressed. Perhaps the biggest concern is the amount of ionizing radiation that the patient is exposed to. Ionizing radiation, such as dental radiographs, has enough energy to damage DNA in cells, which may lead to cancer. Furthermore, dental radiography has also been associated with low infant birth weight.[15]

The American Dental Association Council on Scientific Affairs recommends that dentists should weigh the benefits of dental radiographs against the consequences of increasing a patient's exposure to radiation and implement appropriate radiation control procedures.[16] The American Association of Endodontists (AAE) has a position paper on the use of CBCT for endodonticts. The AAE recommends using the ALARA

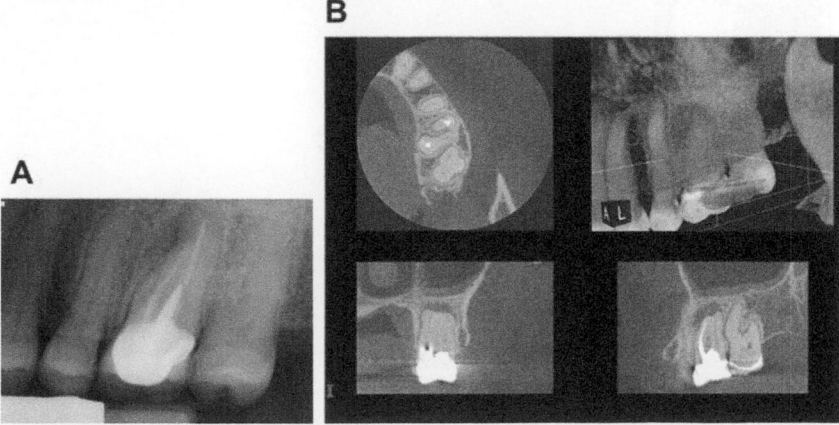

Fig. 3. (*A*) Conventional PAR of tooth number 14. (*B*) CBCT images show unobturated distal buccal and mesiolingual canals.

principle, which stands for as low as reasonably achievable.[17] I use CBCT in approximately 10% of all cases. However, if the device had no ionizing radiation output, I would use this technology for every case.

OCT

OCT is essentially an optical ultrasound that emits no radiation yet provides detailed information to the operator. It is widely used to obtain high-resolution images of the retina and the anterior segment of the eye.

OCT was first mentioned in the proceedings of the International Conference on Optics in Life Sciences in 1990, with the first in vivo images published in 1993.[17] OCT is indicated for morphologic tissue imaging at a high resolution (better than 10 μm). This strategy gives it an advantage over ultrasound and magnetic resonance imaging, which are not ideal for tissue imaging.

OCT was first mentioned in the dental literature in 1998.[18] Since then, more than 50 articles have been published on the benefits of OCT in dentistry. It is used to image hard and soft dental tissue,[19] enamel demineralization and remineralization,[20,21] and early caries.[22] OCT is useful for a noninvasive approach on periodontal diagnosis,[23] and to help visualize periodontal ligament changes in orthodontic movement.[24]

Shemesh and colleagues[25] obtained OCT scans with a Lightlab imaging M2-CV system in combination with an ImageWire 2 catheter. This system is designed for intracoronary imaging in atherosclerotic plaque diagnosis. It is commercially available for clinical use in cardiac catheterization laboratories (**Fig. 4**). Shemesh and colleagues[26] also reported that OCT is a promising nondestructive imaging method for the diagnosis of vertical root fractures (**Fig. 5**), and holds promise for full in vivo endodontic imaging to assess intercanal anatomy, cleanliness of the canal after preparation, and perforations.[25] OCT scans can help determine the interface of the human pulp-dentin complex, and may be used in the future to prevent iatrogenic exposures of the pulp.[27] Optical occurrence tomography was used in the laboratory to investigate apical microleakage after laser-assisted endodontic treatment.[28]

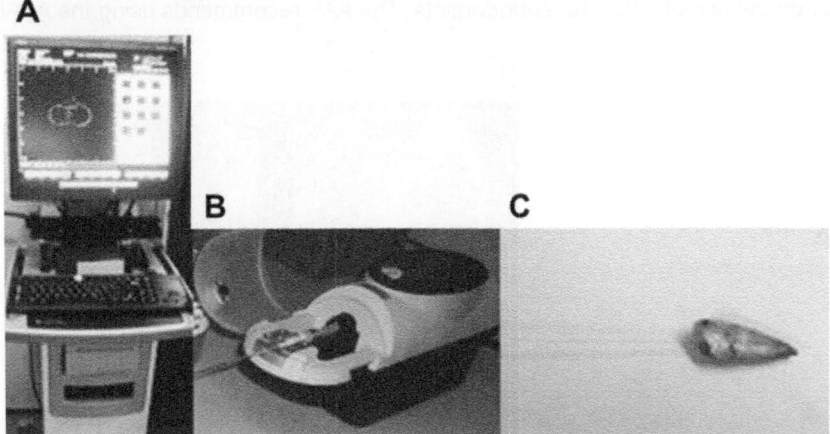

Fig. 4. (*A*) The OCT screen and machine. (*B*) The motor connected to the catheter. (*C*) The activated OCT catheter inside the root canal. (*From* Shemesh H. The ability of optical coherence tomography to characterize the root canal walls. J Endod 2007;33:1370; with permission.)

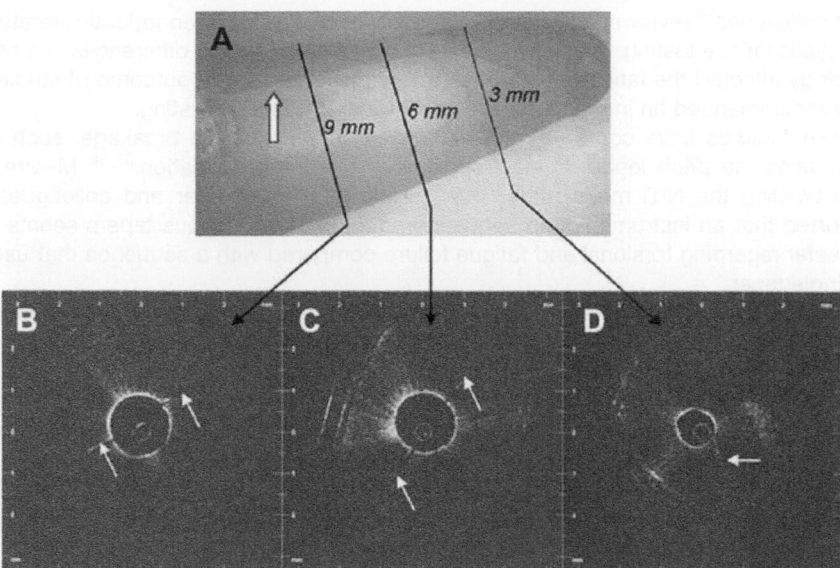

Fig. 5. Root sample (*A*) where the fracture is marked by an arrow, and the corresponding OCT images at 9 mm (*B*), 6 mm (*C*), and 3 mm (*D*) from the apex. OCT visualization of the vertical root fracture is marked by arrows. (*From* Shemesh H. Diagnosis of vertical root fractures with OCT. J Endod 2008;34:741; with permission.)

OCT is an optical signal acquisition and processing method. It captures micrometer resolution and three-dimensional images from within optical scattering media. It is commercially available for ophthalmologic medicine, and used in art conservation. There is no commercially available product for use in dentistry. Future applications in dentistry may include caries detection, periodontal probing, digital impression taking, cancer screening, and endodontic imaging.

Instrumentation

The ideal endodontic instrument has yet to be invented. Ideally, it would be a single instrument that would navigate the canal to working length with ease. It would not break, ledge, or perforate the canal, as well as remove all the canal contents and preserve the dentin. Until approximately 20 years ago, endodontics relied on carbon and stainless steel instruments. NiTi rotary instrumentation has forever changed endodontic instrumentation. This is not a new technology. It is a modern technology proved in the dental literature, but it has limitations.

Perhaps the most frustrating shortcoming of NiTi instruments is file breakage. Torsional stress and cyclic fatigue are 2 frequently studied components of instrument separation. Torsional failure, which may be caused by using too much apical force during instrumentation, occurs more frequently than flexural fatigue, which may result from use in curved canals.[29] Cyclic failure increases with increasing cross-sectional area.[30] When the working end of a NiTi rotary file was bound, smaller files broke with less torque, as did files in more acute curvatures.[31] Clinical use significantly reduces cyclic fatigue.[32] Zhang and colleagues[33] concluded that the cross-sectional design has a greater effect than taper or size of the instrument on the stresses developed in the instrument under either torsion or bending. Certain cross-sectional configurations are prone to fracture by excess torsional stress. Plotino and colleagues[34] reviewed several devices that were used in the endodontic literature for cyclic fatigue testing. These investigators discovered that the differences in methodology affected the fatigue behavior of rotary instruments and outcome of studies, and recommended an international standard for cyclic fatigue testing.

Manufactures have come up with novel ways to prevent file breakage, such as increasing the pitch length,[35] electropolishing,[36] thermal nitridation,[37,38] M-wire,[39] and twisting the NiTi metal rather than milling it.[40,41] Schrader and colleagues[42] reported that an instrumentation sequence encompassing various tapers seems to be safer regarding torsional and fatigue failure compared with a sequence that used 1 single taper.

Hundreds of studies were performed testing NiTi rotary files, but this metal has limitations. We need to move away from NiTi and investigate other metals.

Ferrous Polycrystalline Shape-memory Alloy

Ferrous polycrystalline shape-memory alloy shows huge superelasticity. The iron alloy has twice the maximum superelastic strain obtained in NiTi alloys. The stress level is high so the alloy can be made into a thin wire that can reach the inner part of the body like the brain to deliver stents.[43] Investigations are under way to determine if this metal has a practical application in endodontic rotary instruments.

Self-adjusting File

Another novel approach is to change the instrument design entirely. The self-adjusting file (SAF) (ReDent-Nova Inc, Ra'anana, Israel) was first introduced in the dental literature in April 2010. It is a hollow, thin cylindrical NiTi lattice that adapts to the longitudinal and cross-section of the root canal (**Fig. 6**).[44] The file is elastically compressible from a diameter of 1.5 mm to dimensions to those of a number 20 stainless steel K-file.[45–47] Rather than a drilling or reciprocating action, the SAF is operated with a transline (in and out) vibrating handpiece with 3000 to 5000 vibrations per minute. This action has a scrubbing, sandpaperlike effect on the canal walls. The hollow design allows for constant irrigation throughout the procedure. Metzger and colleagues[46] showed that the SAF operation resulted in root canal walls that were free of debris

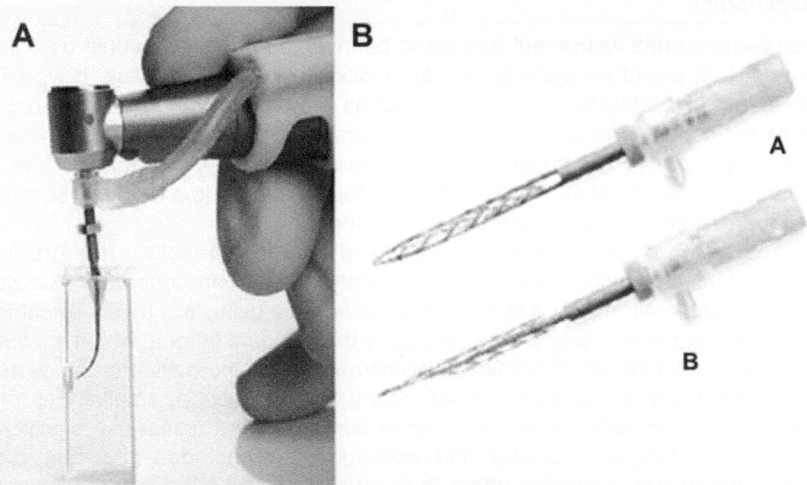

Fig. 6. (*A*) SAF file in a plastic block. (*B*) The SAF file. (*From* Metzger Z. The self-adjusting file, part I. J Endod 2010;36:683–4; with permission.)

in all thirds of the canal in all (100%) of the samples. In addition, smear layer-free surfaces were observed in 100% and 80% of the coronal and middle thirds of the canal, respectively. In the apical third of the canal, smear layer-free surfaces were found in 65% of the root canals.[45]

More research needs to be undertaken on this new file system. A limitation is the preestablishment of a glide path equivalent to a size 20 K-file before using the SAF. Overall, the SAF seems to have an advantage in cleaning and shaping oval canals, and may be a great adjunct to existing NiTi rotary instrumentation technologies.

Apexum Device

A new device developed by Apexum Ltd (Or-Yehuda, Israel) is based on minimally invasive removal of periapical chronically inflamed tissues through a root canal access. The Apexum device consists of 2 instruments: an Apexum NiTi ablator and an Apexum polyglycolic acid (PGA) ablator. The Apexum NiTi ablator is composed of a hollow tube, a sheath (**Fig. 7**A), and a NiTi precurved metal wire (see **Fig. 7**B). The hollow tube and sheath are inserted into the canal to within 1 mm of the tooth apex. The NiTi precurved metal wire goes through the hollow tube into the periapical lesion (see **Fig. 7**C). When the Apexum NiTi ablator is rotated at 250 revolutions per minute (rpm) using a slow handpiece it breaks up the periapical tissues. The second instrument, the Apexum PGA ablator, is a bioabsorbable filament, which is inserted through the sheath into the periapical tissues (see **Fig. 7**D). This instrument whips into the periapical lesion at 7000 rpm for 30 seconds and liquefies its contents to be rinsed and then suctioned out.

This technology is presented after only 1 publication in the *Journal of Endodontics*. Metzger and colleagues[48] showed that removing or debulking of the periapical inflamed tissue, using the Apexum procedure, seems to enhance healing kinetics with no adverse effect. More research needs to be completed to establish this technique as a viable treatment modality.

The Apexum device requires the root canal preparation to be open to a number 40 master apical file. A study by Usman and colleagues[49] showed that a size 20 apical preparation with greater taper (GT) rotary instruments left more bacteria and debris in

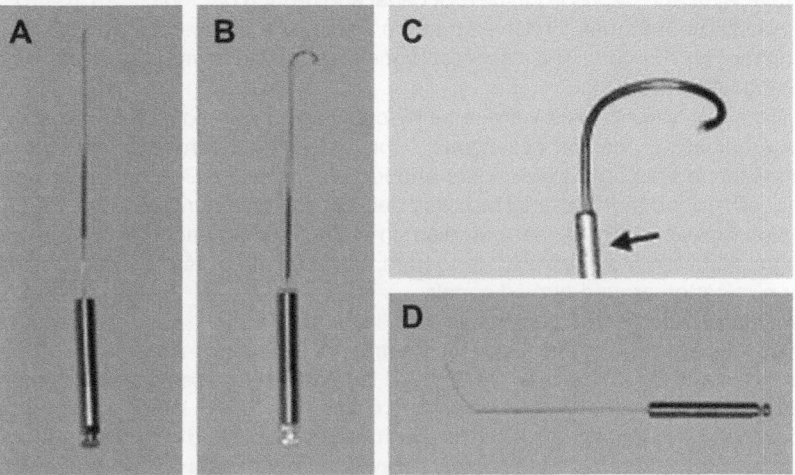

Fig. 7. (*A–D*) Apexum device. (*From* Metzger Z. Healing kinetics of periapical lesions enhanced by the apexum procedure. J Endod 2009;35:155; with permission.)

the apical third than a size 40 GT preparation. The conclusion was that apical third cleanliness could be predicted mainly by instrument size. Kvist and Reit[50] studied the results of endodontic retreatment and concluded that even although the surgical retreatment seemed to result in a more rapid periapical bone fill after 4 years, results were similar between the 2 treatment modalities.

Lin and colleagues[51] found it is not necessary to completely curette out all the inflamed periradicular tissues during surgery, because this granulationlike tissue is incorporated into the new granulation tissue as part of the healing process. Controlling the source of irritants in the root canal is more important than removing all periradicular tissues affected by the irritants.

The idea of having another instrument in our armamentarium that can help even 1 more patient heal faster, with low morbidity, makes this an instrument worthy of more study.

Lasers

No article on the technologic advances in endodontics is complete without the mention of lasers. A search of dental lasers in the US National Library of Medicine National Institute of Health (http://www.pubmed.gov/) resulted in more than 4000 entries dating back to 1964 on the use of lasers in dentistry.

In the endodontic literature the neodymium:yttrium-aluminum-garnet (Nd:YAG), erbium:chromium:yttrium-scandium-gallium-garnet (Er:Cr:YSGG), and the erbium: yttrium-aluminum-garnet (Er:YAG) are the lasers that are most studied. The Nd:YAG laser has been shown to significantly reduce the number of bacteria,[52,53] and reduced apical leakage after root canal obturation.[54] Another study stated that there were no significant differences between laser-irradiated and nonlaser-irradiated groups.[55] The Nd:YAG laser can soften gutta percha for retreatment[56] and is an effective tool for the removal of root canal obturation materials.[57] In addition, temperature rises on the root surface ranging from 17°C to 27°C can occur.[58] A temperature increase greater than 10°C can be detrimental to the attachment apparatus.[59,60]

The Er:Cr:YSGG laser is developed and manufactured by Waterlase MD (Biolase Technology, Irvine, CA, USA). This laser is equipped with a 200-μm radially emitting laser tip. The tip diameter is equivalent to a number 20 file. It can be used to remove the smear layer and debris from the root canal and reduce bacteria.[61] An in vitro study by Rahimi and colleagues[62] showed that the laser could be used for an apical preparation in root end surgery. The laser preparation resulted in fewer cracks and chipping compared with ultrasonics.

Conflicting in vitro studies were recently published in the *Journal of the American Dental Association*. Jha and colleagues[63] concluded that neither the laser nor rotary instrumentation was able to eliminate endodontic infection. Contrarily, Gordon and colleagues[64] found that bacterial recovery decreased when duration or power of laser irradiation increased. These last 2 studies simulated straight canals that were opened to a large diameter. More research is needed, especially to determine bacterial reduction or elimination around curved canals.

The Er:YAG laser might be suitable for clinical application, as a suppressive and removal device of biofilms in endodontic treatments,[65] and it can be a potential therapy for human infected root canals.[66] An Er:YAG laser that has recently been marketed in dentistry is the Powerlase (Lares Research, Chico, CA, USA). It has photon-induced photoacoustic streaming that has not been studied or published in the dental literature.

Because pulsed lasers create pressure waves in irrigant fluids within the root canal, the potential for extrusion of fluid from the apex should be considered when assessing intracanal laser treatments in endodontics.[67]

Research has not proved that lasers are superior to other treatment modalities. The practitioner has to decide if the cost and risks associated with a dental laser outweigh its benefits. Most endodontic studies have used the laser for cleaning, shaping, and disinfection of the root canal system. There are no published case-controlled studies that show that the laser yields a higher degree of success than current endodontic procedures.

Irrigation

The goal of root canal treatment is total eradication of all bacteria from the canal system before obturation. A study by Nair and colleagues[68] showed that 88% of teeth that were instrumented with stainless steel and NiTi rotary instruments, irrigated with 5.25% sodium hypochlorite (NaOCl), rinsed with 17% ethylenediaminetetraacetic acid and obturated with gutta percha and zinc oxide eugenol cement, still contained viable bacteria in the apical one-third of the root. In a study by Peters and colleagues,[69] a microcomputed tomography scan was used to determine that a large portion of canal surfaces remained unchanged during NiTi preparation. Irrigation helps with the removal of debris, destruction of microorganisms, dissolution of organic debris, removal of the smear layer, and disinfecting areas inaccessible to endodontic instruments.[70] There is no single irrigating solution that alone sufficiently covers all of the functions required from an irrigant.[71] This section discusses 3 new ways to help reduce the number of viable organisms in the root canal system using adjuncts to irrigation alone.

EndoActivator

The EndoActivator (Advanced Endodontics, Santa Barbara, CA, USA) is a device that agitates solutions subsonically (**Fig. 8**). Thirty seconds of NaOCl subsonic agitation with the EndoActivator seems to be slightly more effective in reducing bacterial load in the root canal compared with NaOCl irrigation alone.[72] The EndoActivator provides a better irrigation of lateral canals compared with traditional needle irrigation alone,[73] and it extrudes statistically less irrigant beyond the apex.[74]

However, there is no statistically significant difference in canal isthmus cleanliness when used as an adjunct to aid in canal debridement compared with irrigation alone.[75] Shen and colleagues[76] showed that the structure of biofilm did not show any obvious change when 2 chlorhexidine solutions, surrounding the biofilm, were exposed to continuous ultrasonic or sonic agitation. Furthermore, Huffaker and colleagues[77] revealed that there is no significant difference in the ability of the EndoActivator and a standard irrigation control group to eliminate cultivable bacteria from root canals.

EndoVac

Unlike conventional irrigation that uses positive pressure; the EndoVac system (Discus Dental, Culver City, CA, USA) is a negative pressure device. It consists of a disposable

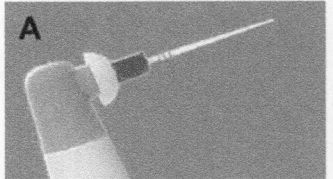
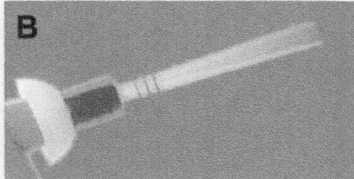

Fig. 8. (*A*) EndoActivator with a blue tip. (*B*) The blue tip sonically activated. (*From* Haapasalo M. Irrigation in endodontics. Dent Clin North Am 2010;54:306; with permission.)

syringe, EndoVac macrocannula, and microcannula. After a complete instrumentation of the root canal system, the EndoVac system is first applied to flush the chamber with an irrigation/suction tip attached to a disposable syringe (**Fig. 9**C). Gross debris in the canal is removed with the macrocannula (see **Fig. 9**A) while the dental assistant continuously adds irrigation into the chamber of the tooth. Subsequently, the microcannula (see **Fig. 9**B) is inserted to the working length; irrigation is again added to the pulp chamber. The irrigation is then suctioned down the canal, through the holes in the microcannula, causing an apical negative pressure (ANP).

A study by Shin and colleagues[78] reported that the EndoVac left significantly less debris behind than conventional needle irrigation methods. ANP removed more debris from narrow isthmi in mandibular mesial roots than manual dynamic irrigation in a closed system.[79] The EndoVac is adept at penetrating NaOCl to the working length in a closed system,[80] and produces less extrusion than needle irrigation.[81] The use of ANP has a significant reduction of postoperative pain levels compared with conventional needle irrigation.[82]

A study by Miller and Baumgartner showed that although there were fewer colony-forming units of *Enterococcus faecalis* bacteria when using the EndoVac, it was not statistically different than a 30-gauge side-vented needle.[83] A study by Brito and colleagues[84] compared NaviTip needles (Ultradent, South Jordan, UT, USA), EndoActivator, and the EndoVac system. The study concluded no evident antibacterial superiority with any technique used.

Light-activated Disinfection

Light-activated disinfection (LAD) is also known as photodynamic antimicrobial chemotherapy, photodynamic therapy, and photo-activated disinfection in the literature. The photosensitizer can be toluidine blue dye, methylene blue dye,[85,86] and

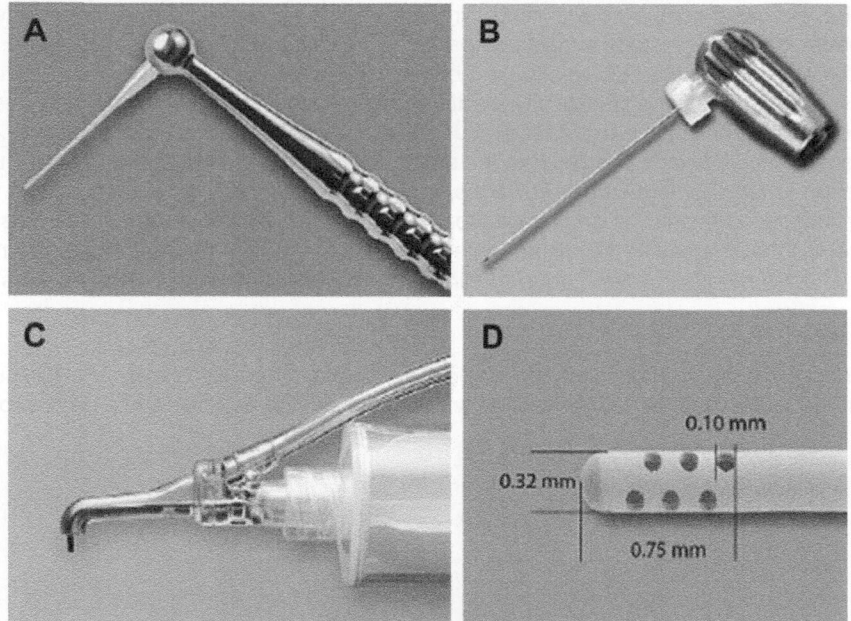

Fig. 9. (*A–D*) Components of the EndoVac system. (*From* Haapasalo M. Irrigation in endodontics. Dent Clin North Am 2010;54:307; with permission.)

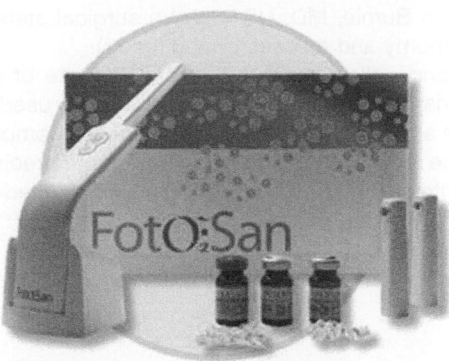

Fig. 10. FotoSan introductory kit. (*Courtesy of* CMS Dental Aps, Copenhagen, Denmark; with permission.)

perfluorodecahydronaphthalene combined with methylene blue dye.[87] Nanoparticle-based endodontic therapy using poly(lactic-co-glycolic acid) (PLGA) nanoparticles loaded with methylene blue are reported in the literature.[88] The photosensitizer binds to the surface of a microorganism. After light activation the photosensitizer absorbs the light, which affects the oxygen present. The oxygen molecule is split into a reactive oxygen specimen that destroys microbial cell walls and other structures. The light source is usually a laser, white light, red light, or a light-emitting diode. Bacterial growth modes play a vital role in influencing the susceptibility to LAD in a dose-dependent manner. The nature of the photosensitizer formulation influences the susceptibility of biofilms to LAD.[84]

The treatment is to fully instrument and irrigate the canal system. The canal is then filled with a photosensitizer and then illuminated with a light source. The root canal is then dried and obturated. The only commercially available unit is the FotoSan (CMS Dental Aps, Copenhagen, Denmark) (**Fig. 10**). Although the unit is not available in the United States, it may serve as an adjunct in a multistep irrigation and disinfection protocol in the future.

Computed Tomography-guided Endodontic Surgery

Dr Stephen Buchanan demonstrated computed tomography (CT)-guided endodontic surgery in the San Diego Convention Center for the American Association of Endodontists annual meeting in April 2010. Using the treatment planning software Simplant R

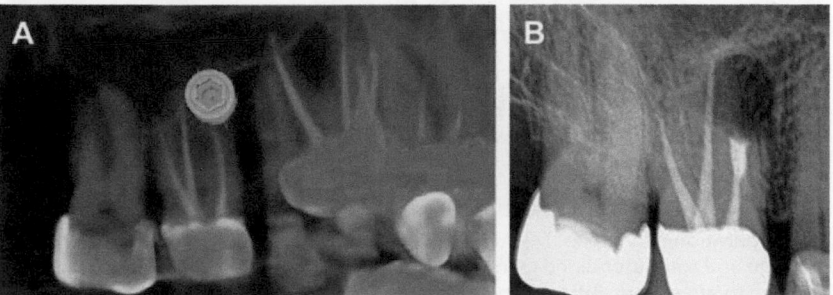

Fig. 11. (*A*) Simplant osteotomy plan. (*B*) Osteotomy, and completed apicoectomy procedure. (*Courtesy of* Stephen Buchanan, DDS, Santa Barbara, CA.)

(Materialise Dental, Glen Burnie, MD, USA) and a surgical stent, Dr Buchanan performed a precise osteotomy and apicoectomy (**Fig. 11**).

A study by Pinsky and colleagues[89] introduced the use of computer-generated surgical guides for periapical surgery. This technique was used to test whether the guide allowed for more accurate localization of the apices, compared with a freehand access preparation. The result was that the apex was more precisely and consistently localized using computer guidance. The study was completed in vitro using stone models and an acrylic surgical guide (**Fig. 12**).

CT-guided endodontic surgery can be particularly useful for performing osteotomies close to anatomic structures, such as the inferior alveolar nerve and mental foramen.

MTA

MTA (Dentsply Tulsa Dental, Tulsa, OK, USA) (**Figs. 13** and **14**), is not a new technology in endodontics. It is a highly researched material that is proving to be successful in more endodontic procedures. MTA, a material that is composed of calcium, silica, and bismuth,[90] comes in a powder form that is activated with the addition of sterile water. MTA has been used in pulp capping, pulpotomies, 1-step apexification, perforation repair, and root canal filling procedures.[91]

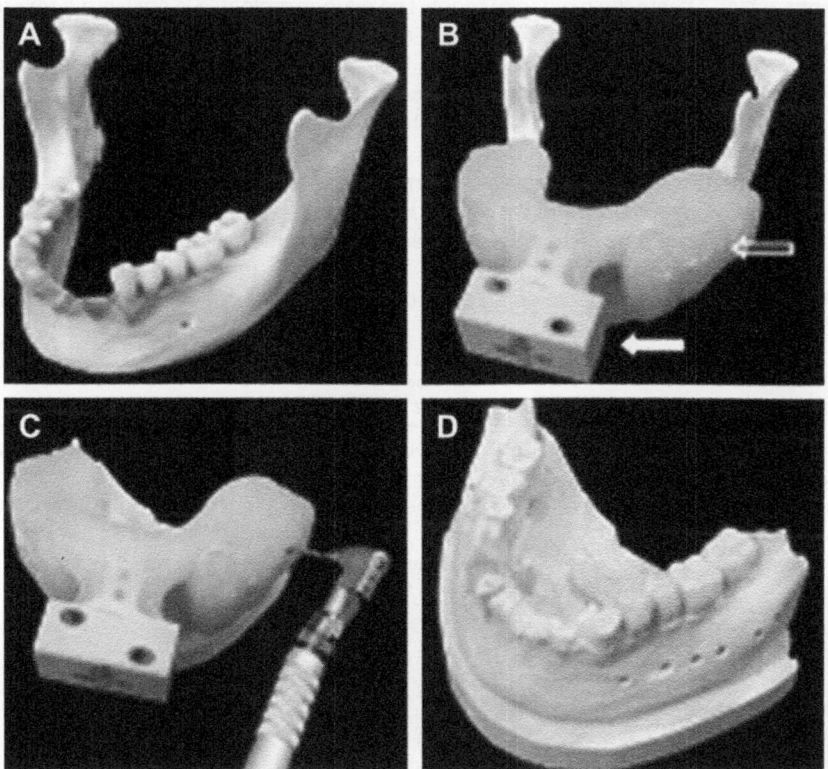

Fig. 12. Preparation of samples. (*A*) After selection of a dentate mandible, (*B*) A computer-aided design and computer-aided manufacturing surgical guide was prepared, using a registration cube (*plain arrow*). Buccal flanges were pierced (*empty arrow*) to guide the surgical drill. (*C*) Test side being drilled. (*D*) Osteotomies after drilling. (*From* Pinsky H. Periapical surgery using CAD/CAM guidance: preclinical results. J Endod 2007;33:149; with permission.)

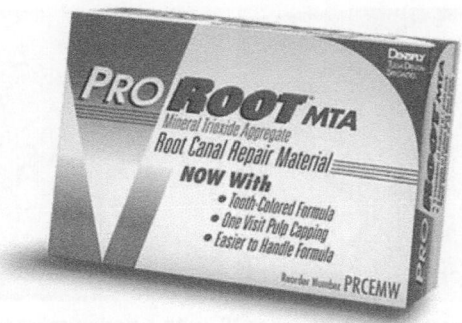

Fig. 13. MTA cement. (*Courtesy of* Dentsply Tulsa Dental, Tulsa, OK; with permission.)

The regenerative procedure of pulp capping and pulpotomy in adult and primary teeth has been reported in the dental literature. MTA is biocompatible and contributes to the possible mechanism of dentin bridge formation and tissue repair.[92] MTA seems to be more effective than calcium hydroxide for maintaining long-term pulp vitality after direct pulp capping.[93] In a study completed by Eghbal and colleagues,[94] fourteen patients having an irreversible pulpitis were treated with an MTA pulpotomy. For 2 months, 12 of 14 MTA pulpotomies performed on individual teeth resulted in an asymptomatic vital pulp. The other 2 patients dropped out of the study. Subramaniam and colleagues[95] showed that MTA pulpotomies in primary teeth had a 95% success rate compared with 85% for formocresol pulpotomies. Doyle and colleagues[96] discovered that, after a 2-year follow-up, MTA pulpotomies in primary teeth presented a better prognosis than ferric sulfate and eugenol-free ferric sulfate pulpotomies. MTA is currently the choice of material for a primary tooth pulpotomy. If more favorable studies are produced, with longer outcomes, and greater sample size, then MTA may be used for the treatment of irreversible pulpitis in adult teeth.

MTA has been used in nonvital pulp therapy as well. Shin and colleagues[97] showed that a revascularization procedure, with MTA cement, has the potential to heal a partially necrotic pulp; this can be beneficial for the continued root development of immature teeth (**Fig. 15**).

MTA has recently been incorporated into a sealer. Camilleri and colleagues[98] concluded that the sealer based on MTA had comparable sealing ability to a Pulp Canal Sealer (Sybron Dental Specialties, Orange, CA, USA). When in contact with a simulated body fluid, the MTA sealer releases calcium ions in solution that encourage the deposition of calcium phosphate crystals. Fluoride doped MTA showed stable sealing during a period of up to 6 months. This finding was significantly better than conventional silicate MTA cements and comparable with AH-Plus (Dentsply International Inc, Johnson

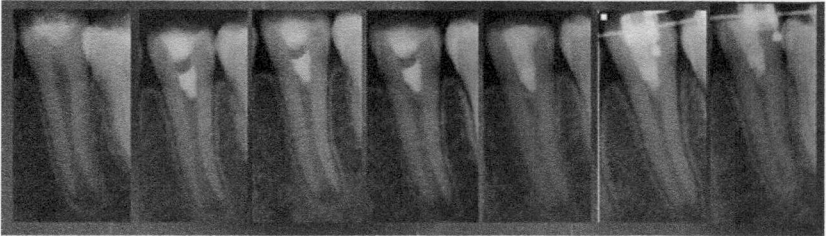

Fig. 14. Apexogenesis with MTA cement. Completed in 3.5 years. (*Courtesy of* Rory E. Mortman, DDS, West Palm Beach, FL.)

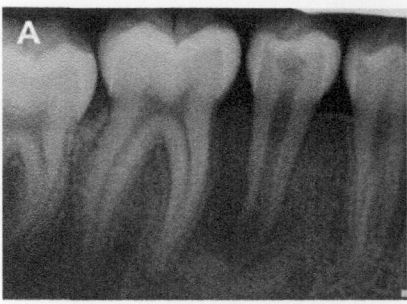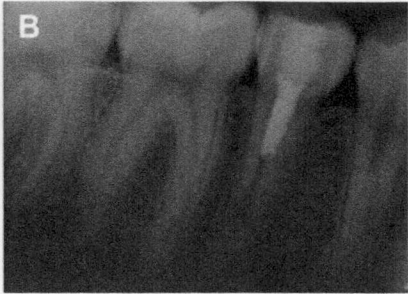

Fig. 15. (*A*) Partially necrotic tooth, number 29, with a periapical radiolucency. (*B*) 9 months after operation showing periapical healing, canal calcification, and root end closure. (*Courtesy of* Sang Y. Shin, DMD, West Palm Beach, FL.)

City, TN, USA).[99] However, more research still needs to be published to determine if this sealer is better than sealers that are currently available.

The main drawbacks of MTA include potential discoloration, presence of toxic elements found in the material makeup, difficult handling characteristics, long setting time, high material cost, absence of a known solvent for this material, and the complexity of its removal after curing.[100]

SUMMARY

This article addresses the technologic advances in endodontics pertaining to new and emerging technology. CBCT and OCT are 2 new imaging technologies that can assist the practitioner in the diagnosis of pulpal disease. The SAF and the Apexum device can be used for instrumentation and bulk debridement of an apical lesion respectively. Nd:YAG laser, Er:Cr:YSGG laser, EndoActivator, EndoVac, and LAD may assist the practitioner in cleaning the root canal system. CT-guided surgery shows promise in making endodontic surgery easier, as does MTA cement for regenerative endodontic procedures.

ACKNOWLEDGMENTS

The author would like to thank the considerate review of Dr Sam Masyr, Dr Sang Shin, Mary Stanley, and Julie Shapiro McSweeney.

REFERENCES

1. Merriam-Webster's Collegiate Dictionary. 10th edition. Springfield (MA): Merriam-Webster Inc; 2010. p. 1206.
2. Hargreaves MK, Cohen S. The core science of endodontics. In: Pathways of the pulp. Elsevier; 2006. p. 36–8.
3. Novelline RA. Squire's fundamentals of radiology. 5th edition. Harvard University Press; 1997.
4. Bender IB, Seltzer S. Roentgenographic and direct observation of experimental lesions in bone: I. 1961. J Endod 2003;29(11):702–6 [discussion: 701].
5. Bender IB, Seltzer S. Roentgenographic and direct observation of experimental lesions in bone: II. 1961. J Endod 2003;29(11):707–12 [discussion: 701].
6. Goldman M, Pearson AH, Darzenta N. Reliability of radiographic interpretations. Oral Surg Oral Med Oral Pathol 1974;38(2):287–93.
7. Garcia de Paula-Silva FW, Wu MK, Leonardo MR, et al. Accuracy of periapical radiography and cone-beam computed tomography scans in diagnosing apical

peridontitis using histopathological findings as a gold standard. J Endod 2009; 35(7):1009–12.

8. Blattner TC, George N, Lee CC, et al. Efficacy of cone-beam computed tomography as a modality to accurately identify the presence of second mesiobuccal canals maxillary first and second molars: a pilot study. J Endod 2010;36(5):867–70.

9. Estrela C, Bueno MR, Sousa-Neto MD, et al. Method for determination of root curvature radius using cone-beam computed tomography images. Braz Dent J 2008;19(2):114–8.

10. La SH, Jung DH, Kim EC, et al. Identification of independent middle mesial canal in mandibular first molar using cone-beam computed tomography imaging. J Endod 2010;36(3):542–5.

11. Ozer SY. Detection of vertical root fractures of different thicknesses in endodontically enlarged teeth by cone-beam computed tomography versus digital radiography. J Endod 2010;36(7):1245–9.

12. Estrela C, Bueno MR, De Alencar AH, et al. Method to evaluate inflammatory root resorption by using cone-beam computed tomography. J Endod 2009; 35(11):1491–7.

13. Rosenberg PA, Frisbie J, Lee J, et al. Evaluation of pathologists (histopathology) and radiologists (cone-beam computed tomography) differentiating radicular cysts from granulomas. J Endod 2010;36(3):423–8.

14. Garcia de Paula-Silva FW, Hassan B, Bezerra da Silva LA, et al. Outcome of root canal treatment in dogs determined by periapical radiography and cone-beam computed tomography scans. J Endod 2009;35(5):723–6.

15. Hujoel PP, Bollen AM, Noonan CJ, et al. Antepartum dental radiography and infant low birth weight. JAMA 2004;291(16):1987–93.

16. American Dental Association Council on Scientific Affairs. The use of dental radiographs: update and recommendations. J Am Dent Assoc 2006;137(9):1304–12.

17. Fercher AF, Hitzenberger CK, Drexler W, et al. In vivo optical coherence tomography. Am J Opthalmol 1993;116(1):113–4.

18. Colston B, Sathyam U, Dasilva L, et al. Dental OCT. Opt Express 1998;3(6): 230–8.

19. Kakuma H, Ohbayashi K, Arakawa Y. Optical imaging of hard and soft dental tissues using discretely swept optical frequency domain reflectometry optical coherence tomography at wavelengths from 1560 to 1600 nm. J Biomed Opt 2008;13(1):014012.

20. Le MH, Darling CL, Fried D. Automated analysis of lesion depth and integrated reflectivity in PS-OCT scans of tooth demineralization. Lasers Surg Med 2010; 42(1):62–8.

21. Manesh SK, Darling CL, Fried D. Polarization-sensitive optical coherence tomography for the nondestructive assessment of the remineralization of dentin. J Biomed Opt 2009;14(4):044002.

22. Li J, Bowman C, Fazel-Rezai R, et al. Speckle reduction and lesion segmentation of OCT tooth images for early caries detection. Conf Proc IEEE Eng Med Biol Soc 2009;2009:1449–52.

23. Xiang X, Sowa MG, Iacopino AM, et al. An update on novel non-invasive approaches for periodontal diagnosis. J Periodontol 2010;81(2):186–98.

24. Na L, Lee BH, Baek JH, et al. Optical approach for monitoring the periodontal ligament changes induced by orthodontic forces around maxillary anterior teeth of white rats. Med Biol Eng Comput 2008;46(6):597–603.

25. Shemesh H, van Soest G, Wu MK, et al. The ability of optical coherence tomography to characterize the root canal walls. J Endod 2007;33(11):1369–73.

26. Shemesh H, van Soest G, Wu MK, et al. Diagnosis of vertical root fractures with optical coherence tomography. J Endod 2008;34(6):739–42.
27. Braz AK, Kyotoku BB, Gomes AS. In vitro tomographic image of human pulp-dentin complex: optical coherence tomography and histology. J Endod 2009; 35(9):1218–21.
28. Todea C, Balabuc C, Sinescu C, et al. En face optical coherence tomography investigation of apical microleakage after laser-assisted endodontic treatment. Lasers Med Sci 2009;25(5):629–39.
29. Sattapan B, Nervo GJ, Palamara JE, et al. Defects in rotary nickel-titanium files after clinical use. J Endod 2000;26(3):161–5.
30. Oh SR, Chang SW, Lee Y, et al. A comparison of nickel-titanium rotary instruments manufactured using different methods and cross-sectional areas: ability to resist cyclic fatigue. Oral Surg Oral Med Oral Pathol Oral Radiol Endod 2010; 109(4):622–8.
31. Booth JR, Scheetz JP, Lemons JE, et al. A comparison of torque required to fracture three different nickel-titanium rotary instruments around curves of the same angle but of different radius when bound at the tip. J Endod 2003; 29(1):55–7.
32. Plotino G, Grande NM, Sorci E, et al. A comparison of cyclic fatigue between used and new Mtwo Ni-Ti rotary instruments. Int Endod J 2006;39(9):716–23.
33. Zhang EW, Cheung G, Zheng YF. Influence of cross-sectional design and dimension on mechanical behavior of nickel-titanium instruments under torsion and bending: a numerical analysis. J Endod 2010;36(8):1394–8.
34. Plotino G, Grande NM, Cordaro M, et al. A review of cyclic fatigue testing of nickel-titanium rotary instruments. J Endod 2009;35(11):1469–76.
35. Diemer F, Calas P. Effect of pitch length on the behavior of rotary triple helix root canal instruments. J Endod 2004;30(10):716–8.
36. Praisarnti C, Chang JW, Cheung GS. Electropolishing enhances the resistance of nickel-titanium rotary files to corrosion-fatigue failure in hypochlorite. J Endod 2010;36(8):1354–7.
37. Rapisarda E, Bonaccorso A, Tripi TR, et al. The effect of surface treatments of nickel-titanium files on wear and cutting efficiency. Oral Surg Oral Med Oral Pathol Oral Radiol Endod 2000;89(3):363–8.
38. Gavini G, Pessoa OF, Barletta FB, et al. Cyclic fatigue resistance of rotary nickel-titanium instruments submitted to nitrogen ion implantation. J Endod 2010;36(7): 1183–6.
39. Alapati SB, Brantley WA, Lijima M, et al. Metallurgical characterization of a new nickel-titanium wire for rotary endodontic instruments. J Endod 2009;35(11): 1589–93.
40. Gambarini G, Grande NM, Plotino G, et al. Fatigue resistance of engine-driven rotary nickel-titanium instruments produced by new manufacturing methods. J Endod 2008;34(8):1003–5.
41. Testarelli L, Grande NM, Plotino G, et al. Cyclic fatigue of different nickel-titanium rotary instruments: a comparative study. Open Dent J 2009;3:55–8.
42. Schrader C, Dent M, Peters AO. Analysis of torque and force with differently tapered rotary endodontic instruments in vitro. J Endod 2005;31(2):120–3.
43. Tanaka Y, Himuro Y, Kainuma R, et al. Ferrous polycrystalline shape-memory alloy showing huge superelasticity. Science 2010;327(5972):1488–90.
44. Metzger Z, Teperovich E, Zary R, et al. The self-adjusting file (SAF). Part 1: respecting the root canal anatomy–a new concept of endodontic files and its-implementation. J Endod 2010;36(4):679–90.

45. Hof R, Perevalov V, Eltanani M, et al. The self-adjusting file (SAF). Part 2: mechanical analysis. J Endod 2010;36(4):691–6.
46. Metzger Z, Teperovich E, Cohen R, et al. The self- adjusting file (SAF). Part 3: removal of debris and smear layer–a scanning electron microscope study. J Endod 2010;36(4):697–702.
47. Patino PV, Biedma BM, Liebana CR, et al. The influence of a manual glide path on the separation rate of NiTi rotary instruments. J Endod 2005;31(2):114–6.
48. Metzger Z, Huber R, Slavescu D, et al. Healing kinetics of periapical lesions enhanced by the apexum procedure: a clinical trial. J Endod 2009;35(2):153–9.
49. Usman N, Baumgartner JC, Marshall JG. Influence of instrument size on root canal debridement. J Endod 2004;30(2):110–2.
50. Kvist T, Reit C. Results of endodontic retreatment: a randomized clinical study comparing surgical and nonsurgical procedures. J Endod 1999;25(12):814–7.
51. Lin LM, Gaengler P, Langeland K. Periradicular curettage. Int Endod J 1996;29(4):220–7.
52. Moshonov J, Orstavik D, Yamauchi S, et al. Nd:YAG laser irradiation in root canal disinfection. Endod Dent Traumatol 1995;11(5):220–4.
53. Doertbudak O, Moritz A, Gutknecht N, et al. Nd:YAG laser irradiation of infected root canals in combination with microbiological examinations. J Am Dent Assoc 1997;128(11):1525–30.
54. Park DS, Lee HJ, Yoo HM, et al. Effect of Nd:YAG laser irradiation on the apical leakage of obturated root canals: an electrochemical study. Int Endod J 2001;34(4):318–21.
55. Meire M, Mavridou A, Dewilde N, et al. Longitudinal study on the influence of Nd:YAG laser irradiation on microleakage associated with two filling techniques. Photomed Laser Surg 2009;27(4):611–6.
56. Viducic D, Jukic S, Karlovic Z, et al. Removal of gutta-percha from root canals using an Nd:YAG laser. Int Endod J 2003;36(10):670–3.
57. Anjo T, Ebihara A, Takeda A, et al. Removal of two types of root canal filling material using pulsed Nd:YAG laser irradiation. Photomed Laser Surg 2004;22(6):470–6.
58. Yu DG, Kimura Y, Tomita Y, et al. Study on removal effects of filling materials and broken files from root canals using pulsed Nd:YAG laser. J Clin Laser Med Surg 2000;18(1):23–8.
59. Eriksson AR, Albrektsson T. Temperature threshold levels for heat-induced bone tissue injury: a vital-microscopic study in the rabbit. J Prosthet Dent 1983;50(1):101–7.
60. Atrizadeh F, Kennedy J, Zander H. Ankylosis of teeth following thermal injury. J Periodontal Res 1971;6(3):159–67.
61. Schoop U, Goharkhay K, Klimscha J, et al. The use of the erbium, chromium: yttrium-scandium-gallium-garnet laser in endodontic treatment: the results of an in vitro study. J Am Dent Assoc 2007;138:949–55.
62. Rahimi S, Yavari HR, Shahi S, et al. Comparison of the effect of Er, Cr-YSGG laser and ultrasonic retrograde root-end cavity preparation on the integrity of root apices. J Oral Sci 2010;52(1):77–81.
63. Jha D, Guerrero A, Ngo T, et al. Inability of laser and rotary instrumentation to eliminate root canal infection. J Am Dent Assoc 2006;137:67–70.
64. Gordon W, Atabakhsh VA, Meza F, et al. The antimicrobial efficacy of the erbium, chromium: yttrium-scandium-gallium-garnet laser with radial emitting tips on

root canal dentin walls infected with *Enterococcus faecalis*. J Am Dent Assoc 2007;138:992–1002.

65. Noiri Y, Katsumoto T, Azakami H, et al. Effects of Er:YAG laser irradiation on biofilm-forming bacteria associated with endodontic pathogens in vitro. J Endod 2008;34(7):826–9.

66. Kimura Y, Tanabe M, Imai H, et al. Histological examination of experimentally infected root canals after preparation by Er:YAG laser irradiation. Lasers Med Sci 2010 Jun 24. [Epub ahead of print].

67. George R, Walsh LJ. Apical extrusion of root canal irrigants when using Er:YAG and Er, Cr:YSGG lasers with optical fibers: an *in vitro* dye study. J Endod 2008; 34(6):706–8.

68. Nair PN, Henry S, Cana V, et al. Microbial status of apical root canal system of human mandibular first molars with primary apical periodontitis after "one-visit" endodontic treatment. Oral Surg Oral Med Oral Pathol Oral Radiol Endod 2005; 99(2):231–52.

69. Peters OA, Schonenberger K, Laib A. Effects of four Ni-Ti preparation techniques on root canal geometry assessed by micro computed tomography. Int Endod J 2001;34(3):221–30.

70. Hargreaves MK, Cohen S. Cleaning and shaping of the root canal system. In: Pathways of the pulp. Elsevier; 2006. p. 315.

71. Haapasalo M, Shen Y, Qian W, et al. Irrigation in endodontics. Dent Clin North Am 2010;54:291–312.

72. Pasqualini D, Cuffini A, Scotti N, et al. Comparative evaluation of the antimicrobial efficacy of a 5% sodium hypochlorite subsonic-activated solution. J Endod 2010;36(8):1358–60.

73. de Gregorio C, Estevez R, Cisneros R, et al. Effect of EDTA, sonic, and ultrasonic activation on the penetration of sodium hypochlorite into simulated lateral canals: an in *vitro* study. J Endod 2009;35(6):891–5.

74. Desai P, Himel V. Comparative safety of various intracanal irrigation systems. J Endod 2009;35(4):545–9.

75. Klyn S, Kirkpatrick T, Rutledge R. *In vitro* comparisons of debris removal of the endoactivator system, the F file, ultrasonic irrigation, and NaOCl irrigation alone after hand-rotary instrumentation in human mandibular molars. J Endod 2010; 36(8):1367–71.

76. Shen Y, Stojicic S, Qian W, et al. The synergistic antimicrobial effect by mechanical agitation and two chlorhexidine preparations on biofilm bacteria. J Endod 2010;36(1):100–4.

77. Huffaker SK, Safavi K, Spangberg LSW, et al. Influence of a passive sonic irrigation system on the elimination of bacteria from root canal systems: a clinical study. J Endod 2010;36(8):1315–6.

78. Shin SJ, Kim HK, Jung IY, et al. Comparison of the cleaning efficacy of a new apical negative pressure irrigating system with conventional irrigation needles in the root canals. Oral Surg Oral Med Oral Pathol Oral Radiol Endod 2010; 109(3):479–84.

79. Susin L, Liu Y, Yoon JC, et al. Canal and isthmus debridement efficacies of two irrigant agitation techniques in a closed system. Int Endod J 2010;43(12): 1077–90.

80. de Gregorio C, Estevez R, Cisneros R, et al. Efficacy of different irrigation and activation systems on the penetration of sodium hypochlorite into simulated lateral canals and up to working length: an *in vitro* study. J Endod 2010;36(7): 1216–21.

81. Mitchell RP, Yang SE, Baumgartner JC. Comparison of apical extrusion of NaOCl using the EndoVac or needle irrigation of root canals. J Endod 2010; 36(2):338–41.

82. Gondim E Jr, Setzer F, Bertelli dos Carmo C, et al. Postoperative pain after the application of two different irrigation devices in a prospective randomized clinical trial. J Endod 2010;36(8):1295–301.

83. Miller TA, Baumgartner JC. Comparison of the antimicrobial efficacy of irrigation using the EndoVac to endodontic needle delivery. J Endod 2010;36(3): 509–11.

84. Brito PR, Souza LC, Machado de Oliveira JC, et al. Comparison of the effectiveness of three irrigation techniques in reducing intracanal *Enterococcus faecalis* populations: an *in vitro* study. J Endod 2009;35(10):1422–7.

85. Souza LC, Brito P, Machado de Oliveira J, et al. Photodynamic therapy with two different photosensitizers as a supplement to instrumentation/irrigation procedures in promoting intracanal reduction of *Enterococcus faecalis*. J Endod 2010;36(2):292–6.

86. Upadya MH, Kishen A. Influence of bacterial growth modes on the susceptibility to light-activated disinfection. Int Endod J 2010;43(11):978–87.

87. George S, Kishen A. Augmenting the antibiofilm efficacy of advanced noninvasive light activated disinfection with emulsified oxidizer and oxygen carrier. J Endod 2008;34(9):1119–23.

88. Pagonis T, Chen J, Fontana CR, et al. Nanoparticle-based endodontic antimicrobial photodynamic therapy. J Endod 2010;36(2):322–8.

89. Pinsky HM, Champleboux G, Sarment DP. Periapical surgery using CAD/CAM guidance: preclinical results. J Endod 2007;33(2):148–51.

90. Parirokh M, Torabinejad M. Mineral trioxide aggregate: a comprehensive literature review- part I: chemical, physical, and antibacterial properties. J Endod 2010;36(1):16–27.

91. Parirokh M, Torabinejad M. Mineral trioxide aggregate: a comprehensive literature review- part II: leakage and biocompatibility investigations. J Endod 2010; 36(2):190–202.

92. Paranjpe A, Zhang H, Johnson JD. Effects of mineral trioxide aggregate on human dental pulp cells after pulp-capping procedures. J Endod 2010;36(6): 1042–7.

93. Mente J, Geletneky B, Ohle M, et al. Mineral trioxide aggregate or calcium hydroxide direct pulp capping: an analysis of the clinical treatment outcome. J Endod 2010;36(5):806–13.

94. Eghbal MJ, Asgary S, Baglue RA, et al. MTA pulpotomy of human permanent molars with irreversible pulpitis. Aust Endod J 2009;35(1):4–8.

95. Subramaniam P, Konde S, Mathew S, et al. Mineral trioxide aggregate as pulp capping agent for primary teeth pulpotomy: 2 year follow up study. J Clin Pediatr Dent 2009;33(4):311–4.

96. Doyle TL, Casas MJ, Kenny DJ, et al. Mineral trioxide aggregate produces superior outcomes in vital primary molar pulpotomy. Pediatr Dent 2010; 32(1):41–7.

97. Shin SY, Albert JS, Mortman RE. One step pulp revascularization treatment of an immature permanent tooth with chronic apical abscess: a case report. Int Endod J 2009;42:1118–26.

98. Camilleri J, Gandolfi MG, Siboni F, et al. Dynamic sealing ability of MTA root canal sealer. Int Endod J 2011;44(1):9–20.

99. Gandolfi MG, Prati C. MTA and F-doped MTA cements used as sealers with warm gutta-percha. Long-term study of sealing ability. Int Endod J 2010; 43(10):889–901.

100. Pariokh M, Torabinejad M. Mineral trioxide aggregate: a comprehensive literature review–part III: clinical applications, drawbacks, and mechanism of action. J Endod 2010;36(3):400–13.

Advances in Local Anesthesia in Dentistry

Orrett E. Ogle, DDS[a,b,*], Ghazal Mahjoubi, DMD[a]

KEYWORDS

- Local anesthesia • Local anesthesia devices
- Reversal of local anesthesia • Safety dental syringes

Local pain management is, without doubt, the most critical aspect of patient care in dentistry. The improvements in agents and techniques for local anesthesia are probably the most significant advances that have occurred in dental science, enabling the profession to make tremendous therapeutic advances that would otherwise not have been possible. Today's anesthetics are safe, effective, and can be administered with negligible soft tissue irritation and minimal concerns for allergic reactions. This article provides an update on the most recently introduced local anesthetic agents as well as new technologies used to deliver local anesthetics.

ARTICAINE

Articaine is the newest addition to the local anesthetic arsenal, and was approved by the Food and Drug Administration (FDA) in April 2000. It is a member of the amino amide class of local anesthetics, and is the most widely used local anesthetic agent in dentistry in several European countries and in Canada. Articaine hydrochloride (HCl) is available in 4% strength with 1:100,000 or 1:200,000 epinephrine.

The amide structure of articaine is, in general, similar to that of other local anesthetics. It is unique, however, among the amide local anesthetics in that it does not contain a benzene ring like the others but instead contains a thiophene ring. The thiophene ring increases its liposolubility, making it more effective in crossing lipid barriers. It also contains an additional ester group, which enables articaine to undergo biotransformation in the plasma (hydrolysis by plasma esterase) as well as in the liver (by hepatic microsomal enzymes).

The authors have nothing to disclose.
[a] Oral and Maxillofacial Surgery, Department of Dentistry, Woodhull Medical and Mental Health Center, 760 Broadway, Brooklyn, NY 11206, USA
[b] Program in Oral and Maxillofacial Surgery, Woodhull Medical and Mental Health Center, 760 Broadway, Brooklyn, NY 11206, USA
* Corresponding author. Oral and Maxillofacial Surgery, Department of Dentistry, Woodhull Medical and Mental Health Center, 760 Broadway, Brooklyn, NY 11206.
E-mail address: Orrett.ogle@woodhullhc.nychhc.org

Dent Clin N Am 55 (2011) 481–499
doi:10.1016/j.cden.2011.02.007
0011-8532/11/$ – see front matter © 2011 Elsevier Inc. All rights reserved.

Articaine HCl does not possess any relevant systemic side effects or gross toxicity, and can be considered a safe local anesthetic.[1] The safety and efficacy of articaine has been studied, and it has been found to be a well-tolerated, safe, and effective local anesthetic for use in clinical dentistry that will meet the clinical requirements for pain control of most dental procedures in most patients.[2,3] Its lower systemic toxicity and wide therapeutic range permits the use of articaine in higher concentrations than other amide-type local anesthetics.[4]

Articaine reaches its peak blood concentration in about 25 minutes following a single-dose dental injection by the submucosal route of a solution containing 1:200,000 epinephrine. It diffuses better through soft tissue and bone than other local anesthetics. The concentration of articaine in the alveolus of a tooth in the upper jaw after extraction was about 100 times higher than that in systemic circulation.[5] Approximately 60% to 80% of articaine HCl is bound to human serum albumin and γ-globulins, and is rapidly metabolized by plasma carboxyesterase to its primary metabolite—articainic acid—which is secreted by the kidneys as an inactive metabolite. The elimination half-life is 20 minutes. The onset of anesthesia is within 1 to 9 minutes after injection, and complete anesthesia lasts approximately1 hour for infiltrations and up to approximately 2 hours for nerve block.

Berlin and colleagues[6] compared the efficiency of articaine to lidocaine in a primary intraligamentary injection administered with a computer-controlled local anesthetic delivery system, and found that the efficacy of 4% articaine with 1:100,000 epinephrine was similar to the efficacy of 2% lidocaine with 1:100,000 epinephrine for intraligamentary injections. No statistically significant differences were seen in the onset and duration of anesthesia between articaine and lidocaine solutions when they were applied for maxillary infiltration anesthesia.[7] However, extraction of maxillary teeth without palatal injection was found to be possible by depositing 2 mL articaine HCl to the buccal vestibule of the tooth rather than lidocaine, possibly due to articaine's better bone and soft tissue penetration and diffusion.[8] Because of its bone-penetrating ability, articaine has become popular for producing profound anesthesia in lower premolars and lower anterior teeth using localized field blocks (infiltrations) without resorting to mandibular blocks. A prospective randomized, double-blind cross-over study looked at articaine and lidocaine mandibular buccal infiltration anesthesia, and found that mandibular buccal infiltration is more effective with 4% articaine with epinephrine than with 2% lidocaine with epinephrine in achieving pulpal anesthesia. Both injections were associated with mild discomfort.[9] Other studies compared the efficacy of articaine and lidocaine for inferior alveolar nerve blocks, showing that 4% articaine with 1:100,000 epinephrine was similar to 2% lidocaine with 1:100,00 epinephrine in inferior alveolar nerve blocks when used for regular dental procedures[10] with no significant difference in patients with irreversible pulpitis.[11] When the two anesthetics were compared in pediatric dental patients, a visual analog score method indicated that articaine is an effective local anesthetic in children but that it was no more effective than lidocaine.[12]

When articaine was compared with mepivacaine 2%, the results indicated that 4% articaine was superior to 2% mepivacaine in depth of anesthesia, mainly over the first 60 minutes.[13]

In the light of its pharmacodynamic properties, articaine can be arranged with local anesthetics similar to lidocaine.

Articaine in Pediatric Patients

The use of articaine in pediatric patients younger than 4 years is not recommended. The quantity to be injected should be determined by the age and weight of the child and the magnitude of the operation. For children younger than 10 years who have a normal lean body mass and normal body development, the maximum dose may be determined by the application of any of the standard pediatric drug formulas. In any case, the maximum dose of 4% articaine HCl should never exceed the equivalent of 7 mg/kg (0.175 mL/kg) or 3.2 mg/lb (0.0795 mL/lb) of body weight.

It is important to be careful when administering articaine to a sedated child, because there is an increased risk of adverse reactions occurring and the sedation may mask the clinical signs. There is a direct link between adverse reactions and local anesthesia volumes.[14]

Articaine and Paresthesia

Persistent paresthesia of the lips, tongue, and oral tissues have been reported with the use of articaine HCl, with slow, incomplete, or no recovery. These adverse events have been reported chiefly following inferior alveolar nerve blocks and seem to involve the lingual nerve most often. Epidemiologic studies of permanent paresthesia following a local anesthetic injection by Haas[15] suggested that the 4% solutions used in dentistry, namely articaine and prilocaine, are more highly associated with this occurrence. Another study by Miller and Haas[16] published in 2000 reported that the incidence of paresthesia from either prilocaine or articaine (the only two 4% drugs on the dental market) was close to 1:500,000 injections, which is relatively low. This result suggests that there may be factors involved other than the drugs themselves.

In a detailed review of paresthesia cases due to nerve blocks evaluated by the Oral and Maxillofacial Surgery Department of the University of California at San Francisco, Pogrel[17] reported that 35% of the cases involved the use of lidocaine and 30% involved the use of articaine. Pogrel concludes that nerve blocks can cause permanent damage to the nerves, independent of the local anesthetic used, and that he did not find any disproportionate nerve involvement from articaine but that articaine is associated with this phenomenon in proportion to its usage.

A 2005 report by the Canada Review Agency (CRA) offered conflicting numbers of paresthesia incidents involving the use of articaine. (The link of articaine with paresthesia was first reported from Canada in 1995.) Like Pogrel, these investigators also concluded that the CRA found no common factor explaining articaine-linked paresthesias.[18]

The operator must therefore look at the evidence of reported articaine-associated paresthesia cases carefully, and be guided by ethical obligations to deliver the most outstanding care possible, without denying patients access to the better care to which they are entitled and yet not expose them to unnecessary risks.

Other Considerations

The metabolism of articaine was found to be age-independent in healthy male volunteers, therefore no change of dosage of articaine in elderly patients should be necessary,[19] but it should be used with caution in patients with heart blocks. It should also be used with caution in patients during or following the administration of potent general anesthetic agents, because cardiac arrhythmias may occur under such conditions. Systematic allergic reactions caused by articaine have been reported.[20] Articaine is classified in Pregnancy Category C, and should be used during pregnancy only if the anticipated benefit justifies the risk to the fetus. It is not known whether the drug is excreted in human milk, and caution should be exercised if it is administered to a nursing woman.

ORAQIX (LIDOCAINE & PRILOCAINE PERIODONTAL GEL 2.5%/2.5%)

Oraqix (Dentsply Pharmaceutical, York, PA, USA) is a topical anesthetic agent introduced in 2004, and is designed primarily for use by dental hygienists. The FDA approved Oraqix for periodontal applications. It is a needle-free subgingival anesthetic for use in adults requiring localized anesthesia in periodontal pockets during scaling and/or root-planing procedures.

Oraqix is an oil at room temperature, so it can be easily applied into periodontal pockets requiring root planing and scaling. Once applied it solidifies at body temperature into an elastic gel, enabling it to remain in place while the anesthetics take effect. It is applied on the gingival margin around the selected tooth using a blunt-tipped Oraqix applicator. Scaling and root planing may begin 30 seconds after the application, and the anesthetic effect has a duration of approximately 20 minutes.[21]

Oraqix offers minimal risk for an allergic reaction, and it may be reapplied to a maximum of 5 treatment cartridges if longer duration of the anesthetic effect is required. Overdose reactions are similar to overdoses from injectable amides (such as lidocaine).[22]

The Oraqix applicator cost about $36.00 (**Fig. 1**).

REVERSING LOCAL ANESTHESIA

In postsurgical patients prolonged soft tissue anesthesia is very desirable, and oral surgeons have combined oral nonsteroidal anti-inflammatories along with the long-acting local anesthetic bupivacaine HCl to successfully manage pain in the postsurgical period.[23] However, many individuals who have had less invasive procedures (eg, routine restorations) have complained to their dentist at follow-up appointments of the inconvenience and annoyance of not being able to eat, drink, or talk normally for several hours after their dental visit because of their lip and/or tongue being numb. In reality, the majority of routine dental treatments are not so invasive that they require a patient to leave the dental office with residual soft tissue anesthesia that lingers for many hours. Patients having these minimally invasive procedures, as well as pediatric patients, could benefit from the reversal of the local anesthetic.

In May 2009, The FDA approved OraVerse (phentolamine mesylate) for the reversal of soft tissue anesthesia and the associated functional deficits resulting from a local dental anesthetic.[24] OraVerse (Novalar Phrmaceuticals Inc, San Diego, CA, USA) is approved for use in both adults and children; however, it is not recommended for use in children younger than 6 years or weighing less than 15 kg (33 lbs).

OraVerse is a formulation of phentolamine, an α-adrenergic antagonist. The hypothesis for the mechanism of action is that phentolamine acts as a vasodilator, resulting in faster diffusion of the local anesthetic into the vascular system and away from the site, thereby reducing the unwanted side effects of lingering lip and tongue numbness.

Tavares and colleagues[25] evaluated the safety and efficacy of a formulation of phentolamine mesylate (OraVerse) as a local anesthesia reversal agent for pediatric patients. These investigators found that the drug was well tolerated and safe in children 4 to 11 years old, and that it accelerated the reversal of soft tissue local

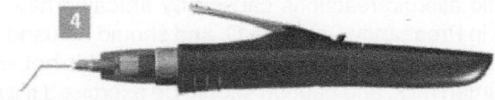

Fig. 1. Oraqix applicator.

anesthesia after a dental procedure in children 6 to 11 years old. The median recovery time to normal lip sensation was 60 minutes for the subjects in the study group versus 135 minutes for subjects in the control group. Tavares and colleagues noted no differences in adverse events, pain, analgesic use, or vital signs.

The phentolamine mesylate must be injected in the same volume and at the same site as the local anesthetic with vasoconstrictor is administered, for example, 1 carpule of lidocaine = 1 carpule of OraVerse. Although tachycardia and cardiac arrhythmia may occur with the parenteral use of α-adrenergic blocking agents, such events are uncommon after submucosal administration, and has not been reported with the use of OraVerse.

DELIVERY DEVICES

While local anesthesia has been great for dentistry and has permitted the introduction of several sophisticated techniques, it is also one of the biggest reasons why people don't go to the dentist: "fear of the needle." To the public, the fear of "the needle" ranks with the fear of "a root canal." These injections can cause pain due to the needle puncture of the oral mucosa, the pressure of the solution entering the area to be anesthetized, and the pH of the anesthetic solution. All of the technologies that have recently been introduced involve devices that try to reduce the pain of anesthetic injection, decrease the failure rates of achieving local anesthesia, and reduce the area anesthetized and thus the residual effects of the anesthesia.

Vibrotactile Devices

Pain relief by vibrotactile stimuli is a well-known phenomenon, and for many years dentists have intuitively used vibrations to decrease the pain from infiltration anesthesia in the upper jaw. The technique of pinching and shaking the cheek in an attempt to distract the brain from the discomfort of the anesthetic shot has been widely utilized with great success. Because the brain (cerebral cortex) is focused on the vibration, the perception of "pain" from the pressure of the liquid entering the tissue is decreased. The gate theory, introduced by Melzac and Wall[26] in 1965, suggested that pain can be reduced by simultaneous activation of nerve fibers that conduct nonnoxious stimuli. Stimulation of larger-diameter fibers (eg, using appropriate pressure or vibration) can close the neural gate so that the central perception of pain is reduced. The proposal is based on the fact that small-diameter nerve fibers carry pain stimuli through a gate mechanism and that larger-diameter nerve fibers going through the same gate can inhibit the transmission of the smaller nerves carrying the pain signal. This aspect led to the theory that the pain signals can be interfered with or modified by stimulating the periphery with nonnoxious stimuli such as pressure and vibrations traveling through the larger-diameter fibers. Some of the newer local anesthetic delivery systems aimed at easing the fear of the needle take advantage of the gate control theory of pain management, which suggests that pain can be reduced by simultaneous activation of nerve fibers through the use of vibration.

Inui and colleagues[27] have shown, however, that pain reduction due to nonnoxious touch or vibration can result from tactile-induced pain inhibition within the cerebral cortex itself and that the inhibition occurs without any contribution at the spinal level, including descending inhibitory actions on spinal neurons. Their study suggested that activation of the tactile pathway at a level higher than that in the spinal cord can inhibit cortical responses to noxious stimuli and does not rely on a gating mechanism.

There are currently 4 devices being marketed in the United States that try to reduce pain at the injection site by relying on vibrations.

VibraJect

VibraJect (Miltex Inc, York, PA) is a small device that aims to block the pain from injections through the use of vibrations (**Fig. 2**). It is a small battery-operated attachment that snaps on to the standard dental syringe. It delivers a high-frequency vibration to the needle that is strong enough for the patient to feel. Nanitsos and colleagues[28] found this device to be effective in decreasing injection site pain and used the gate control theory to explain their findings. Research regarding the effectiveness of VibraJect, however, has been mixed. Nanitsos and colleagues (2009),[28] Murray and colleagues (2003),[29] and Blair (2002)[30] reported the device to be effective whereas Saijo and colleagues (2005)[31] and Yoshikawa and colleagues[32] (2003) reported no significant pain reduction when VibraJect was applied to a conventional dental syringe.

VibraJect was introduced in 2002, and is now in the general price range of US$289 to $359 (it has been seen on certain Web sites for $269). The dental retailers of this device advertise that both the VibraJect and VibraJect R3 dental syringes are equipped with rechargeable batteries with long durability. Several dentists in private practice blogs have complained about short battery life, however.

DentalVibe

DentalVibe (BING Innovations LLC, Crystal Lake, IL, USA) is a recently introduced cordless, handheld injection system, which also uses vibration diversion based on the pain gate theory (**Fig. 3**). The device delivers a pulsed, percussive vibration with enhanced amplitude, which gently taps the mucosa in a synchronized, changing pattern.[33] The changing pattern is supposed to keep the A-β nerve fibers activated. The DentalVibe consists of a U-shaped vibrating tip attached to a microprocessor-controlled Vibra-Pulse motor. The activated U-shaped vibrating tip is first applied to the injection site, and the dental needle may be inserted anywhere in the vibrational zone. It also lights the injection area and has an attachment to retract the lip or cheek.

The DentalVibe sells for approximately $795.00.

Accupal

The Accupal is a cordless device made specifically for palatal injections. It uses both vibration and pressure to precondition the palatal mucosa (**Fig. 4**). Accupal (Accupal, Hot Springs, AR, USA) provides pressure and vibrates the injection site 360° proximal

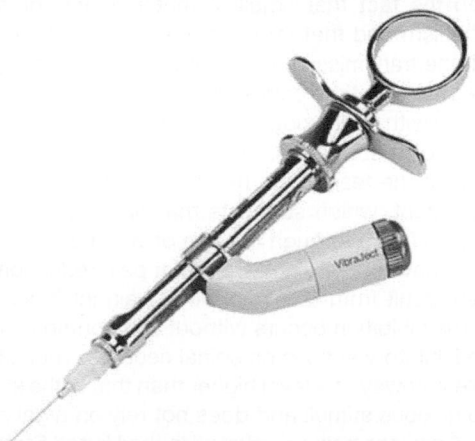

Fig. 2. VibraJect.

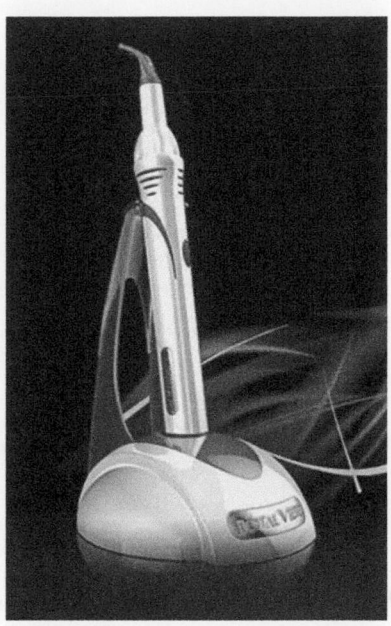

Fig. 3. DentalVibe.

to the needle penetration, which shuts the "pain gate," according to the manufacturer. After placing the device at the injection site and applying moderate pressure, the unit lights up the area and begins to vibrate.[34] The needle is placed through a hole in the head of the disposable tip, which is attached to the motor. It uses one AAA standard battery.

The company has recently expanded its product line with the I/A model, designed for inferior alveolar nerve blocks. The device is the same except for a special tip designed for mandibular injections. According to the company it improves success in inferior alveolar blocks. Accupal devices retails for $499.00 but have been seen online for $399.00. Tips cost about $2.00 apiece.

Single Tooth Anesthesia/CompuDent (WAND)
The STA (Single Tooth Anesthesia) system (Milstone Scientific Inc, Livingston, NJ, USA), introduced in 2007, also uses vibrational technology to decrease pain (**Fig. 5**).

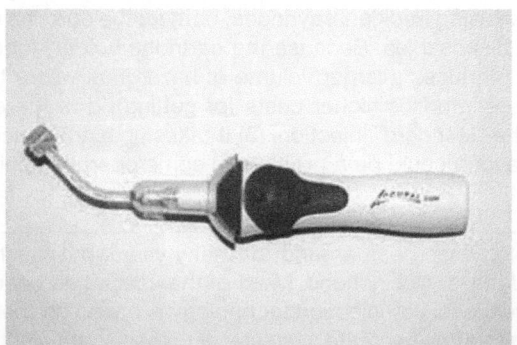

Fig. 4. Accupal.

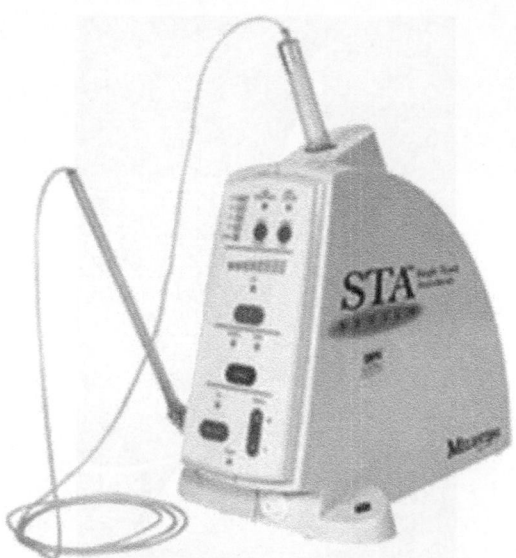

Fig. 5. Single Tooth Anesthetic delivery system. (*Courtesy of* Milestone Scientific, Inc; with permission.)

In addition, it "tells" the dentist if the needle has been positioned properly via real-time visual and audible feedback, providing information on the exit pressure of the anesthetic and the type of tissue encountered. It also uses a computer program to control the anesthesia flow to provide low-pressure injections resulting in pain-free, precise anesthetic delivery, regardless of required pressures[35] (loose connective vs firm connective palatal mucous membrane). The "hardware" looks similar to a miniature computer tower connected to a cartridge containing the local anesthetic. A tube connects this to a pen-like handpiece with a very tiny needle. The cartridge holder, tube, and "wand" handpiece are all single-use disposables. The unit is designed to do intraligamentary periodontal ligament (PDL) injections, replacing the dreaded needle that is used for inferior alveolar blocks with a smaller one for single-tooth anesthesia. The PDL injection allows the dentist to start working immediately after the injection is administered, resulting in uninterrupted treatment. The STA sells for about $1995.00.

Some complaints about the STA have been made. (1) Regarding cost, it is more expensive than using traditional syringes, both for the purchasing of the machine and the necessary disposables. Because the cartridge holder, tube, and handpiece are disposables, it produces a larger volume of hazardous waste than the standard syringe and therefore imposes higher costs for getting rid of the extra waste. (2) It takes longer than the "standard" injection. (3) It takes up extra space which, depending on space and layout, could be a problem in some operating suites.

Jet Injections

Jet-injector technology has been around for many years, but has had rather limited clinical use beyond mass vaccinations. Most of the usage has been mainly confined to intramuscular injections. Jet-injection technology is based on the principle of using a mechanical energy source to create a release of pressure sufficient to push a dose of liquid medication through a very small orifice, creating a thin column of fluid with enough force that it can penetrate soft tissue into the subcutaneous tissue without a needle.

Jet injectors are believed to offer advantages over traditional needle injectors by being fast and easy to use, with little or no pain, less tissue damage, and faster drug absorption at the injection site. Needle-free injectors also offer the advantage of preventing infections that can result from a needle procedure. The big disadvantage in dentistry is that only enough volume can be expressed to anesthetize the soft tissue, and the devices may therefore be used only for topical anesthesia and not for pulpal anesthesia.

Controlled studies evaluating efficacy are lacking, and reports are primarily anecdotal. To date, the effectiveness of the technique in dentistry has been reported to be limited.[36] Soft tissue anesthesia seems to be adequate but pulpal anesthesia inadequate. The main use with current available devices seems to be limited to pedodontics because of less bone density. In oral surgery under intravenous sedation or general anesthesia, it is often desirable to deposit local anesthetic solution with a vasoconstrictor at multiple sites for the purposes of vasoconstriction and postoperative analgesia. The jet injector makes it possible to accomplish this with a minimum of effort and time. Other uses would be in the removal of fracture arch bars or ligature wires in oral surgery, the application of bands in orthodontics, which is often somewhat painful, and for small punch biopsies.

Syrijet

The Syrijet Mark II (Keystone Industries [aka Mizzy], Cherry Hill, NJ, USA) has been on the market for nearly 40 years and has had some minor improvements over the years (**Fig. 6**). The main reason for including it here is because it is the most widely used jet injector in dentistry. Some good features of the device is that it accepts the standard 1.8-mL cartridges of local anesthetic solution (thereby ensuring sterility of the solution), permits the administration of a variable volume of solution from 0 to 0.2 mL, and is completely autoclavable.

The Syrijet Mark II has a nozzle pressure of 2000 pounds per square inch (psi), and at this pressure it was found that jet injection of local anesthetic solutions provides penetration and infiltration nearly comparable to that produced by needle injection to near 1 cm depth, with quantities up to 0.2 mL per injection.[37] The Syrijet retails for $2279.00 (Patterson Dental Systems). Cost and limited clinical application appear to be the drawbacks of this device in dental practice. The marketing is mainly aimed at pedodontists.

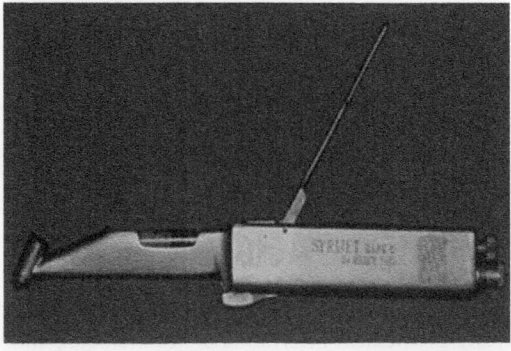

Fig. 6. Syrijet.

Med-Jet

Med-Jet (Medical International Technologies, Montreal, QC, Canada) is a device that is not yet on the market at the time of writing (**Fig. 7**). In February 2010 Medical International Technology announced via a PR Newswire (PR Newswire is a vendor headquartered in New York City that is hired by companies and agencies to send out text press releases to the media) their plan to introduce their needle-free injection technology to dentistry with their "Med-Jet model MIT-H-VI" needleless syringe between March and July 2011.[38] The device was patented in Canada in 2002[39] and the company is currently awaiting FDA approval to launch its needleless injector onto the United States dental market. Initial premarket reports of this device are very promising, but no real clinical information is available. The price for the Med-Jet model MIT-H-VI has not yet been published; however, the Med-Jet MBX model, which is used in medicine, sells for about $5000.00.

Intraosseous Injection

The intraosseous (IO) injection involves placement of a local anesthetic directly into the cancellous bone adjacent to the tooth to be anesthetized, and is used primarily in endodontic practice. Clinical experience has shown that local anesthetics seem to be significantly less effective in endodontic pain patients who present with signs and symptoms of irreversible pulpitis and/or acute periradicular inflammation, secondary to either an apical extension of pulpal inflammation or pulpal necrosis and bacterial invasion. Clinical studies have reported that a single inferior alveolar nerve (IAN) block injection of local anesthetic (1.8 mL) is ineffective in 30% to 80% of patients with irreversible pulpitis.[40] Khan and colleagues[41] stated that patients with irreversible pulpitis had an eightfold higher failure of local anesthetic injections in comparison with nonendodontic patients. For patients who are comfortable until the pulp is exposed or nearly exposed, the intrapulpal injection, which delivers the solution directly into inflamed pulpal tissues, is generally used as the final option to control pain during the endodontic procedure.[42] Some individuals, however, will not be able to tolerate the pulp exposure procedure and can be helped by supplemental anesthesia via an IO technique that delivers the anesthetic to the cancellous bone surrounding the apices of injected teeth. The IO route offers the ability to deliver higher doses closer to the apex, and clinical trials have indicated that the IO route of injection significantly enhances pulpal anesthesia after IAN block injection in endodontic pain patients.[43] There is no evidence that the IO injection provides effective pulpal anesthesia to teeth with irreversible pulpitis when the anesthetic is administered in an IO manner alone. IO injections provide pulpal anesthesia for a duration of less

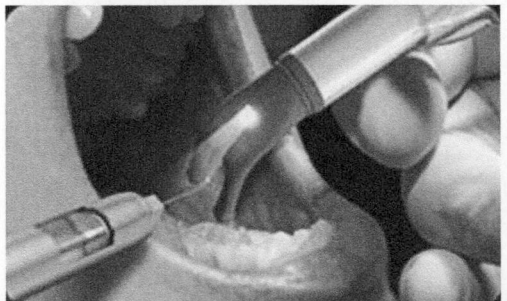

Fig. 7. MedJet. (*Courtesy of* Medical International Technologies, Montreal, QC, Canada; with permission.)

than 60 minutes with vasoconstrictor and approximately 15 to 30 minutes without vasoconstrictor.[44] Although primarily used as a device for supplemental anesthesia, the Stabident IO injection system has been evaluated as a primary injection. Chamberlain and colleagues[45] found that 95% of patients were successfully anesthetized for operative dentistry procedures when using the Stabident IO injection technique, and Leonard[46] reported that a majority of extractions were successful with the system.

Stabident
The Stabident (Fairfax Dental Inc, Miami, FL, USA) device has been available for several years (**Fig. 8**). The system was first marketed in the United Kingdom in February 1991, and introduced to the United States in November of the same year. This system is composed of:

1. Perforator. a solid stainless-steel needle of 27 gauge (0.43 mm), beveled at the free end to enable it to drill through cortical bone, and mounted at the other end on a plastic shank with the standard grooved head of slow-speed dental burrs enabling it to be driven by the standard latch-type contra-angle handpiece. A protective cap enclosing the needle is removable from the plastic shank prior to use. When activated, the perforator drills a small hole through the cortical plate without creating a large-diameter opening that would allow backflow of the anesthetic solution.
2. Injection needle. This is a conventional 27-gauge injection needle but of ultra-short (8 mm) length, which is placed in the hole made by the perforator. The ultra-short needle is used to facilitate the reinsertion of the needle into the opening made by the perforator. The combination of a very short needle and holding the syringe like a pen gives point control over the needle.

There are 2 kit sizes: the standard kit comprises 20 perforators and 20 injection needles and the economy kit comprises 100 perforators and 100 injection-needles. The economy kit costs about $100.00.

The alternative Stabident comprises a perforator of slightly larger diameter than that of the regular perforator, a manually insertable guide sleeve, and a 30-gauge injection needle. The guide sleeve is a metal tube having a wide funnel entrance at one end, surrounded by a plastic part that includes a blade-shaped finger-grip to which is attached a safety cord. The free end of the metal tube does not terminate in a sharp point or in beveling, but is slightly cone-shaped to act as a lead-in. The plastic cap is removed before using the guide sleeve.

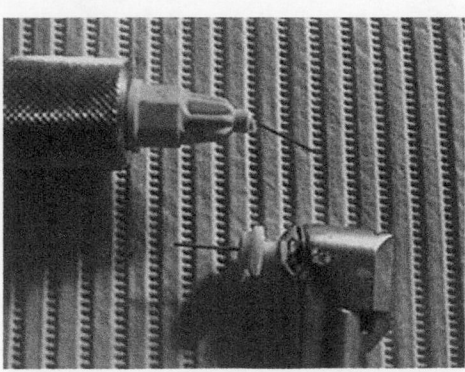

Fig. 8. Stabident.

Numerous studies have shown the Stabident system to be safe and effective when used as directed.[47] The advantages of the product are that it is relatively inexpensive and can be used with equipment already existing in a dental office: a slow-speed handpiece with a latch contra-angle for the perforator and a standard dental anesthetic syringe for the needle.

The main disadvantage of the device is that the perforation needs to be made in a reasonably accessible and visible location in the attached gingiva distal to the tooth to be anesthetized. If the penetration zone is located in alveolar mucosa that moves once the perforator is withdrawn, it can be extremely difficult to locate the perforation site with the anesthetic needle. Even in attached gingiva, it can sometimes be difficult to relocate the perforation site. It is not unusual for the clinician to have to make a second or even a third perforation. Posterior teeth often require that the 9-mm long needle be bent at a 45° angle at the hub in order to obtain a comfortable path of insertion, thus running the risk of breakage.

X-Tip

The X-Tip anesthetic system (Dentsply International Inc, Tulsa, OK, USA) was designed to eliminate the big weakness of Stabident (**Fig. 9**). The problem with the Stabident system is finding the hole that is made to inject the anesthetic solution. The X-Tip solves this problem by making the pilot drill itself a hollow tube through which a 27-gauge needle can pass. The initial drill stays in place, allowing the anesthetic to be placed without hunting for the hole that was just created.

The X-Tip system consists of 2 parts: (1) a drill made of a solid, beveled piece of stainless steel, and (2) a guide-sleeve component, a special funnel-shaped hollow needle that remains in the bone after perforation to facilitate injection needle placement. The solid drill leads the guide sleeve through the cortical plate, where it is separated and withdrawn, leaving the guide sleeve in the cortical bone. The guide sleeve stays in place for the entire procedure, allowing for more anesthetic to be placed if necessary. The hollow guide sleeve is designed to accept a 27-gauge needle to inject the anesthetic solution. The X-Tip drill and guide sleeve is used with a slow-speed handpiece of 15,000 to 20,000 rpm.

The X-Tip is available as a 10-pack starter system of 10 X-Tip guide sleeves, 10 27-gauge needles, directions for use, instructional video, and technique card. There

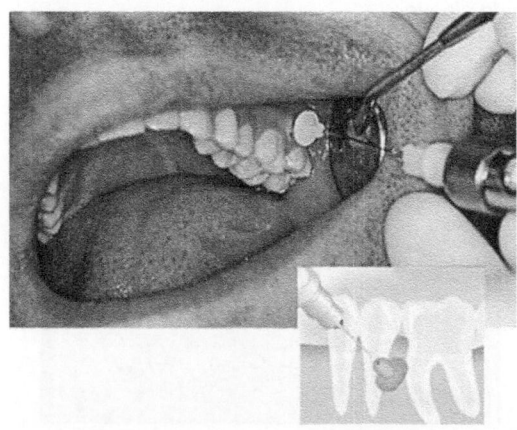

Fig. 9. X-Tip.

is also the 50-pack refill, 50 X-Tip guide sleeves and 50 27-gauge needles. The 10-tip starter kit costs $33.00 and the 50-tip kit $133.00.

The big advantage of the system is that the guide sleeve remains in place to identify the perforation location for needle placement. Like the Stabident system, the X-Tip also does not require additional specialized equipment and has been comparably effective in providing profound anesthesia. Disadvantages of the X-Tip are that the drill and guide sleeve occasionally remain "stuck" together after perforation, and in attempting to remove the drill the guide sleeve also comes out of the hole. The use of a small hemostat to hold the sleeve is sometimes useful. It is also sometimes more difficult to perforate thick or dense bone in the posterior mandible with the X-Tip than with the Stabident perforator. The X-Tip has been reported to have more postoperative pain in males, 1 to 3 days after the procedure, which may be contributed to by increased heat formation during perforation because of the X-Tip's wider diameter of the drill and guide sleeve.[48]

Tulsa Dental (Dentsply International Inc, Tulsa, OK, USA) informed us in September 2010 that they are no longer making the X-Tip. As of mid-September 2010 it was still available at Henry Schein Inc (Melville, NY, USA) and Darby Dental (Jericho, NY— which had a 2010 third-quarter special on the X-Tip). Patterson Dental (St Paul, MN, USA) was no longer selling this product. The authors are unaware if the Assignee of the patent (D438303: 2/27/2001), X-Tip Technologies LLC (Lakewood, NJ, USA) (inventors: Michael Feldman [Toms River, NJ, USA] and Moshe Meller [Haifa, IL, USA]) will try to get another company to produce the X-Tip.

IntraFlow

The IntraFlow Anesthesia System (Pro-Dex Medical Devices, Irvine, CA, USA) is designed to be used as a primary or supplemental means of delivering anesthesia

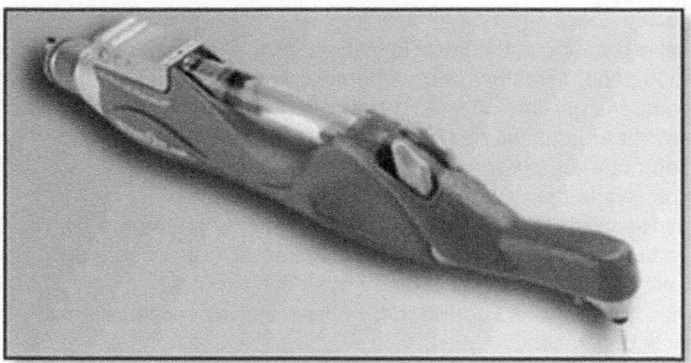

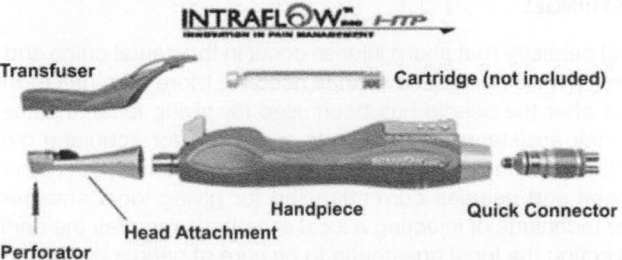

Fig. 10. IntraFlow. (*Courtesy of* Pro-Dex, Inc; with permission.)

(Fig. 10). The manufacturer indicates that it can be used for general dental procedures, endodontic therapy, oral surgery, cosmetic and restorative procedures, and implantology.

The IntraFlow Anesthesia System is composed of 4 core components:

1. The handpiece with a seat for the anesthetic carpule and quick disconnect: a rheostat and a coupling
2. The head attachment
3. The perforator: 24-gauge hollow stainless steel needle
4. The transfuser: ABS Shell & Slider with 20-gauge stainless steel cannula attaches to the head attachment and carries solution from the standard 1.8-mL dental cartridge to the perforator.

After assembling the device according to manufacturer's instructions it is connected to the standard slow-speed line. The rheostat is depressed at full speed, and the perforator is pushed through the gingiva, cortex, and into the cancellous spaces. It should take about 3 to 4 seconds to perforate. To carry out the injection, the rheostat is depressed again (this time more lightly), and 0.9 mL (half a cartridge) of the local anesthetic is slowly injected. Unlike the X-Tip or Stabident, the device is not withdrawn. It is a one-step procedure.

The IntraFlow system starter kit includes:

1× IntraFlow handpiece
1× head attachment
1× quick disconnect
20× disposable transfuser and perforator assemblies
1× recapping stand
1× soaking tub
1× practice book.

The biggest advantage of the IntraFlow anesthesia system is that it allows entry into the penetration zone, injection, and withdrawal in one continuous step, without the need to relocate the perforation site. This single-step method can be helpful in penetration zones that are difficult to visualize or access, such as the second and sometimes the first molar areas, or where there is horizontal bone loss or a limited band of attached gingiva in the desired penetration zone.

Disadvantages of the IntraFlow are start-up and maintenance costs, and that the device can occasionally leak anesthetic, especially if not assembled properly. The handpiece sells for about $900 and the needles for about $2 apiece. The efficacy of this device has not yet been supported by peer-reviewed research; however, studies are presently in progress.

SAFETY DENTAL SYRINGES

It is a fact of clinical dentistry that sharp injuries occur in the dental office and that 25% of the sharp injuries involve anesthetic syringe needles. More than half of the needle-stick injuries occur after the needle has been used for giving local anesthesia in the mouth. Dentists, their assistants, and patients are at risk for acquiring blood-borne infections transmitted via sharp hollow-bore steel needles from one person to another through the syringes and needles currently used for giving local anesthesia in the mouth. The proper technique of injecting a local anesthetic requires the dentist to first aspirate before injecting the local anesthetic to be sure of needle position. Aspiration contaminates the bore of the needle with the patient's blood. After the anesthetic is given, dental office personnel must remove the needle from the syringe by recapping the needle and using its cap to disengage the needle from the syringe before disposal. This entire process poses a risk for needle-stick injuries.

The majority of needle-stick injuries that occur in dental offices do so at a point in the work flow at which safety syringes, in addition to recapping systems, could contribute to injury prevention. Cleveland and colleagues[49] analyzed percutaneous injuries reported by dental health care personnel in the Centers for Disease Control and Prevention (CDC) National Surveillance System for Health Care Workers (NaSH) from December 1995 through August 2004. The investigators found a total of 360 reported percutaneous injuries of which 36% were reported by dentists, 34% by oral surgeons, 22% by dental assistants, and 4% each by hygienists and students. Almost 25% involved anesthetic syringe needles. Of 87 needle-stick injuries, 53% occurred after needle use with possible exposure to hepatitis B (HBV) or C (HCV) or human immunodeficiency virus (HIV). Detailed reports showed that the injuries occurred during activities in which a safety feature could have been activated (such as during passing and handling) or a safer work practice used.

Occupational exposure to pathogenic organisms via needle-stick injury is a common concern among all health care workers, including dental professionals. In 1991 the Occupational Safety and Health Administration (OSHA) issued a standard regulating occupational exposure to blood-borne pathogens, including HIV, HBV, and HCV, and both OSHA and the CDC recommend that health care personnel adopt safer work practices and consider using medical devices with safety features. In response to OSHA regulations, the One Hundred Sixth Congress of the United States of America enacted the Needlestick Safety and Prevention Act, H.R.5178 (Law 106 430, Nov 6, 2000). The Needlestick Safety and Prevention Act (H.R. 5178) mandated that the 1991 OSHA Bloodborne Pathogens Standard (29 CFR 1910.1030) be revised to strengthen the requirements related to the use of safety-engineered sharp devices. It also required state legislatures to pass regulations mandating the use of safety-enhanced devices, including dental anesthetic safety needles, to prevent needle-stick injuries. By law, therefore, the use of sharps with engineered sharps injury protection is now required.

{The law and revised standard do not cover public—ie, state and municipal facilities—in federal OSHA states. However, of the 27 states that are under federal OSHA, 9—Georgia, Maine, Massachusetts, Missouri, New Hampshire, Ohio, Rhode Island, Texas and West Virginia—have passed needle safety laws covering their publicly owned health care facilities. The 23 states under state OSHA must have regulations that are at least as effective as those of federal OSHA. These states were mandated to have a revised blood-borne pathogens standard that is equivalent to federal OSHAs by October 18, 2001}.

After the enactment of H.R. 5178, several devices appeared on the market. Surveys reported wide user dissatisfaction with many of the safety devices, however. Some had poor clinical performance and clinicians found the majority to be cumbersome and not user-friendly, and many dentists were unable to adapt to using them effectively. Results of a review and bench tests indicate that the devices tested were no safer than traditional anesthetic needles.[50] Most have disappeared from the market. In 2006, for example, Med Design Corporation (Ventura, CA, USA) stopped selling the 1 SHOT Safety Syringe (introduced in 2003) and in 2008, MedPro Safety Products, Inc (Lexington, KY, USA) announced that it was no longer selling its Safe-Mate Safety Needle.

There is still a need for safety syringes that will protect providers from needle-stick injury, and some are available on the market.

Ultra Safety Plus XL Syringe

The Ultra Safety Plus XL syringe (Septodont, Lancaster, PA, USA) has a sterile disposable protective shield that is fitted with a dental needle into which anesthetic carpules are placed. The plunger assembly is reusable and autoclavable. The Ultra Safety Plus XL syringe provides protection from the needle because the needle is covered both before and after injection, and the needle does not have to be disassembled prior to disposal, which further protects the worker who is cleaning the dental tray. Providers who used this type of syringe reported that there was more time required for changing anesthetic carpules.

UltraSafe Syringe

The UltraSafe syringe (Safety Syringes Inc, Carlsbad, CA, USA) is a disposable syringe and needle with a transparent, plastic syringe barrel, which has a retractable needle sheath. Providers can view the carpule contents through the clear plastic syringe barrel; this is further helpful in aspiration and in viewing anesthetic content, and also protects the provider from injury because the needle is covered before and after injection. The difference between this type of syringe and the Ultra Safety Plus XL syringe is that in the UltraSafe syringe the entire assembly is disposable and is not autoclavable.

HypoSafety Syringe

The HypoSafety syringe (Dentsply MPL Technologies, Susquehanna, PA, USA) is a translucent disposable plastic syringe and needle combination. The needle can be retracted into the barrel of the syringe after the injection. Therefore, the needle is covered before and after injection, which will minimize the chance of needle-stick injury for providers. The obstacle with this type of syringe is that the dentist is not able to reexpose the safety shield in order to administer a second injection if the needle has been bent; this can therefore delay the procedure and will require use of a second syringe in the case of a bent needle technique having been used.

SafetyWand

The SafetyWand is a device specifically made for the STA/CompuDent (WAND). It is a specially designed wand handpiece with a self-retracting needle. The manufacturer (Milestone Scientific Inc, Livingston, NJ, USA) claims that it is the first patented injection device to be fully compliant with OSHA regulations under the federal Needlestick Safety Act. The SafetyWand provides a fully automated single-handed activation as well as the ability to reuse the device repeatedly during a single patient session.

SUMMARY

Articaine and the combination drug Oraqix (lidocaine & prilocaine periodontal gel 2.5%/2.5%) are the only new anesthetic agents that have been introduced over the past decade. Several innovative devices aimed at decreasing the discomfort associated with the standard injection of local anesthetic in the mouth are now available. This article presents these devices in what the authors believe to be an objective fashion without bias toward any product. Where evidence is available regarding the efficacy of a device, this is also stated.

This overview should enlighten the practicing dentist regarding newer methods of rendering pain control, the possibility of reversing the unpleasant feeling of prolonged numbness following restorative procedures, and safety syringes designed to protect staff involved in direct patient care.

ACKNOWLEDGMENTS

The authors wish to acknowledge the assistance of Dr Manaf Saker for the literature research on the section on articaine.

REFERENCES

1. Leuschner J, Leblanc D. Studies on the toxicological profile of the local anaesthetic articaine. Arzneimittelforschung 1999;49:126–32.
2. Malamed SF, Gagnon S, Leblanc D. Articaine hydrochloride: a study of the safety of a new amide local anesthetic. J Am Dent Assoc 2001;132:177–85.
3. Malamed SF, Gagnon S, Leblanc D. Efficacy of Articaine: a new amide local anesthetic. J Am Dent Assoc 2000;131:635–42.
4. Oertel R, Ebert U, Rahn R, et al. The effect of age on pharmacokinetics of the local anesthetic drug articaine. Clin Pharmacokinet 1997;33:417–25.
5. Vree TB, Gielen MJ. Clinical pharmacology and the use of articaine for local and regional anaesthesia. Best Pract Res Clin Anaesthesiol 2005;19:293–308.
6. Berlin JA, Nusstein J, Reader A, et al. Efficacy of articaine and lidocaine in a primary intraligamentary injection administered with a computer-controlled local anesthetic delivery system. Oral Surg Oral Med Oral Pathol Oral Radiol Endod 2005;99:361–6.
7. Vahatalo K, Antila H, Lehtinen R. Articaine and lidocaine for maxillary infiltration anesthesia. Anesth Prog 1993;40:114–6.
8. Uckan S, Dayangac E, Araz K. Is permanent maxillary tooth removal without palatal injection possible? Oral Surg Oral Med Oral Pathol Oral Radiol Endod 2006;102:733–5.
9. Kanaa MD, Whitworth JM, Corbett IP, et al. Articaine and lidocaine mandibular buccal infiltration anesthesia: a prospective randomized double-blind crossover study. J Endod 2006;32:296–8.
10. Mikesell P, Nusstein J, Reader A, et al. A comparison of articaine and lidocaine for inferior alveolar nerve blocks. J Endod 2005;31:265–70.
11. Claffey E, Reader A, Nusstein J, et al. Anesthetic efficacy of articaine for inferior alveolar nerve blocks in patients with irreversible pulpitis. J Endod 2004;30:568–71.
12. Malamed SF, Gagnon S, Leblanc D. A comparison between articaine HCl and lidocaine HCl in pediatric dental patients. Pediatr Dent 2000;22:307–11.
13. Bortoluzzi M, Manfro R, Kafer G, et al. Comparative study of the efficacy of articaine and mepivacaine: a double-blind, randomized, clinical trial. The Internet Journal of Dental Science 2009;7(1). Available at: http://www.ispub.com/journal/the_internet_journal_of_dental_science/volume_7_number_1_28/article/comparative-study-of-the-efficacy-of-articaine-and-mepivacaine-a-double-blind-randomized-clinical-trial.html. Accessed August, 2010.
14. Wright GZ, Weinberger SJ, Friedman CS, et al. The use of articaine local anesthesia in children under 4 years of age—a retrospective report. Anesth Prog 1989;36:268–71.
15. Haas DA. Articaine and paresthesia: epidemiological studies. J Am Coll Dent 2006;73:5–10.

16. Miller PA, Haas DA. Incidence of local anaesthetic-induced neuropathies in Ontario from 1994-1998 [special issue]. J Dent Res 2000;79:627.
17. Pogrel MA. Permanent nerve damage from inferior alveolar nerve blocks—an update to include articaine. J Calif Dent Assoc 2007;35(4):271–3.
18. Articaine HCL 4% with epinephrine 1:100,000—Update '05. Canada Review Agency Newsletter 2005;29(6):1–2.
19. Oertel R, Ebert U, Rahn R, et al. The effect of age on pharmacokinetics of the local anesthetic drug articaine. Reg Anesth Pain Med 1999;24:524–8.
20. El-Qutob D, Morales C, Peláez A. Allergic reaction caused by articaine. Allergol Immunopathol (Madr) 2005;33(2):115–6.
21. Available at: http://www.drugs.com/oraqix.html. Accessed August, 2010.
22. Basset KB, DiMarco AC, Naughton DK. Local anesthesia for dental professionals. Upper Saddle River (NJ): Pearson Education, Inc; 2010.
23. Malamed SF. Handbook of local anesthesia. 5th editon. St Louis (MO): C.V. Mosby; 2004. p. 277–8.
24. Available at: http://www.drugs.com/oraverse.html. Accessed August, 2010.
25. Tavares M, Max Goodson J, Studen-Pavlovich D, et al. Reversal of soft-tissue local anesthesia with phentolamine mesylate in pediatric patients. J Am Dent Assoc 2008;139(8):1095–104.
26. Melzac R, Wall PD. Pain mechanisms: a new theory. Science 1965;19:971–9.
27. Inui K, Tsuji T, Kakigi R. Temporal analysis of cortical mechanisms for pain relief by tactile stimuli in humans. Cereb Cortex 2006;16(3):355–65.
28. Nanitsos E, Vartuli A, Forte A, et al. The effect of vibration on pain during local anaesthesia injections. Aust Dent J 2009;54(2):94–100.
29. Murray P, Terrett K, Lynch E, et al. Efficacy of a vibrating dental syringe attachment on pain levels [abstract: 1177]. In: 81st General Session of the Int Assoc for Dent Research. Göteborg (Sweden), June 25–28, 2003. Available at: http://iadr.confex.com/iadr/2003Goteborg/techprogram/. Accessed February 15, 2011.
30. Blair J. Vibraject from ITL dental. Dent Econ 2002;92:90.
31. Saijo M, Ito E, Ichinohe T, et al. Lack of pain reduction by a vibrating local anesthetic attachment: a pilot study. Anesth Prog 2005;52(2):62–4.
32. Yoshikawa F, Ushito D, Ohe D, et al. Vibrating dental local anesthesia attachment to reduce injection pain. J Jpn Dent Soc Anesthesiol 2003;31:194–5.
33. Available at: http://www.Dentalvibe.com. Accessed August, 2010.
34. Available at: http://www.accupal.com. Accessed August, 2010.
35. Available at: http://www.stais4U.com/technology.html. Accessed August, 2010.
36. Dabarakis N, Alexander V, Tsirlis A, et al. Needle-less local anesthesia: clinical evaluation of the effectiveness of the jet anesthesia Injex in local anesthesia in dentistry. Quintessence Int 2007;38(10):572–6.
37. Bennett CR, Mundell RD, Monheim LM. Studies on tissue penetration characteristics produced by jet injection. J Am Dent Assoc 1971;83(3):625–9.
38. PR Newswire (February 8, 2010—9:30 AM EST) Denver, CO source: Medical International Technologies Inc. Available at: http://mitneedlefree.com/en/news/99-medical-international-technology-mit-inc. Accessed August, 2010.
39. Canadian patent # 2,021,567, Canadian intellectual property office, Gatineau, Quebec K1A 0C9, Canada.
40. Nusstein J, Reader A, Nist R, et al. Anesthetic efficacy of the supplemental intraosseous injection of 2% lidocaine with 1:100,000 epinephrine in irreversible pulpitis. J Endod 1998;24:487–91.
41. Khan A, Ren K, Hargreaves K. Neurochemical factors in injury and inflammation of orofacial tissues. In: Sessle B, Lavigne G, Lund J, et al, editors. Orofacial pain: basic

sciences to clinical management. Chicago: Quintessence Publications; 2001. p. 45–52 Section 1.

42. Smith GN, Smith SA. Intrapulpal injection: distribution of an injected solution. J Endod 1983;9:167–70.
43. Dunbar D, Reader A, Nist R, et al. Anesthetic efficacy of the intraosseous injection after an inferior alveolar nerve block. J Endod 1996;22:481–6.
44. Replogle K, Reader A, Nist R, et al. Anesthetic efficacy of the intraosseous injection of 2 percent lidocaine (1:100,000 epinephrine) and 3 percent mepivacaine in mandibular first molars. Oral Surg Oral Med Oral Pathol Oral Radiol Endod 1997; 83(1):30–7.
45. Chamberlain TM, Davis RD, Murchison DF, et al. Systemic effects of an intraosseous injection of 2% lidocaine with 1:100,000 epinephrine. Gen Dent 2000;48: 299–302.
46. Leonard MS. The efficacy of an intraosseous injection system of delivering local anesthetic. J Am Dent Assoc 1995;126(1):81–6.
47. Reader A, Nusstein L. Local anesthesia for endodontic pain. Endod Top 2002;3: 14–30.
48. Guglielmo A, Reader A, Nist R, et al. Anesthetic efficacy and heart rate effects of the supplemental intraosseous injection of 2% mepivacaine with 1:20,000 levonordefrin. Oral Surg Oral Med Oral Pathol Oral Radiol Endod 1999;87(3):284–93.
49. Cleveland J, Barker L, Cuny E, et al. Preventing percutaneous injuries among dental health care personnel. J Am Dent Assoc 2007;138(2):169–78.
50. Cuny E, Fredeknd R, Budenz A. Dental safety needles' effectiveness: results of a one-year evaluation. J Am Dent Assoc 2000;131(10):1443–8.

Technological Advances in Extraction Techniques and Outpatient Oral Surgery

Adam Weiss, DDS*, Avichai Stern, DDS, Harry Dym, DDS

KEYWORDS

• Powered periotome • Polyurethane foam • Piezosurgery
• Immediate implants • Orthodontic extrusion • Bone grafting
• Physics forceps

There have been several exciting technological advances in extraction techniques and outpatient oral surgery within the last decade. A variety of new instruments and techniques are revolutionizing the fields of oral and maxillofacial surgery and dentistry. A powered periotome has been developed to atraumatically extract teeth. This instrument is particularly useful for immediate or delayed implant placement. In addition, a technique using implant drills has been developed to extract teeth in preparation for immediate implant placement. Piezosurgery is also being increasingly used for outpatient oral surgery techniques. The precise and effortless nature of piezosurgery has been used in the removal of certain third molars and in bone grafting. Moreover, the Physics Forceps has been created, which uses class 1 lever mechanics to extract teeth without having to use excessive force or squeezing motion. Lasers are also being used for a wide variety of outpatient procedures such as removal of impacted teeth and excision of oral lesions. Orthodontic techniques are also being used by some practitioners to help facilitate extraction of impacted teeth near the inferior alveolar nerve. The use of polyurethane foam to help close oral antral communications may offer a simple technique of handling this fairly common occurrence following dental extractions.

POWERED PERIOTOME

The traditional means of extracting teeth often involving creation of a mucoperiosteal flap, elevation, and luxation with forceps often results in fracture or deformation of the dentoalveolar complex.[1] This trauma could lead to ridge defects, making the

Department of Dentistry and Oral and Maxillofacial Surgery, The Brooklyn Hospital Center, 121 Dekalb Avenue, Brooklyn, NY 11201, USA
* Corresponding author.
E-mail address: aweissdds@gmail.com

Dent Clin N Am 55 (2011) 501–513
doi:10.1016/j.cden.2011.02.008
0011-8532/11/$ – see front matter © 2011 Elsevier Inc. All rights reserved.

dental.theclinics.com

placement of implants very difficult or even impossible in some cases. Also, elevation of the mucoperiosteum may compromise the periosteal blood supply to the alveolus, leading to loss of marginal alveolar bone even in relatively atraumatic extractions. In addition, if the adjacent teeth to the tooth to be extracted have extensive restorations or crown coverage, the powered periotome eliminates the need to elevate against and possibly damage these restorations.

A powered periotome (Powertome 100S, WestPort Medical, Salem, OR) as shown in **Fig. 1** has been developed that allows for the precise extraction of a tooth while producing minimal or no alveolar bone loss. This atraumatic means of dental extraction preserves bone and gingival architecture and gives the clinician the option of placing future or even immediate implants. The powered periotome functions by using the mechanisms of "wedging" and "severing" to aid in tooth extraction.[2] As shown in **Fig. 2**, these instruments are made of very thin metal blades that are gently wedged down the periodontal ligament space in a circumferential manner. This device severs Sharpey's fibers, which function to secure the tooth within the alveolar socket. After most of the Sharpey fibers have been severed from the root surface, gentle rotational movement with minimal lateral pressure will facilitate tooth removal.

A powered periotome is an electric unit that contains a handpiece with a periotome that is activated by a foot control. This device allows precise control over the quantity of force that the periotome tip exerts and the distance it travels into the periodontal ligament space. The instrument has a microprocessor-run actuator that eliminates uncertainty while extracting a tooth. As shown in **Fig. 1**, this device comes with a controller box that can be adjusted to 10 different power settings. In addition, the use of the Powertome 100S system frequently allows flapless removal of teeth, decreasing postoperative pain and discomfort while maintaining the periosteal blood supply to the alveolus.[3] The automated powered periotome system also reduces concern for fracture of lingual bone or buccal plate during difficult extractions. The use of a standard periotome is a much more tedious process and can actually cause unneeded discomfort for the patient, especially if a mallet is also needed to separate the tooth from bone.

When using the powered periotome, the authors have found that starting interproximally seems to work most efficiently because of the thickness of the interproximal bone. It is important to keep the blade parallel along the long axis of the tooth being removed. The blade should follow the tooth anatomy circumferentially in an apical direction in 2- to 3-mm increments. When extracting a multirooted tooth, the authors have found it most efficient to section the tooth and treat each sectioned root as a single-rooted tooth.[4] This instrument has a very small learning curve, and has been

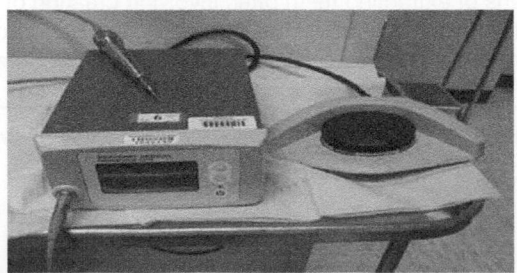

Fig. 1. Powered periotome.

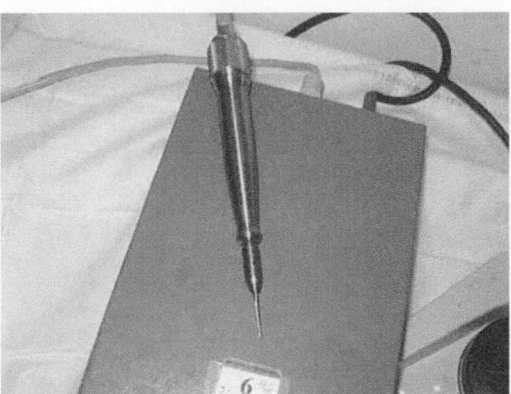

Fig. 2. Powered periotome instrument.

used by both general practice and oral surgery residents for tooth extractions. Photographs from a clinical case taken in the authors' clinic are shown in **Figs. 3** to **6**.

Clinical use by investigators[5] has shown that this product works efficiently to deliver an intact extraction socket with excellent patient acceptance, while at the same time adding little to no additional time as compared with other surgical extraction techniques. Regardless of whether an implant is placed immediately after extraction or if the socket is grafted in preparation for future implant placement, the preservation of alveolar bone allows for more esthetic and functional implant restorations. Millimeters do count when it comes to implants.

USING IMPLANT DRILLS FOR EXTRACTIONS PRIOR TO IMMEDIATE IMPLANT PLACEMENT

The placement of implants for the restoration of lost dentition is becoming commonplace as a treatment option. Immediate implants are in high demand, due to the rising requests for prompt restoration. As mentioned earlier, the key to placing successful and long-lasting immediate implants is preserving as much bone as possible by extracting the tooth as atraumatically as possible. Yalcin and colleagues[6] presented a novel, minimally invasive technique to aid in the extraction of the tooth. To avoid traumatizing the surrounding bone during elevation, implant drills were placed in the root canals to thin the root walls giving way to extraction with the application of much less force, thereby decreasing the chance of traumatizing the thin buccal bone. The thinning of the walls of the roots prior to elevation made it easier to remove

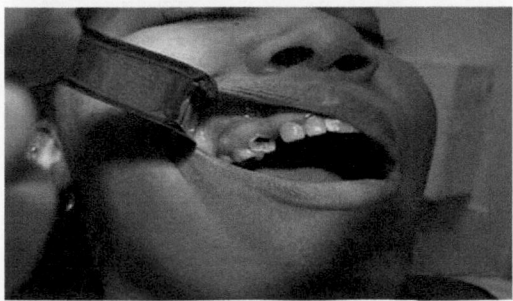

Fig. 3. Preoperative photograph.

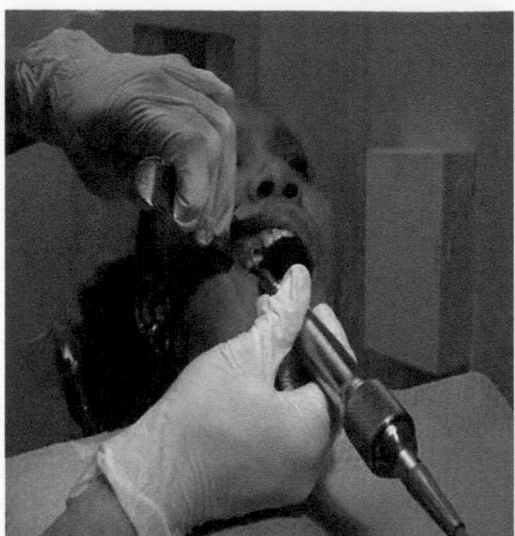

Fig. 4. Intraoperative photograph.

the teeth and minimized the risk of damaging the thin labial wall, especially in root fractures where the fracture line was deep in the socket in immediate implant cases. The investigators were able to successfully complete this procedure with no incisions and without having to reflect any flaps. There was no damage to the labial plate in all of their presented cases. The successful use of this technique may decrease the need for regenerative techniques that could result in graft-related or membrane-related complications.

PIEZOSURGERY

Piezosurgery was introduced in 1988 and has been improved upon since then. Piezosurgery is an innovative bone surgery technique that produces a modulated ultrasonic frequency of 24 to 29 kHz, and a microvibration amplitude between 60 and 200 mm/s.[7] The amplitude of the vibrations created allows a very clean and precise surgical cut. Piezosurgery is very effective in the creation of osteotomies because it works

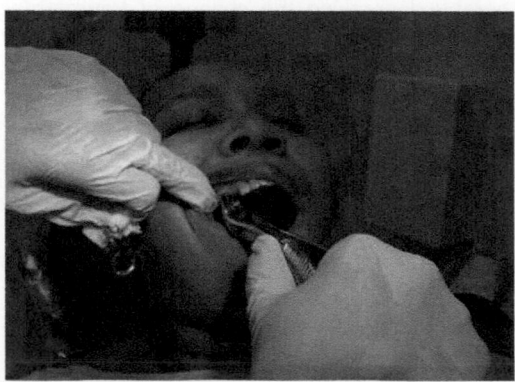

Fig. 5. Intraoperative photograph.

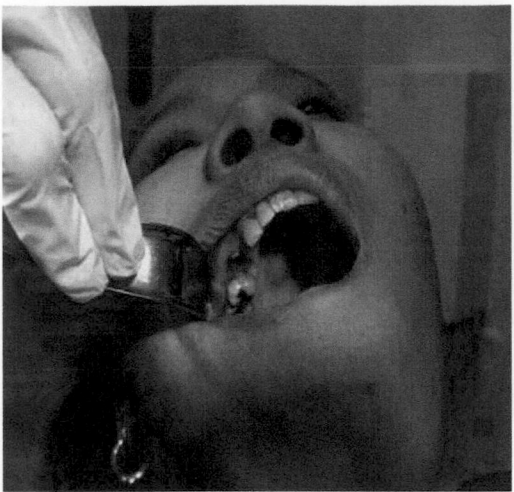

Fig. 6. Postoperative photograph.

selectively, without harming soft tissues such as nerves and blood vessels even with accidental contact with the cutting tip.[8] Piezosurgery thus has a tremendous advantage over the use of burrs and surgical saws that have the potential to cause destruction to soft tissue. When compared with oscillating microsaws, the oscillation of the piezosurgery scalpel tip is very small and therefore able to perform more precise and safe ostetomies.[9] Traditional burrs and microsaws do not distinguish hard and soft tissue.[10] Piezosurgery also gives the operator a clearer field of vision by producing a very restricted bloody region. In addition, as shown in **Figs. 7** and **8**, the surgical control of the device is effortless compared with rotational burrs or oscillating saws because there is no need for an additional force to oppose rotation or oscillation of the instrument[11]

In a recent study by Sortino and colleagues,[7] rotary and piezoelectric techniques were compared in terms of postoperative outcome. The average time of surgery

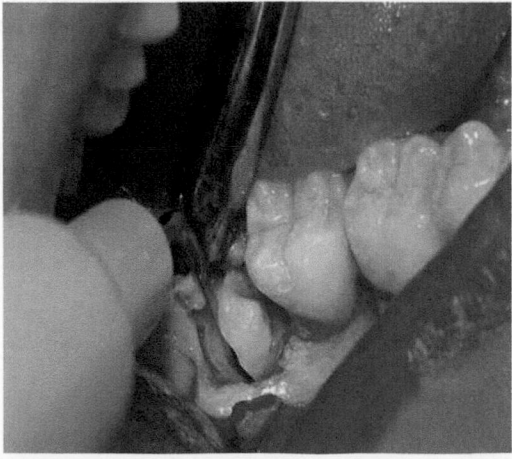

Fig. 7. Piezosurgery used to extract impacted wisdom tooth.

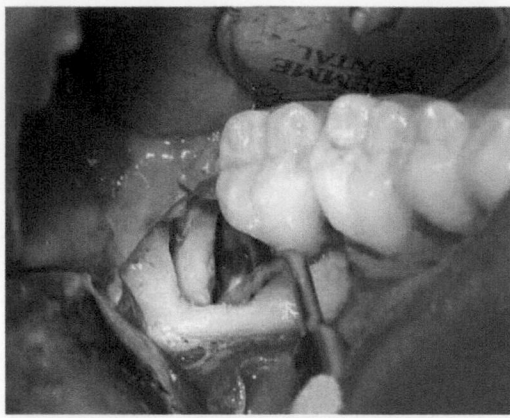

Fig. 8. Piezosurgery used to extract impacted wisdom tooth.

was 25.83% higher with the piezoelectric technique in comparison with the rotary technique. Despite the longer time of the procedure, the investigators also noted that the piezoelectric osteotomy reduced postoperative facial swelling and trismus.

The ability of piezosurgery to allow precise and selective cuts makes this a useful technique when performing surgery close to the inferior alveolar neurovascular bundle and/or the roots of adjacent teeth. The removal of the body of the mandible lateral cortical bone with piezoelectric instrumentation allows adequate access to the surgical area, excellent visibility, minimal bone loss, and precise cutting ability, and allows the protection of the inferior alveolar nerve (IAN) by sparing the soft tissue when osteotomy is performed blind.[12] Because the bone-cutting ability is so precise with minimal bone loss, investigators using this technique have found it easy to readapt the bone windows to their former location and fixate them.[11] Similarly, piezosurgery can be used to perform sinus lifts in a very precise and controlled manner, as shown in **Figs. 9** and **10**.

By contrast, manual and/or mechanical instruments used in the close proximity of delicate structures (vascular, nervous tissue) do not allow for control of the cutting depth and can damage these structures by accidental contact.[7] This new bone lid technique described uses the piezosurgery device to cut and elevate a precisely defined bone lid on the lateral cortex of the mandible to provide access to the teeth needing extraction or even a lesion that needs to be excised. The bone window is then elevated with the help of a curved osteotome. The tooth or lesion can then be

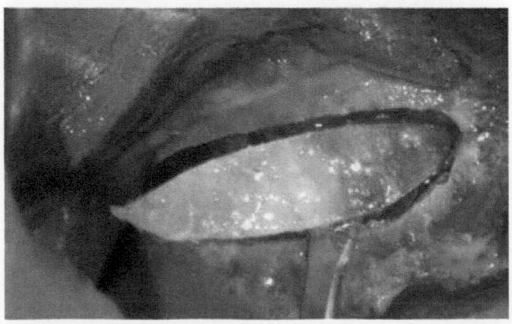

Fig. 9. Piezosurgery used for sinus lift procedure.

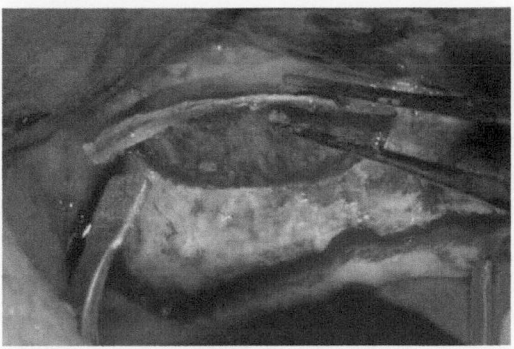

Fig. 10. Piezosurgery used for sinus lift procedure.

seen and subsequently removed atraumatically by either sectioning with piezosurgery or by circular piezo-osteotomy. After the visual confirmation of an undamaged IAN and adjacent tissues, the bone lid is placed back into its original position and fixated with absorbable miniplates.

Bone-Grafting Technique Distal to Second Molar After Third Molar Exo-Piezosurgery

Besides being a useful in exodontias and lesion excision, piezosurgery is now being used in bone grafting. A periodontal pocket distal to the second molar often leads to increased dental sensitivity, increased difficulty in attaining proper oral hygiene in the zone, and the gradual loss of bone support distal to the second molar.[13] Kugelberg and colleagues[14] studied 215 cases and found that 2 years after third molar removal, 43.3% of the patients had probe depths of greater than 7 mm distal to the adjacent second molar.

Penarrocha and colleagues[15] presented a technique in which a bone block is harvested from the retromolar zone distal to the defect using a piezosurgery instrument along with abundant sterile physiologic saline irrigation. The bone block is then placed strategically distal to the second molar, in the area of the defect. After stable graft placement within the walls of the defect is confirmed, 3-0 silk sutures are then placed. The investigators noted that the bone block prevented soft tissue collapse, and no membrane was required in this procedure.

USE OF PHYSICS FORCEPS FOR TOOTH EXTRACTION

The Physics Forceps[16] (**Fig. 11**) uses first-class level mechanics to atraumatically extract a tooth from its socket. One handle of the device is connected to a "bumper," which acts as a fulcrum during the extraction. This "bumper" is usually placed on the facial aspect of the dental alveolus, typically at the mucogingival junction. The beak of the extractor is positioned most often on the lingual or palatal root of the tooth and into the gingival sulcus.[17] Unlike conventional forceps, only one point of contact is made on the tooth being extracted. Together the "beak and bumper" design acts as a simple first-class lever. A squeezing motion should not used with these forceps. By contrast, the handles are actually rotated as one unit using a steady yet gentle rotational force with wrist movement only. Once the tooth is loosened, it may be removed with traditional instruments such as a conventional forceps or rongeur. If considering immediate implant placement, the clinician should consider reducing the buccal aspect of the tooth to be extracted a couple of millimeters with a surgical bur subgingivally, or consider using a periotome before using the Physics Forceps.

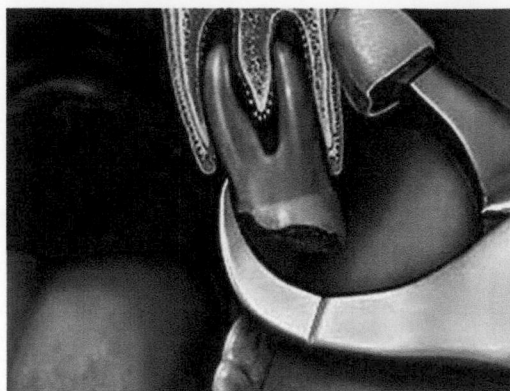

Fig. 11. Physics Forceps.

LASERS FOR EXTRACTION OF IMPACTED TEETH

The use of lasers in outpatient oral and maxillofacial surgeries is becoming more and more popular. Lasers provide a useful alterative and/or adjunct to traditional techniques. The laser osteotomy for removal of impacted teeth offers noncontact and low-vibration bone cutting to allow precise bone ablation without any visible, negative, thermal side effects.[18] Stubinger and colleagues[18] presented a comparison of techniques using Er:YAG lasers, using either a fiber-optic delivery system or an articulated arm delivery system to remove impacted teeth in 30 patients. In 20% of the cases in which the articulated arm delivery laser was used to section teeth, a conventional dental drill was needed to finish the procedure. For the surgical extraction of the teeth, the covering bone was first ablated, layer by layer, using the Er:YAG laser. In the case of the fiber-optic Er:YAG laser the fiber was closely guided around the teeth, creating a narrow gap with minimal bone loss. After uncovering the teeth, they were extracted conventionally by means of standard forceps. However, 4 impacted teeth required separation using the laser, taking care not to damage the adjacent soft tissue, which was protected by elevators. Despite the encouraging clinical results, Er:YAG laser osteotomies tend to be time consuming, and some patients complained about the sound and smell of the laser surgical procedure. Another disadvantage of the laser application was insufficient operative suction, which significantly inhibited the laser cutting because of the overall volume of irrigation and blood covering the bone surface. Another disadvantage of both systems was the lack of a feedback system for depth control. As a result, the technique involves a learning curve, and ultimate success may be dependent on the experience of the surgeon.

LASERS FOR BIOPSY AND TREATMENT OF ORAL LESIONS

Many oral and maxillofacial surgeons are now using laser therapy for a variety of outpatient surgical procedures. As an example, the physical properties of the laser and its effect on tissue make it ideal for incisional or excisional removal of intraoral pathologic lesions. Laser therapy provides for excellent hemostasis and has a low propensity for postoperative scarring.[19] Ben-Bassat and colleagues[20] first described laser therapy for the treatment of oral leukoplakia in 1978. Since then, several studies have found it to be a safe and effective treatment option. Many different laser types have been used in the treatment of oral leukoplakias, including the carbon dioxide

(CO_2), neodymium:yttrium-aluminum garnet (Nd:YAG), argon, and potassium-titanylphosphate (KTP) lasers.[21] In a large retrospective study, van der Hem and colleagues[22] used the CO_2 laser to treat 282 leukoplakias in 200 patients and achieved a cure rate of 89% during a mean follow-up period of 52 months. The benefits of laser therapy include the creation of a bloodless surgical field and thus improved visualization during surgery, decreased postoperative pain, and limited scarring and contraction.[23] The disadvantages of laser treatment include the inability to obtain samples for histologic analysis when ablative techniques are used, and the need for additional time-consuming safety measures during surgical treatment.

NEW TECHNIQUE TO DECREASE PARESTHESIA RISK WITH EXTRACTION OF IMPACTED THIRD MOLARS (HORIZONTALLY OR MESIALLY IMPACTED THIRD MOLARS)

The risk of paresthesia is one of the most feared complications when removing third molars that have radiographic signs of proximity to the IAN. If there is close proximity between the IAN and the roots of the third molar, the incidence of paresthesia may be as high as19%.[24] Landi and colleagues[25] present a current case series demonstrating a technique that surgically removed the mesial aspect of the anatomic crown of the third molar (M3) to create enough space for mesial M3 migration. After the migration of the M3 had occurred; the extraction could then be performed in a second surgical procedure while minimizing neurologic risks. The investigators noted that all M3s moved mesially within 6 months (mean 174.1 days, range 92–354 days) and could be successfully removed without any neurologic consequences. The goal of this technique was to allow spontaneous mesial migration of the impacted M3 by sectioning the portion of the M3 crown in contact with the distal aspect of the second molar. Three to 4 months after the surgery, all M3s moved forward and reached the distal aspect of the second molars. It is important to keep in mind that every effort should be made, at least during the first operative procedure, to not to interfere with tooth vitality. In the worst-case scenario, a pulpotomy procedure can be done and the procedure can continue as planned.

ORTHODONTIC TECHNIQUE: EXTRACTION OF IMPACTED MANDIBULAR THIRD MOLARS

The use of orthodontics in a multidisciplinary approach to perform safe tooth extraction is another advancement worthy of discussion. Third molars in close proximity to the IAN have a significant negative impact on recovery for pain and oral function.[26] Bonetti and colleagues[27] described an orthodontic-surgical procedure that has proven useful for safe extraction of impacted third molars in the presence of high risks (such as neurologic complications) resulting from the tooth's close location to the mandibular canal. This technique involved assessment of surgical risks, creation of the orthodontic anchorage, surgical exposure of the third molar crown, orthodontic extrusion of the third molar as shown in (**Fig. 12**), clinical and radiographic assessment of the extrusion level, and finally third molar extraction. The advantage of this technique is that the risk of direct trauma to the nerve is eliminated, due to both the increased distance between the roots and the mandibular canal and the decreased need for surgical manipulation during the extraction. A potential problem with this technique is soft tissue damage from impingement on the mucosa of the cheek and the gingiva. This type of damage is often unavoidable because of the location of the orthodontic device. In addition, working in this area of the mouth presents great difficulty, and the action of the masseter muscle leads to cheek compression against the orthodontic appliances. Often this procedure is also more time consuming than simple

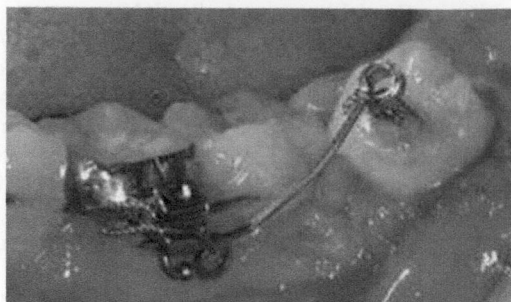

Fig. 12. Orthodontic bracketing to facilitate third molar removal.

extraction techniques. Each clinical case should be judged individually. For example, this technique will be of no value for a tooth that cannot move because of ankylosis. This technique should be used only in carefully selected cases in conjunction with an orthodontist, being certainly difficult, time consuming, and not always successful.

CLOSURE OF ORAL ANTRAL COMMUNICATIONS WITH POLYURETHANE FOAM

Oral antral communications (OACs) are a commonly seen clinical complication treated by oral and maxillofacial surgeons. If less than 5 mm, these communications will often close spontaneously,[28] though the actual size of an OAC is often difficult to determine clinically. Frequently these defects are surgically closed using multiple varied techniques to avoid the development of chronic sinusitis and the development of a fistula.[29] A variety of soft tissue flaps such as the buccal sliding flap and the rotational palatal

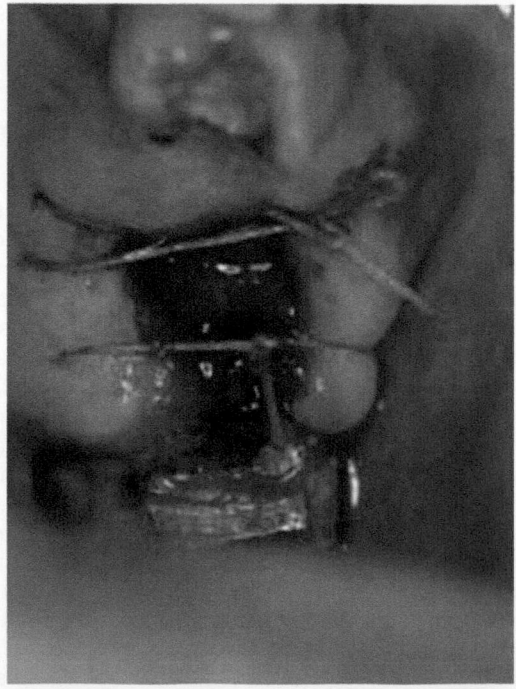

Fig. 13. Closure of oral antral communication with polyurethane foam.

flap have been presented in the literature as a means of closing OACs. Visscher and colleagues[30] presented a new and easy to perform method of closing OACs with use of a biodegradable polyurethane foam, without the need for surgical flap rotations. It is believed that the polyurethane foam provides reinforcement for the blood clot and protects it from being displaced. Ten consecutive patients with OACs were treated with this foam (as shown in **Fig. 13**) and evaluated at 2 weeks and 8 weeks after closure. In this feasibility study, 7 of the 10 patients achieved closure without further surgical intervention. This technique allows the closure of OACs without any other additional training or special equipment. Although more studies on this technique will need to be performed, this procedure possibly provides a valuable alternative to surgical closure OACs.

DISCUSSION

Outpatient oral and maxillofacial surgical techniques have come a long way in recent years. A variety of new instruments and techniques are enabling surgeons to provide services to patients in a shorter period of time with higher accuracy. The powered periotome functions by aiding the surgeon in atraumatically extracting teeth, which allows for either immediate or delayed implant placement into a preserved socket. A technique using implant drills has also been developed to extract teeth in preparation for possible immediate implant placement. Piezosurgery is also being used, as many surgeons are taking advantage of its precise and effortless nature. This type of surgery provides the patient with safe and accurate procedure because soft tissue remains unharmed. Also, the Physics Forceps has been invented, which allows its operator to remove teeth without the use of excessive force or squeezing motion. Lasers are now being used for extraction of impacted teeth and excision of oral lesions. Orthodontic techniques are also being introduced to help minimize nerve damage when a tooth that is near the IAN needs to be extracted. The use of polyurethane foam to help close OACs remains a new possible treatment alternative to more complicated treatment that is possibly just as effective. Technology has allowed extraction techniques and outpatient oral and maxillofacial surgery to evolve, and both surgeons and patients are benefiting.

REFERENCES

1. Dym H, Ogle O. Atlas of minor oral surgery. Philadelphia: W.B. Saunders Company; 2001.
2. White J, Holtzclaw D, Toscano N. Powertome assisted atraumatic tooth extraction. J Implant Advanced Clin Dent 2009;1:6.
3. Levitt D. Atraumatic extraction and root retrieval using the Periotome: a precursor to immediate placement of dental implants. Dent Today 2001;20(11):53–7.
4. Misch CE, Perez H. Atraumatic extractions: a biologic rationale. Dent Today 2008; 27(8):100–1.
5. Kang J, Dym H, Stern A. Use of the Powertome Periotome to preserve alveolar bone during tooth extraction—a preliminary study. Oral Surg Oral Med Oral Pathol Oral Radiol Endod 2009;108:4.
6. Yalcin S, Aktas I, Emes Y, et al. A technique for atraumatic extraction of teeth before immediate implant placement. Implant Dent 2009;18:6.
7. Sortino F, Pedulla E, Masoli V. The piezoelectric and rotatory osteotomy technique in impacted third molar surgery: comparison of postoperative recovery. J Oral Maxillofac Surg 2008;66:2444–8.

8. Kotrikova B, Wirtz R, Krempien R, et al. Piezosurgery—a new safe technique in cranial osteoplasty? Int J Oral Maxillofac Surg 2006;35:461–5.
9. Stubinger S, Kuttenberger J, Filippi A, et al. Intraoral piezosurgery: preliminary results of a new technique. J Oral Maxillofac Surg 2005;63:1283–7.
10. Grenga V, Bovi M. Piezoelectric surgery for exposure of palatally impacted canines. J Clin Orthod 2004;38:446–8.
11. Eggers G, Klein J, Blank J, et al. Piezosurgery: an ultrasound device for cutting bone and its use and limitations in maxillofacial surgery. Br J Oral Maxillofac Surg 2004;42:451–3.
12. Degerliyurt K, Akar V, Denizci S, et al. Bone lid technique with piezosurgery to preserve inferior alveolar nerve. Oral Surg Oral Med Oral Pathol Oral Radiol Endod 2009;108:e1–5.
13. Motamedi MH. A technique to manage gingival complications of third molar surgery. Oral Surg Oral Med Oral Pathol Oral Radiol Endod 2000;90:140.
14. Kugelberg CF, Ahlström U, Hugoson A, et al. The influence of anatomical, pathophysiological and other factors on periodontal healing after impacted lower third molar surgery. J Clin Periodontol 1991;18:37.
15. Penarrocha M, Gomez D, Garcia B, et al. Treatment of bone defects produced by lower molar extraction using ultrasound-harvested autologous bone grafts. J Oral Maxillofac Surg 2008;66:189–92.
16. Golden RM. Dental plier design with offsetting jaw and pad elements for assisting in removing upper and lower teeth utilizing the dental plier design. US patent 6,910,890. GoldenMisch Inc; 2005.
17. Misch C, Perez H. Atraumatic extractions: a biomechanical route. Dent Today 2008;27:8.
18. Stubinger S, von Rechenberg V, Zeilhofer HF, et al. Er:YAG laser osteotomy for removal of impacted teeth: clinical comparison of two techniques. Lasers Surg Med 2007;39:583–8.
19. Strauss RA. Lasers in oral and maxillofacial surgery. Dent Clin North Am 2000; 44(4):851–73.
20. Ben-Bassat M, Kaplan I, Shindel Y, et al. The CO_2 laser in surgery of the tongue. Br J Plast Surg 1978;31:155.
21. Ishii J, Fujita K, Komori T. Laser surgery as a treatment for oral leukoplakia. Oral Oncol 2003;39:759.
22. van der Hem PS, Nauta JM, van der Wal JE, et al. The results of CO_2 laser surgery in patients with oral leukoplakia: a 25 year follow up. Oral Oncol 2005;41:31.
23. Meltzer C. Surgical management of oral and mucosal dysplasias: the case for laser excision. J Oral Maxillofac Surg 2007;65:293.
24. Renton T, Hankins M, Sproate C, et al. A randomized controlled clinical trial to compare the incidence of injury to the inferior alveolar nerve as a result of coronectomy and removal of mandibular third molar. Br J Oral Maxillofac Surg 2005;43:7.
25. Landi L, Manicone P, Piccinelli S, et al. Novel surgical approach to impacted mandibular third molars to reduce the risk of paresthesia: a case series. J Oral Maxillofac Surg 2010;68:969–74.
26. White RP. Recovery after third-molar surgery. Am J Orthod Dentofacial Orthop 2004;126:289.
27. Bonetti GA, Bendandi M, Laino L, et al. Orthodontic extraction: riskless extraction of impacted lower third molars close to the mandibular canal. J Oral Maxillofac Surg 2007;65:2580–6.
28. von Wowern N. Correlation between the development of an orantral fistula and the size of the corresponding bony defect. J Oral Surg 1973;31:98.

29. von Wowern N. Frequency of oro-antral fistulae after perforation to the maxillary sinus. Scand J Dent Res 1970;78:394.

30. Visscher S, van Minnen B, Rudolf RM. Closure of oroantral communications using biodegradable polyurethane foam: a feasibility study. J Oral Maxillofac Surg 2010;68:281–6.

Cone Beam Computed Tomography–assisted Treatment Planning Concepts

Scott D. Ganz, DMD[a,b,*]

KEYWORDS

- Cone beam computed tomography
- Dental implants • Computed tomography
- Interactive treatment planning applications

Computed tomography (CT) and cone beam CT (CBCT) technology allows for an unprecedented three-dimensional (3D) evaluation of each patient's individual anatomy. The advent of this technology has evolved into an indispensable diagnostic tool that can be used for a variety of different clinical applications that include, but are not limited to: dental implant receptor site evaluation; alveolar bone defect and bone augmentation procedures; impacted teeth; orthodontics; endodontics; temporomandibular (TM) joint diagnostics; sinus augmentation procedures; and orthognathic surgical interventions. The presurgical planning phase of these applications that benefit from CBCT technology starts with the accumulation of data for which educated treatment decisions can be accurately determined. Adapting to the ALARA (as low as reasonably achievable) principle, the radiation dosages from CBCT have been minimized through the process of collimation, and reduction in scan time, yet maintaining a high degree of diagnostic accuracy. The benefits versus the risks should be considered when determining the need for a scan. The purpose of this article is to show the benefits of using CBCT technology for dental implant applications.

A myriad of CBCT scanning machines are available in the United States and around the world that claim to deliver high-quality diagnostic images with machine-specific variations on how this can be achieved. In addition, each machine is driven by

Portions of this text were published previously in Ganz SD. Case Report: CBCT-assisted treatment of the failing long span bridge with staged and immediate load implant restoration. DentalTown, Volume 11, Issue 11. Nov 2010 pp 82–86. Reprinted with permission of Dentaltown Magazine and Dentaltown.com.

[a] Department of Restorative Dentistry, University of Medicine and Dentistry, New Jersey, New Jersey Dental School, 110 Bergen Street, Newark, NJ 07103, USA
[b] Private Practice, 158 Linwood Plaza, Suite 204, Fort Lee, NJ 07024, USA
* Department of Restorative Dentistry, University of Medicine and Dentistry, New Jersey, New Jersey Dental School, 110 Bergen Street, Newark, NJ 07103.
E-mail address: drganz@drganz.com

Dent Clin N Am 55 (2011) 515–536
doi:10.1016/j.cden.2011.02.019
0011-8532/11/$ – see front matter © 2011 Elsevier Inc. All rights reserved.

dental.theclinics.com

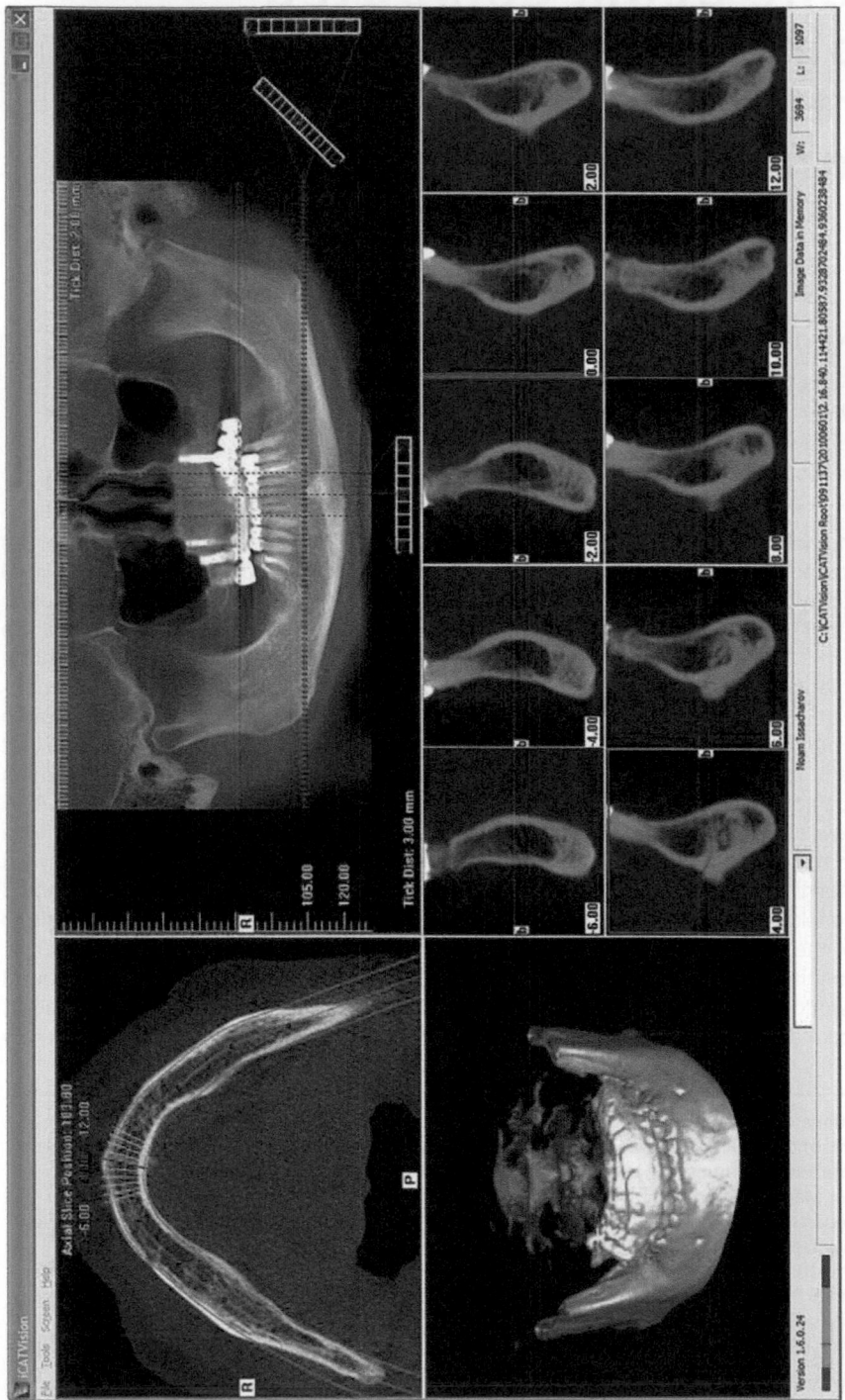

Fig. 1. i-CAT CBCT provides 4 important image views: cross-sectional, panoramic, axial, and 3D volume reconstruction.

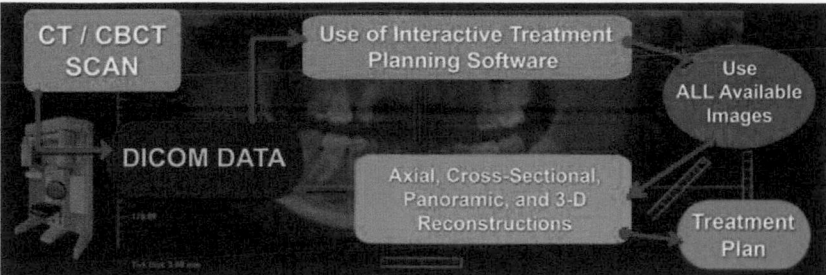

Fig. 2. The flow of information from the i-CAT CBCT scan data to the final treatment plan using interactive treatment planning software.

proprietary software to obtain and visualize the 3D dataset. Once a scan has been taken, the interpretation process begins regardless of which software is used. Each manufacturer allows clinicians to visualize and interact with the data for the purposes of diagnosis and treatment planning. There are 4 important 3D views; (1) axial, (2) cross-sectional, (3) panoramic, and (4) 3D reconstructions (**Fig. 1**) (i-CAT Vision, Imaging Sciences Inc, Hatfield, PA). Each of these views is individually important, providing unique levels of detail. When assimilated in total as a result of the interactive nature of the CBCT native software, these views provide the ultimate overview of the patient's anatomic presentation. The data can also be exported into DICOM (digital imaging and communications in medicine) files that can be visualized through third-party interactive treatment planning software applications that have innovative tools to enhance the diagnosis and treatment planning process. The author has long advocated the concept that "It's not the scan, it's the plan," meaning that the clinician must evaluate and interpret the data provided by the CBCT machine to establish accurate treatment options using innovative state-of-the-art digital tools. Once the scan is taken, it can be viewed on the computer workstation using the native software (ie, i-CAT Vision), or the DICOM data can be exported into an interactive treatment planning software such as SimPlant (Materialise Dental, Glen Burnie, MD, USA), Nobel-Guide (Nobel Biocare, Göteborg, Sweden), Invivo5 (Anatomage, San Jose, CA, USA), (VIP Software, BioHorizons Inc, Birmingham, AL, USA), Straumann coDiagnos-tiX (Straumann USA, Andover, MA, USA), Blue Sky Plan (BlueSkyBio Grayslake, IL, USA), where all available images can be processed and manipulated interactively to create an excellent diagnostic environment (**Fig. 2**).

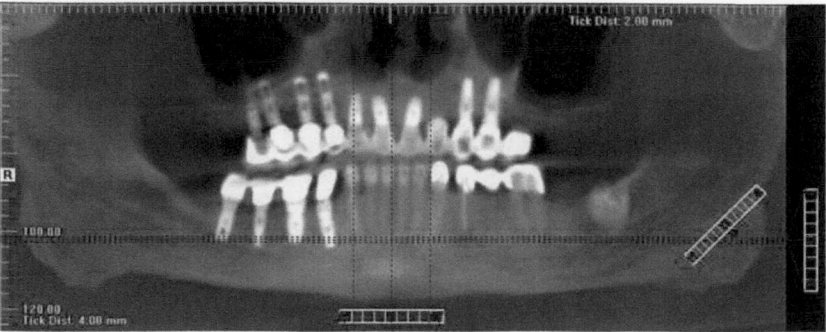

Fig. 3. Panoramic view revealing the maxillary-mandibular relationship, and 3 stages of implant reconstruction.

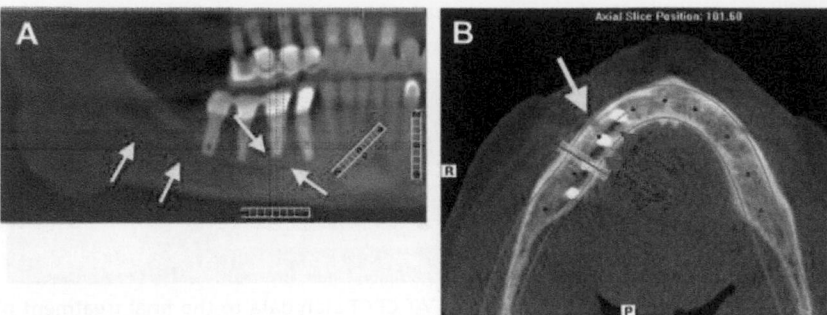

Fig. 4. (*A*) Focusing the field of view to the right mandible illustrates the proximity of the implants near the path of the inferior alveolar nerve (*arrow*). (*B*) The axial view reveals the break in the cortical bone that indicates the mental foramen (*yellow arrow*). The red arrows show an artifact known as beam hardening.

BENEFITS VERSUS RISKS

During the evolution of CT and CBCT, clinicians worldwide discovered what the author has labeled the "reality of anatomy" or the patient's individual anatomic 3D presentation. When a preoperative scan is not performed, potential complications can occur, and issues are then discovered with a postoperative scan. A postsurgical, postreconstruction CBCT scan (i-CAT) was performed after the mandibular right paresthesia did not resolve. The panoramic reconstruction revealed implants placed in 3 quadrants, the right, left, and anterior maxilla, and right mandible (**Fig. 3**). The image can be enlarged to focus on the area of interest such as the path of the inferior nerve and

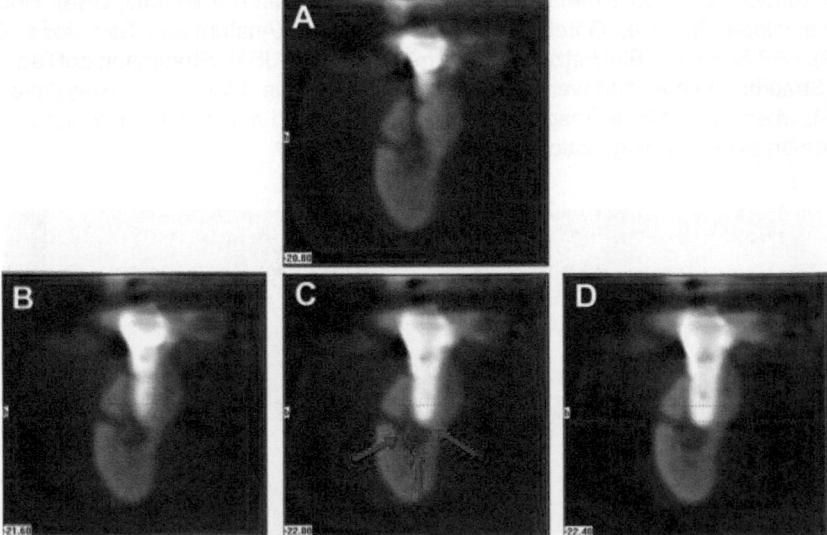

Fig. 5. (*A–D*) A series of cross-sectional slices reveal an implant that perforated into the inferior alveolar nerve, and mental nerve complex (*red arrows*).

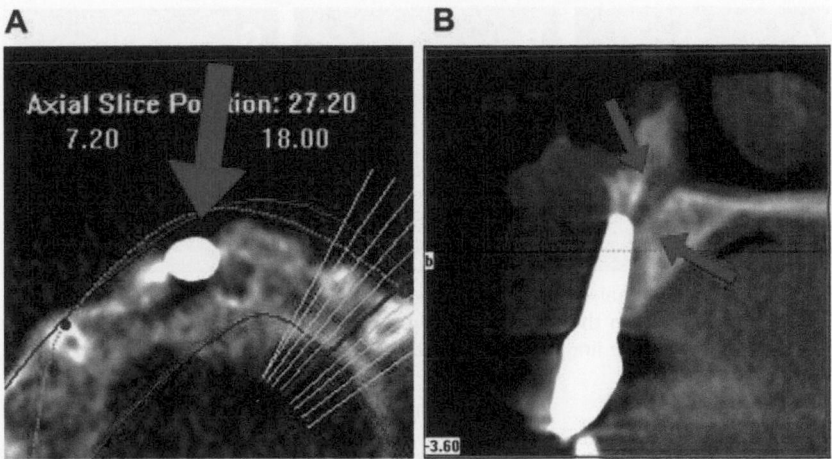

Fig. 6. (*A, B*) The axial view reveals an implant located in the area of the right central incisor tooth that seems to perforate the facial cortical plate (*A, red arrow*). The cross-sectional view was helpful in identifying the apical position of the implant invading the space of the incisal canal (*B, red arrows*).

the proximity of the previously placed implants (**Fig. 4**A). To gain a great appreciation of the local anatomy, the axial slice created perpendicular to the panoramic slice reveals the break in the facial cortical bone (see **Fig. 4**B, yellow arrow), which indicates the mental foramen. The radiolucent areas between the implants could represent the inferior alveolar nerve, or it could also be a phenomenon called beam hardening, which turns the pixels in proximity to dense objects radiolucent (see **Fig. 4**B, red arrows). To differentiate, it is necessary to review the cross-sectional slices. Cross-sectional slices revealed that the implant closest to the mental nerve penetrated into the inferior alveolar nerve canal (**Fig. 5**). If a CBCT scan had been taken before the implant placement either a shorter implant could have been used, or a different receptor site might have been used.

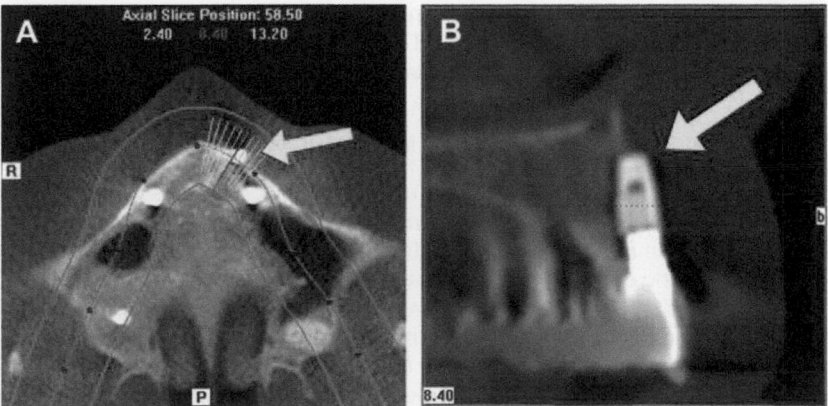

Fig. 7. (*A, B*) This axial view reveals an implant located in the area of the left lateral incisor tooth that significantly perforates the facial cortical plate (*A, yellow arrow*). The cross-section further shows that 50% of the implant is not located within the bone (*B, yellow arrow*).

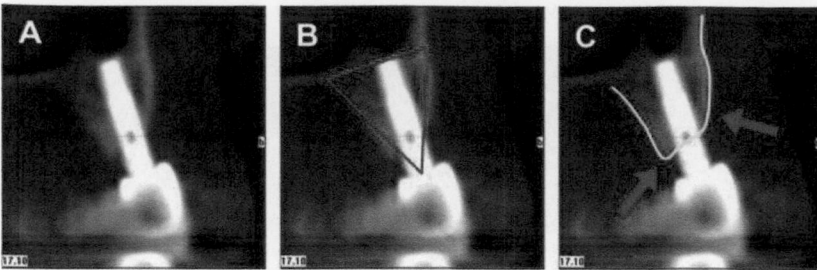

Fig. 8. (*A–C*) Cross-sectional view of an implant that has functioned for 10 years. (*A*) The implant was placed within the triangle of bone (*B*), showing typical receptor bone levels (*yellow line*) higher on the lingual, lower on the facial (*C, red arrows*).

Another paresthesia case resulted from a perforation into the incisal canal. An axial view revealed an implant placed in the area of the right maxillary central incisor (**Fig. 6**A). The implant appeared to perforate through the facial cortical plate (see **Fig. 6**A, large red arrow). The cross-sectional slices clearly illustrated the apical extent of the implant that invaded the incisal canal space causing long-lasting postoperative complications (see **Fig. 6**A, arrows).

A third example of a malpositioned implant can be visualized in the axial slice of a left maxillary lateral incisor (**Fig. 7**A, yellow arrow). The implant significantly perforates through the facial cortical bone. The cross-sectional view further illustrates that 50% of the implant is not located within the alveolar housing (see **Fig. 7**B). The yellow arrow reveals the apical portion of the implant is located within the soft-tissue vestibule. When a preoperative scan is used, implants can be positioned where they are surrounded with a good volume of bone. A cross-sectional slice of an implant in function for 10 years can be visualized in **Fig. 8**A. The implant was positioned within the zone that the author has defined as the "triangle of bone," providing the most volume of surrounding bone (see **Fig. 8**B). The maxillary topography reveals a typical pattern where the bone is higher on the palate or lingual, and lower on the buccal or facial (see **Fig. 8**C). This bone pattern and implant placement are defined as transitional placement. Therefore there are known risks in placing implants without 3D diagnosis and surgical guidance with CT-derived templates. Potential serious complications can be avoided when 3D imaging tools are used, as is shown later.

CASE PRESENTATION: FAILING LONG-SPAN MANDIBULAR BRIDGE

Treating failed long-span bridges presents unique challenges for the clinician and the patient. When anchor abutment teeth fail, and it is recommended that the bridge be removed, often it can no longer be supported by natural teeth. The treatment option to replace the missing dentition consists of a removable-type prosthesis, or an implant retained restoration. Most patients do not want to be without teeth for an extended amount of time and desire the option that most closely replaces their missing teeth: a fixed prosthesis. Many patients are now aware of treatment options that allow for removal of the failing bridge and anchor teeth followed by the immediate placement of dental implants to maintain an immediate transitional restoration. However, in order to present this treatment option to the patient, proper diagnosis and treatment planning are essential for a complete understanding of the available bone, soft tissue, opposing occlusion, vertical dimension, and surrounding vital structures. Current

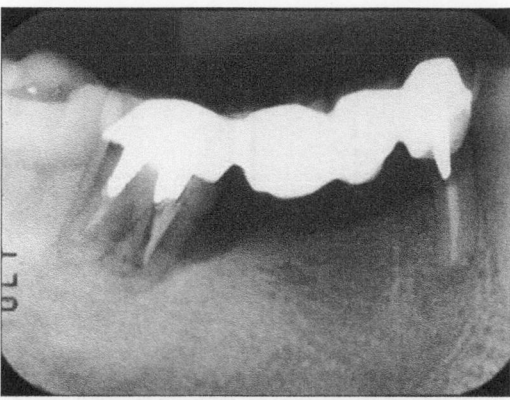

Fig. 9. Preoperative radiograph showing area of bone loss and decay.

two-dimensional panoramic and periapical radiographs can no longer be considered the most accurate diagnostic imaging modalities available.

To properly assess the patient's anatomy, the author recommends 3D assessment using CBCT technology, which empowers the clinician with new tools to make educated decisions regarding the plan of treatment.

A 61-year-old male patient presented with pain and mobility in an existing posterior right mandibular long-span fixed bridge. A routine diagnostic workup was completed, including periapical radiographs and study casts. The patient had a history of bruxism, which may have been contributory to the root fractures and mobility of the bridge. Radiographic loss of bone was evident around the mandibular second molar tooth, the terminal abutment for the fixed bridge, which showed a significant angular defect on the mesial (**Fig. 9**). The first bicuspid had previously been treated with root canal therapy, and appeared to be fractured from the stress of the restoration and/or recurrent decay along the margins. To determine the potential treatment alternatives a CBCT scan was ordered to allow complete inspection of the 3D bony topography, and the relationship of adjacent vital structures. Two-dimensional imaging modalities could not provide an adequate interpretation of the patient anatomy, raising the risk of treatment and potential injury to vital structures.

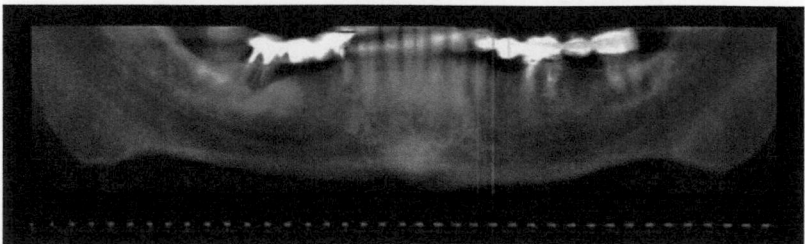

Fig. 10. Panoramic reconstruction reveals the failing right fixed bridge, and the path of the inferior alveolar nerve.

A   B

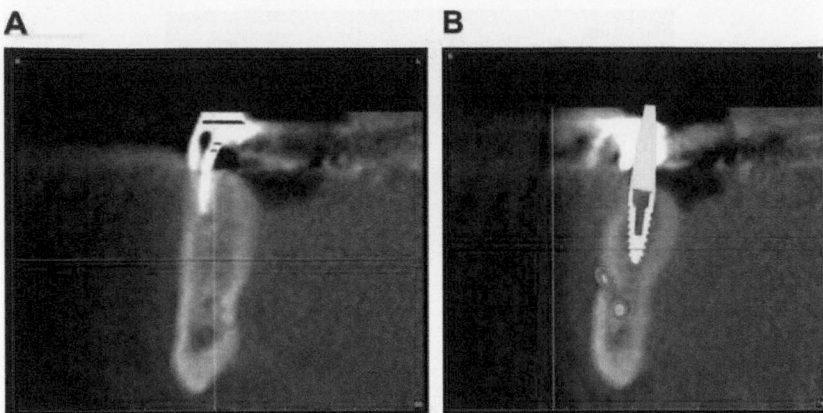

Fig. 11. (*A, B*) A cross-sectional image reveals the facial and lingual cortical bone, the intermedullary bone, and the relative density (*A*), and a simulated implant placed over the mental foramen (*B*).

3D PLANNING

The panoramic image reconstructed from the CBCT dataset differs substantially from a conventional panoramic radiograph. This nondistorted image can be viewed interactively using the incorporated viewing software to assess the broader aspects of the arches (**Fig. 10**). The cross-sectional image is excellent for defining a slice of the mandible where the height and width of the bone can be accurately evaluated. Within an individual slice, the spatial location of the tooth and root can be appreciated (**Fig. 11**A). The facial, lingual cortical, and intermedullary bone can be visualized based on their radiopacity or gray-scale density values. Nuances within the anatomic presentation can be assessed with greater accuracy than with any other imaging modality. Simulated implants can be placed in a position to effectively support the desired restoration, even with close proximity to the mental foramen (see **Fig. 11**B). The

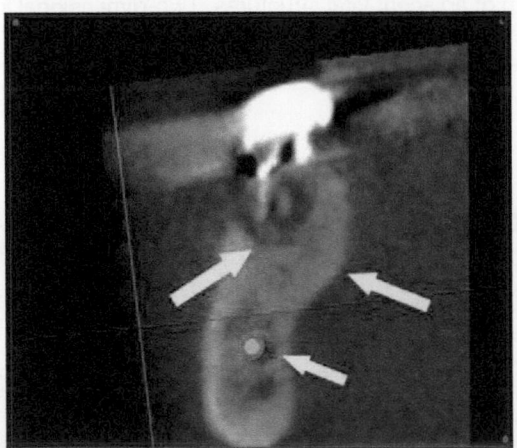

Fig. 12. The cross-sectional slice of the molar reveals the extent of the bone defect, the lingual concavity, and the inferior alveolar nerve (*orange*).

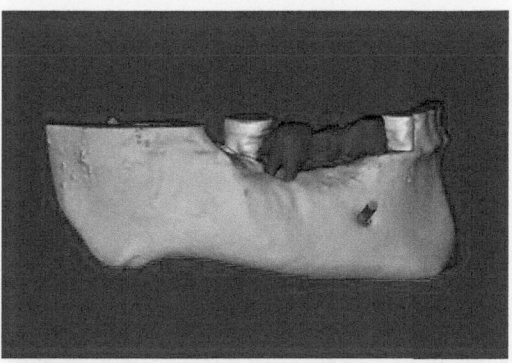

Fig. 13. A 3D reconstructed volume shows the existing bridge (*magenta*), the bone topography, and the mental foramen.

cross-sectional slice of the posterior molar reveals the significant bone defect surrounding the apical roots (**Fig. 12**). A significant lingual concavity was noted with the pattern of cortical bone visualized below the root apex (see **Fig. 12**, yellow arrows). The inferior alveolar nerve can be carefully traced through the mandible to determine proximity to the tooth roots and potential implant receptor sites (see **Fig. 12**, orange). Although there was good-quality bone above the location of the nerve, there was insufficient bone to adequately fixate an implant after immediate extraction. It was therefore elected to remove the molar tooth and fill the defect with grafting material in anticipation of placing an implant after the new bone had matured.

Creating a fully interactive 3D reconstruction from the CBCT scan data allows the clinician further insight into the patient's existing anatomic presentation. Using advanced software masking or segmentation enables the various anatomic entities to be separated for improved diagnostic capabilities (SimPlant). The preexisting bridge has been colorized (**Fig. 13**, magenta), as have the adjacent molar and cuspid teeth (see **Fig. 13**, white). Simulated implants were positioned within the bone to support a new fixed restoration based on the abutment projections that extended above the occlusal table (**Fig. 14**). Note the planned parallelism of the 4 simulated implants. Using advances in interactive software, "selective transparency" as defined

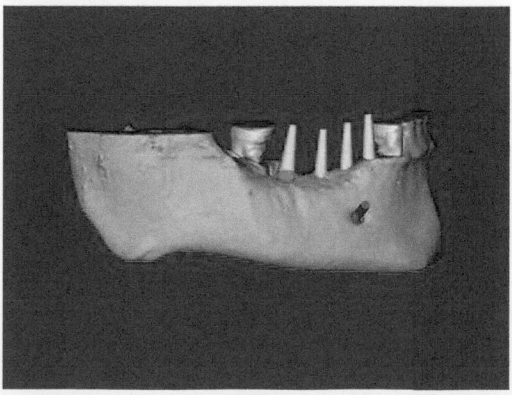

Fig. 14. Simulated implants were positioned within the available space, with abutment projections in yellow.

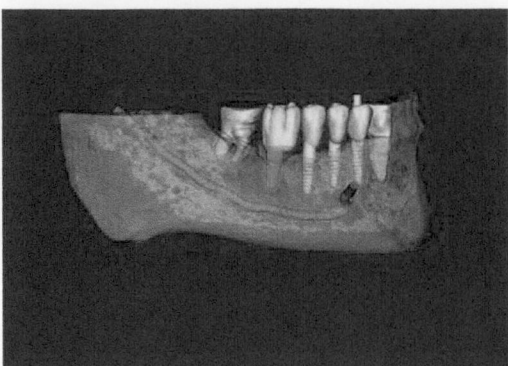

Fig. 15. "Selective transparency" allows close inspection of the implants placed within the virtual teeth, and the proximity to the nerve.

by the author, can be applied to change the opacity of various structures to aid in the diagnosis and planning phase. Accurate placement of realistic implants is enhanced by masking the adjacent tooth roots. The path of the inferior alveolar nerve can also be fully appreciated (**Fig. 15**). If the preexisting restoration could not be physically removed before CT/CBCT imaging and the old occlusion was found to be unfavorable, through further masking or segmentation, it is now possible to build a virtual occlusion using interactive treatment planning software. Virtual teeth (seen in yellow in **Fig. 15**) can correct discrepancies, and allow for an ideal simulated morphology fabrication. The large defect around the molar was significant, and it was determined that it could not be used as a receptor site initially. It was elected to graft this site, and return in 5 months to place a single implant in the molar site. Once the plan has been verified in all 4 available 3D views a virtual template can be fabricated based on the simulated implant positions (**Fig. 16**). Therefore, the final surgical template is only as good as the virtual plan, and therefore, it is advisable to check each view carefully.

Three basic CT-derived template types are available that can be fabricated for dental implant placement: (1) bone borne, (2) tooth borne, and (3) soft-tissue/mucosal borne. Based on the fact that there were adjacent teeth in the region it

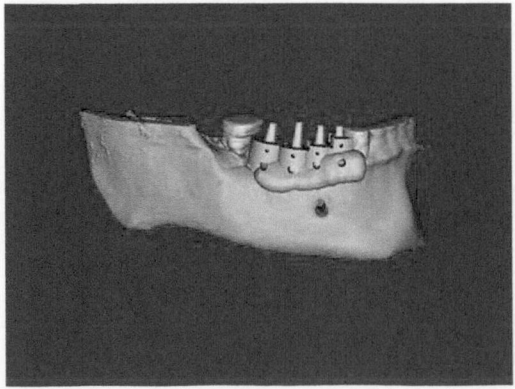

Fig. 16. The 3D plan allows for a virtual template, which is then fabricated by the process of stereolithography.

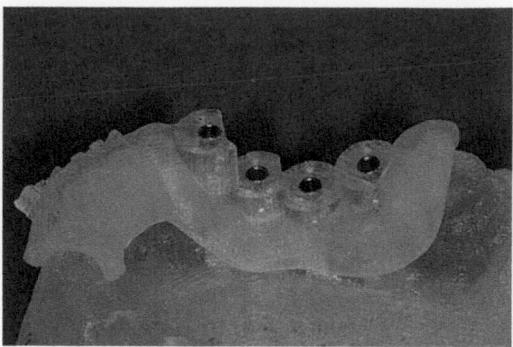

Fig. 17. The stereolithographic tooth-borne template and mandibular model of the patient's anatomy.

was elected to use a tooth-borne template stabilized by the existing occlusion. The CBCT scan data were sent via email for fabrication of a stereolithographic model (**Fig. 17**) (Materialise Dental, Lueven, Belgium). This resin-type model is a replica of the patient's anatomy at the time that the images were acquired. The preexisting bridge was virtually removed via the software before fabrication of the surgical guide. The ability to separate anatomic and other structures from the reconstruction is known as segmentation and is not available in all software applications. The template adapts well to the surrounding dentition and does not require further fixation to prevent movement. The stainless steel tubes are two-tenths of a millimeter wider than the manufacturers' sequential osteotomy drills, allowing accurate guidance during the drilling process. For fully edentulous cases, either bone-borne or mucosal-borne applications, it is advisable to use fixation pins or screws to stabilize the surgical template.

A novel modality pioneered by the author uses a CT-derived stereolithographic model-based approach to link the implant placement and the eventual restoration. Implant replicas, or analogues, were placed in predesignated implant receptors on the stereolithographic partially edentate mandible (**Fig. 18**). To accommodate the immediate restoration, manufacturers' specific abutments were placed on the implant replicas. Note the interimplant distances for proper embrasure design, and appreciation of biologic width. A diagnostic wax-up was accomplished and a clear matrix fabricated to facilitate the fabrication of a provisional prosthesis. Stock, 3inOne titanium

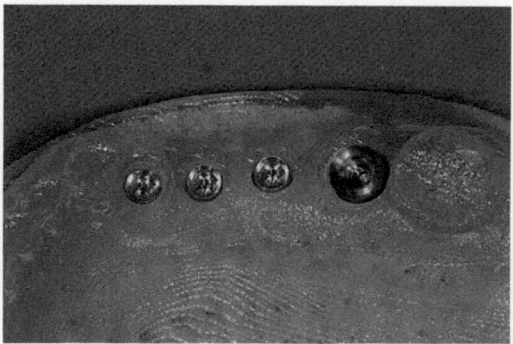

Fig. 18. Implant replicas were placed in the mandibular stereolithographic model.

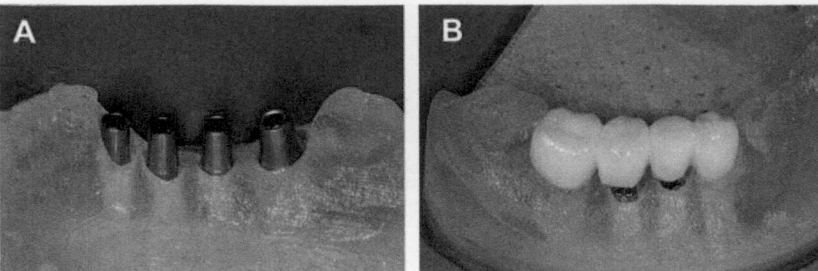

Fig. 19. (*A*) Stock, 3inOne abutments positioned on the implant replicas to support the temporary bridge. (*B*) The processed 4-unit transitional acrylic bridge supported by the abutments.

abutments (BioHorizons) were positioned on the implant replicas to support the temporary restoration (**Fig. 19**A). The processed 4-unit transitional acrylic bridge was supported by the implant abutments (see **Fig. 19**B). Because the molar site would not receive an implant immediately, a distal cantilever pontic was required. The actual implants as simulated in the virtual plan were chosen in advance, as well as how to best position the implants to take advantage of the reverse buttress thread design, coronal microchannels, and internal hexagonal connection design features. The manufacturer has indicated that the Tapered Internal implants (BioHorizons) with the Laser-Lok (BioHorizons) microchannels allow the implants to be vertically placed in 3 potential positions relative to the height of bone. As with most bone-level implants, the implant can be placed at the crest of the bone (**Fig. 20**A). Because of the specific properties of the Laser-Lok microchannels the implant can also be placed supracrestal, or in a transitional position where the lingual cortical plate is higher than the facial cortical plate of bone) (see **Fig. 20** B, C). As indicated earlier, receptor sites often show asymmetry in the bone topography, which cannot be determined with conventional two-dimensional imaging. Regardless of which company manufactured the implants, there are design considerations that can benefit from presurgical prosthetic 3D planning concepts.

SURGICAL INTERVENTION

The preoperative lateral view of the original failing fixed bridge illustrating the ridge-lap pontic design (**Fig. 21**A). The occlusal view of the long-span bridge can be seen in **Fig. 21**B. Once the failed restoration was removed, the underlying fractured tooth roots were assessed. The volumetric change in the pontic areas was assessed by

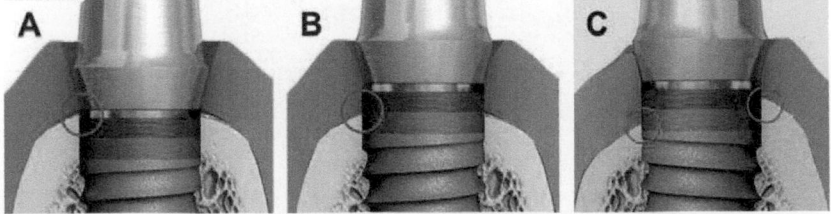

Fig. 20. (*A*) Crestal placement of an implant within the mandibular bone. (*B*) If an implant is placed above the crest it is considered supracrestal placement. (*C*) If bone levels are not even, it is considered transitional placement.

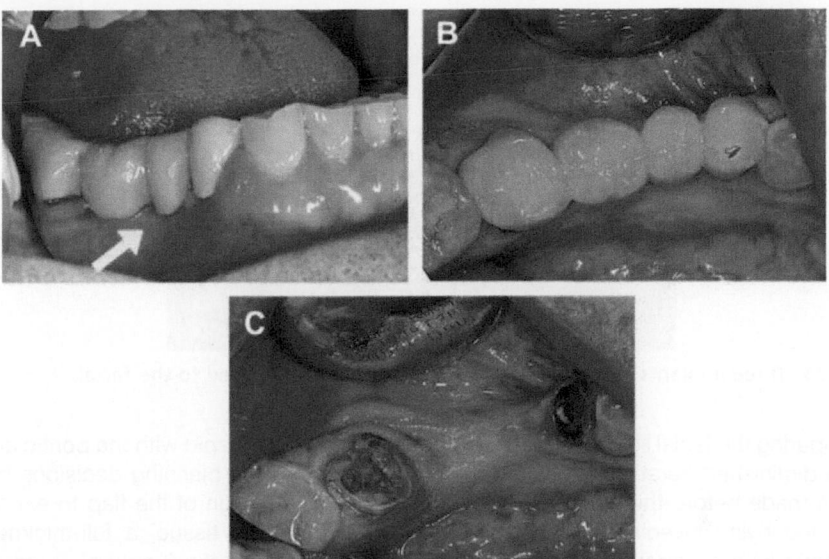

Fig. 21. (*A*) Preoperative lateral view of the original failing fixed bridge showing the ridge-lap design pontics (*A, yellow arrow*). (*B*) Preoperative occlusal view of the original failing fixed bridge. (*C*) Preoperative occlusal view after the bridge had been removed revealing the roots, and diminished bone volume.

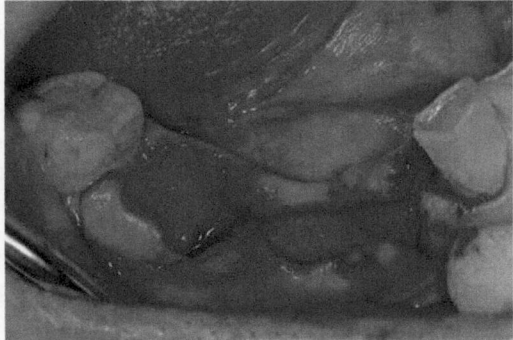

Fig. 22. The full-thickness flap revealed the underlying deficient alveolar ridge.

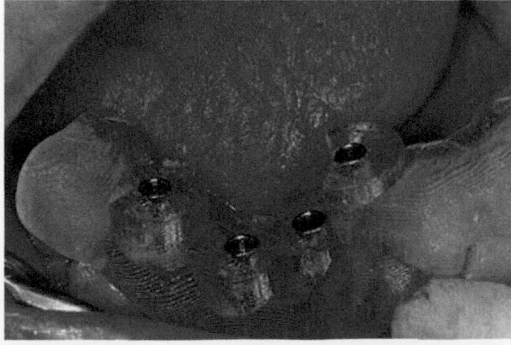

Fig. 23. The tooth-borne template in position to guide the implants.

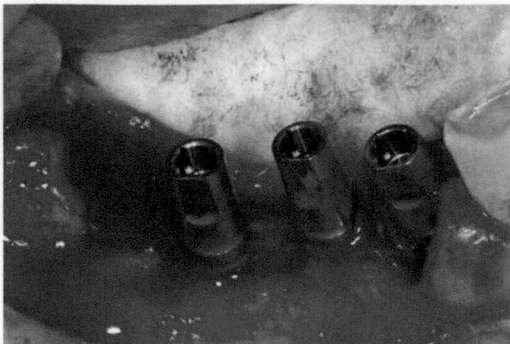

Fig. 24. Three implants placed with the 3inOne abutments rotated to the facial.

comparing the facial lingual dimensions of the molar and bicuspid with the pontic area with diminished keratinized tissue (see **Fig. 21**C). All of the planning decisions had been made before the surgical intervention except the design of the flap to expose the underlying alveolar ridge. To preserve the keratinized tissue, a full-thickness mucoperiosteal flap was required, followed by extraction of the 2 natural abutment teeth (**Fig. 22**). The tooth-borne template was then placed over the site and examined for fit (**Fig. 23**). As per the CBCT-derived plan and template, the first 3 implants were placed (Tapered Internal). The implants were well fixated, allowing for immediate restoration by aligning the internal hexagonal connection to the facial to allow for proper seating of the 3inOne abutments (**Fig. 24**). The posterior molar extraction socket was filled with a corticocancellous mineralized bone graft material (MinerOss, BioHorizons), and covered with a collagen membrane.

The prefabricated 4-unit provisional restoration was seated and relined to fit the 3 anterior implant fixtures. The distal-extension cantilever replaced the missing molar, with care taken not to place pressure on the underlying graft. The soft tissue was sutured to allow for near primary closure as they were wrapped around the abutment projection, helping to establish embrasures (**Fig. 25**). The postoperative periapical radiograph confirms the placement of the anterior 3 implants and the bone graft in the molar defect (**Fig. 26**). The transitional restoration was cemented retained, and left in place for more than 2 months. Once the posterior molar bone graft had matured, the fourth implant was placed according to the original CBCT plan. When the fourth implant had integrated after 8 weeks in function, an abutment was connected, and

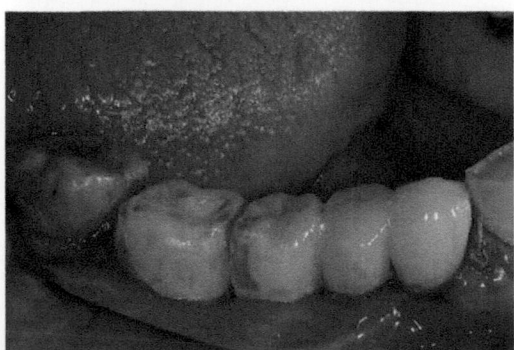

Fig. 25. The transitional 4-unit immediate restoration with soft-tissue closure.

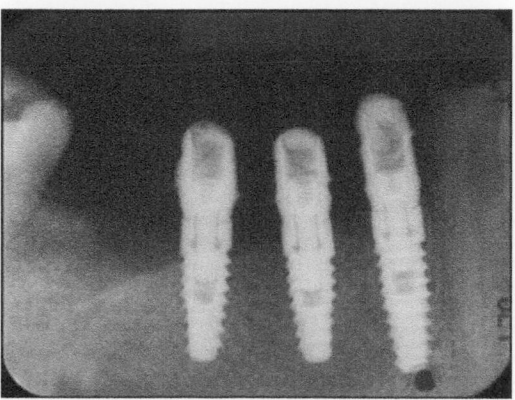

Fig. 26. The postoperative radiograph showing 3 Tapered Internal implants with abutments to support the temporary.

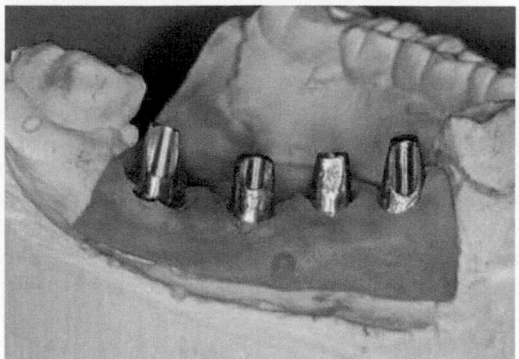

Fig. 27. The final prepared abutments on the working cast after the final implant was loaded.

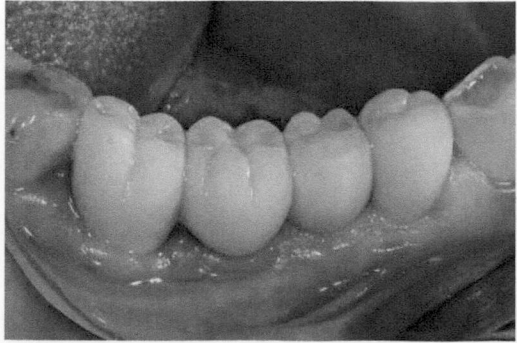

Fig. 28. The bisque bake try-in reveals the new soft-tissue contours and emergence profile established.

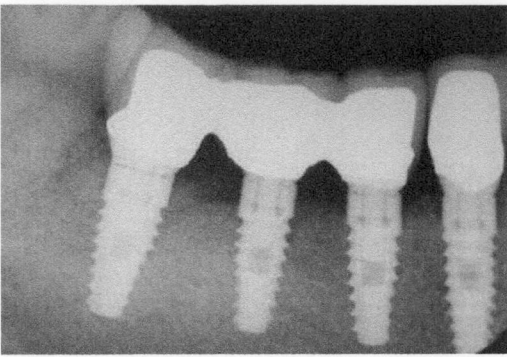

Fig. 29. The postoperative radiograph showing all 4 implants supporting the definitive restoration.

the existing transitional restoration was relined. Impressions were made and a soft-tissue working cast fabricated for the laboratory process. The favorable parallelism afforded by the CBCT-derived planning required only minor preparation of the implant abutments to allow for adequate clearance for the metal alloy and porcelain veneer (**Fig. 27**).

Because of the patient's bruxism, it was elected to splint the posterior 3 units within the framework of the ceramometal restoration, whereas the anterior, longer implant was fabricated as a single unit. The bisque-bake try-in revealed improved soft-tissue contours and emergence profile (**Fig. 28**).

The completed ceramometal units seen in the periapical radiographs show satisfactory parallelism and interimplant distances (**Fig. 29**). The emergence profile of each implant illustrates a smooth transition important to long-term maintenance. The final glaze and porcelain characteristics of the posterior 4 units blend in with the surrounding dentition and soft tissue (**Fig. 30**). Note the excellent adaptation of the embrasures.

POSTOPERATIVE CBCT SCAN EVALUATION

Approximately 2 years after the initial implants were placed in the mandible, the patient returned to the office with a fractured bridge in the left posterior maxilla. Extraction of

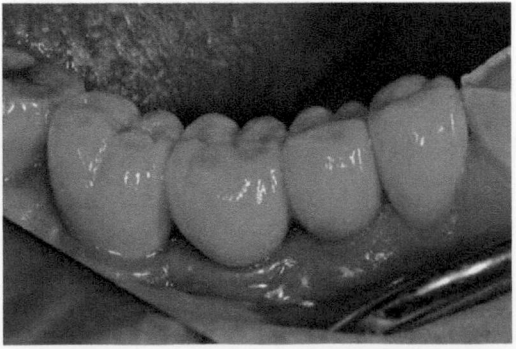

Fig. 30. The postoperative radiograph showing all 4 implants supporting the definitive restoration.

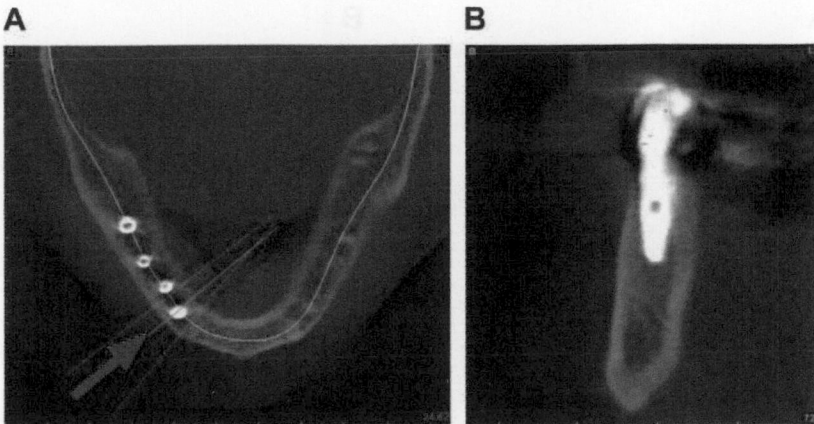

Fig. 31. (*A*) The postoperative CBCT scan axial slice at cross-section of the anterior implant (*red arrow*). (*B*) The cross-sectional slice showing the ideal position of the implant within the bone supporting the tooth.

the necessary teeth would have resulted in a lack of support for a new fixed bridge. It was therefore determined that the area was unrestorable by conventional means. To further evaluate this area it was necessary to gain additional 3D data from a CBCT scan. During the image acquisition, and with the patient's permission, a larger field of view was incorporated to help validate the previous placement of the 4 implants in the posterior right mandible. The results of the CBCT for the mandible helped to substantiate that the initial plan was well executed. Each of the 4 receptor sites was evaluated separately using axial and cross-sectional views. The postoperative CBCT scan axial view indicated the position of the 4 implants (**Fig. 31**A). Starting with the most anterior implant (see **Fig. 31**A, red arrow), a cross-sectional slice indicated an ideal position of the implant within the supporting bone (see **Fig. 31**B). Continuing to the second implant site, the axial and cross-sectional views showed that the implant was positioned with adequate clearance above the inferior alveolar nerve, avoiding potential complications that were reviewed earlier (**Fig. 32**).

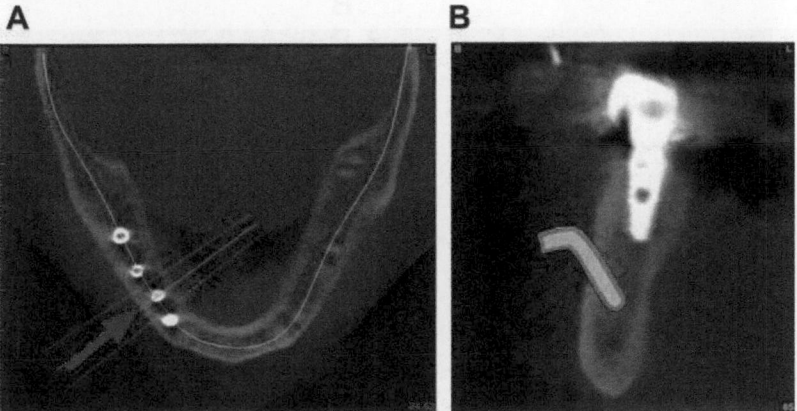

Fig. 32. (*A*) The postoperative CBCT scan axial slice at cross-section of the second implant (*red arrow*). (*B*) The cross-sectional slice showing the position of the implant above the mental nerve and foramen (*orange*).

A   B

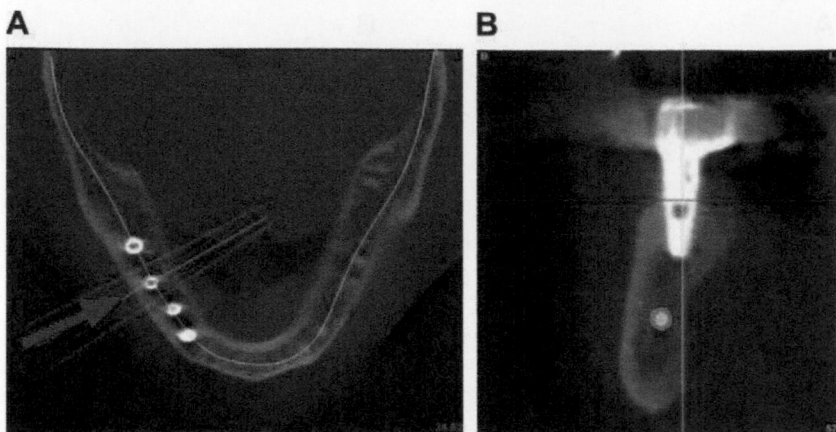

Fig. 33. (*A*) The postoperative CBCT scan axial slice at cross-section of the third implant (*red arrow*). (*B*) The cross-sectional slice showing the ideal position of the implant well above the nerve, avoiding the lingual concavity.

Compare the original plan (see **Fig. 11**B) with the 2-year follow-up scan in **Fig. 32**B. The implants were placed according to the desired position of the restoration.

The postoperative location of the third implant in the series can be seen in the axial view (**Fig. 33**A). The cross-sectional slice (number 57) illustrated the ideal implant positioned to support the tooth and avoid proximity to the path of the inferior alveolar nerve (see **Fig. 33**B). The implant was placed based on the transitional topography of the crestal and cortical bone on the facial and lingual. It was also important to prevent perforation through the lingual concavity, and this was accomplished with the advanced 3D planning and use of the CT-derived template. The final implant had been placed in a delayed method after the large-diameter molar extraction socket was grafted with mineralized bone. The postoperative CBCT scan revealed total bone fill with sufficient volume to support the implant and the restoration (**Fig. 34**). The cross-sectional slice illustrated the vertical relationship between the implant,

A   B

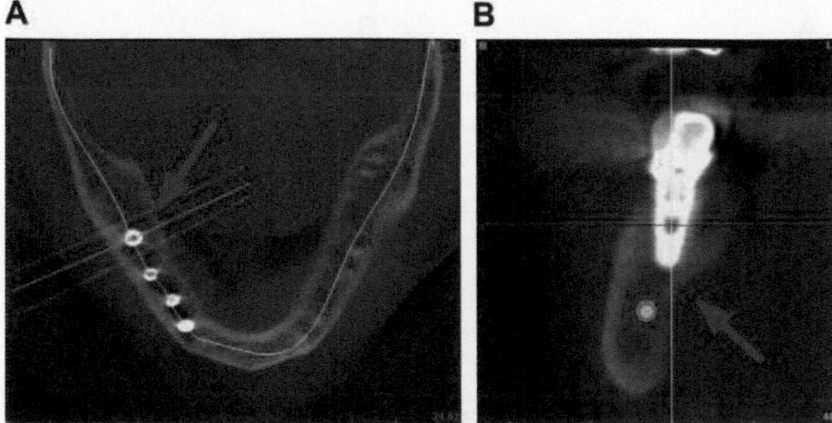

Fig. 34. (*A*) The postoperative CBCT scan axial slice at cross-section of the posterior molar. (*B*) The cross-sectional slice showing the postgraft placement of the implant and the proximity to the lingual concavity (*arrow*).

the abutment, and the crown. The severe concavity was avoided with careful planning and the use of a tapered design implant body style (see **Fig. 34**B, red arrow).

The purpose of this clinical case example was to illustrate the enhanced diagnostic and treatment planning capabilities of CBCT data combined with interactive treatment planning software. The combination of careful diagnosis with proper planning aids the clinician in understanding existing bone topography, bone density, adjacent tooth roots, lingual concavities, occlusion, and the path of the inferior alveolar nerve. Once the information has been gathered, an accurate plan can be established. This plan is then transferred to a surgical guide, allowing for precise implant placement. In a phased approach, 3 initially placed implants were immediately loaded with a transitional cantilever restoration, avoiding the lingual concavity and within a zone of safety above the inferior alveolar nerve. The posterior molar tooth with resulting socket defect was found to be unfavorable for implant fixation, and therefore site development was accomplished with bone grafting. This situation was anticipated and documented preoperatively after interpretation of the CBCT data. Once matured, the molar area became an excellent implant receptor site. The patient was given a transitional restoration the day of surgery, although there was a staged approach and delayed implant placement in the molar area. This case represented one treatment alternative to replacing a failed long-span mandibular and bridge, which was made possible through CBCT scan technology, interactive treatment planning software, and CT-derived surgical templates to guide the placement of the implants based on the restorative needs of the patient. Postoperative CBCT scan data at 2 years validated that the plan had been successfully achieved.

SUMMARY

CT and CBCT scan technologies have played a major role in the evolution of diagnostic imaging for dental applications. The ability to visualize each individual patient's anatomy with an interactive 3D assessment takes the guesswork out of the equation, and allows clinicians to make truly educated decisions regarding treatment. Using the ALARA principle, newer CBCT imaging machines have achieved the delivery of this information with a significant reduction in radiation, and smaller in-office machines that provide almost instant access to enhanced diagnostic imaging. The benefits versus the risks should be considered when determining the need for a scan. Several case examples illustrated complications that occurred when CBCT was not used presurgically. Postoperative scanning can also prove to be a useful application of this technology to help validate the 3D placement of implants, or to evaluate healing progress of bone grafts, or other procedures when warranted.

The advent of this technology has evolved into an indispensable diagnostic tool that can be used for a variety of different clinical applications which include, but are not limited to: dental implant receptor site evaluation; alveolar bone defect and bone augmentation procedures; impacted teeth; orthodontics; endodontics; TM joint diagnostics; sinus augmentation procedures; and orthognathic surgical interventions. The use of the CBCT native software, or when the DICOM dataset is imported and visualized through third-party interactive treatment planning software applications, enhance the diagnosis and treatment planning process. This article highlights the presurgical planning phase of dental implant applications that benefit from CBCT technology so that educated treatment decisions can be accurately determined through a careful evaluation of all 4 3D views: (1) axial, (2) cross-sectional, (3) panoramic, and (4) 3D reconstructions. It is important for clinicians to gain an understanding of how each of these views is individually significant, and how each slice can provide unique levels of detail to provide a comprehensive overview of the patient's anatomic presentation. The use of this technology will help clinicians to avoid potential complications and costly remakes and will result in decreased patient morbidity through improved pre-surgical planning. The digital world will continue to evolve with new and improved tools, with the ultimate goal of benefiting the patients we treat.

SUGGESTED READINGS

Angelopoulos C, Aghaloo T. Imaging technology in implant diagnosis. Dent Clin North Am 2011;55(1):141–58.

Berco M, Rigali PH Jr, Miner RM, et al. Accuracy and reliability of linear cephalometric measurements from cone-beam computed tomography scans of a dry human skull. Am J Orthod Dentofacial Orthop 2009;136(1):17.e1–9 [discussion 17–8].

Chan HL, Misch K, Wang HL. Dental imaging in implant treatment planning. Implant Dent 2010;19(4):288–98.

Dreiseidler T, Mischkowski RA, Neugebauer J, et al. Comparison of cone-beam imaging with orthopantomography and computerized tomography for assessment in presurgical implant dentistry. Int J Oral Maxillofac Implants 2009;24(2):216–25.

Froum S, Casanova L, Byrne S, et al. Risk assessment before extraction for immediate implant placement in the posterior mandible: a computerized tomographic scan study. J Periodontol 2011;82(3):395–402.

Ganz SD. CT scan technology–an evolving tool for predictable implant placement and restoration. International Magazine of Oral Implantology 2001;1:6–13.

Ganz SD. The triangle of bone–a formula for successful implant placement and restoration. Implant Soc 1995;5(5):2–6.

Ganz SD. Mandibular tori as a source for on-lay bone graft augmentation: a surgical procedure. Pract Periodontics Aesthet Dent 1997;9(9):973–82. The Implant Report.

Ganz SD. Use of stereolithographic models as diagnostic and restorative aids for predictable immediate loading of implants. Pract Proced Aesthet Dent 2003; 15(10):763–71.

Ganz SD. Presurgical planning with CT-derived fabrication of surgical guides. J Oral Maxillofac Surg 2005;63(9 Suppl 2):59–71.

Ganz SD. The reality of anatomy and the triangle of bone. Inside Dent 2006;2(5):72–7.

Ganz SD. Techniques for the use of CT imaging for the fabrication of surgical guides. Atlas Oral Maxillofac Surg Clin North Am 2006;14:75–97.

Ganz SD. Using interactive technology: "in the zone with the triangle of bone." Dent Implantol Update 2008;19(5):33–8 [quiz: p1].

Ganz SD. Computer-aided design/computer-aided manufacturing applications using CT and cone beam CT scan technology. Dent Clin North Am 2008;52(4): 777–808.

Ganz SD. Restoratively driven implant dentistry utilizing advanced software and CBCT: realistic abutments and virtual teeth. Dent Today 2008;27(7):122, 124, 126–7.

Ganz SD. Advanced case planning with SimPlant. In: Tardieu P, Rosenfeld A, editors. The art of computer-guided implantology. Chicago: Quintessence; 2009. p. 193–210.

Ganz SD. Case Report: CBCT-assisted treatment of the failing long span bridge with staged and immediate load implant restoration. DentalTown 2010;11(11):82–6.

Ganz SD. The use of CT/CBCT and interactive virtual treatment planning and the triangle of bone: defining new paradigms for assessment of implant receptor sites. In: Babbush C, Hahn J, Krauser J, et al, editors. Dental implants–the art and science. Maryland Heights (MO): Saunders; 2010. p. 146–66.

Ganz SD. Implant complications associated with two- and three dimensional diagnostic imaging technologies. In: Froum SJ, editor. Dental implant complications–etiology, prevention, and treatment. West Sussex (UK): Wiley-Blackwell; 2010. p. 71–99.

Greenstein G, Tarnow D. The mental foramen and nerve: clinical and anatomical factors related to dental implant placement: a literature review. J Periodontol 2006;77(12):1933–43.

Guerrero ME, Jacobs R, Loubele M, et al. State-of-the-art on cone beam CT imaging for preoperative planning of implant placement. Clin Oral Investig 2006;10(1):1–7.

Hassan B, Couto Souza P, Jacobs R, et al. Influence of scanning and reconstruction parameters on quality of three-dimensional surface models of the dental arches from cone beam computed tomography. Clin Oral Investig 2010;14(3):303–10.

Hassan B, van derStelt P, Sanderink G. Accuracy of three-dimensional measurements obtained from cone beam computed tomography surface-rendered images for cephalometric analysis: influence of patient scanning position. Eur J Orthod 2009;31(2):129–34.

Hatcher DC, Dial C, Mayorga C. Cone beam CT for pre-surgical assessment of implant sites. J Calif Dent Assoc 2003;31(11):825–33.

Howard-Swirzinski K, Edwards PC, Saini TS, et al. Length and geometric patterns of the greater palatine canal observed in cone beam computed tomography. Int J Dent 2010; Article ID: 292753.

Lau SL, Chow J, Li W, et al. Classification of maxillary central incisors-implications for immediate implant in the esthetic zone. J Oral Maxillofac Surg 2011;69(1):142–53.

Ludlow JB, Laster WS, See M, et al. Accuracy of measurements of mandibular anatomy in cone beam computed tomography images. Oral Surg Oral Med Oral Pathol Oral Radiol Endod 2007;103(4):534–42.

Mandelaris GA, Rosenfeld AL. The expanding influence of computed tomography and the application of computer-guided implantology. Pract Proced Aesthet Dent 2008;20(5):297–305 [quiz: 306].

Mol A, Balasundaram A. In vitro cone beam computed tomography imaging of periodontal bone. Dentomaxillofac Radiol 2008;37(6):319–24.

Moreira CR, Sales MA, Lopes PM, et al. Assessment of linear and angular measurements on three-dimensional cone-beam computed tomographic images. Oral Surg Oral Med Oral Pathol Oral Radiol Endod 2009;108(3):430–6.

Mraiwa N, Jacobs R, van Steenberghe D, et al. Clinical assessment and surgical implications of anatomic challenges in the anterior mandible. Clin Implant Dent Relat Res 2003;5(4):219–25.

Naitoh M, Nabeshima H, Hayashi H, et al. Postoperative assessment of incisor dental implants using cone-beam computed tomography. J Oral Implantol 2010;36(5): 377–84.

Nevins M, Nevins ML, Camelo M, et al. Human histologic evidence of a connective tissue attachment to a dental implant. Int J Periodontics Restorative Dent 2008; 28(2):111–21.

Nevins M, Kim DM, Jun SH, et al. Histologic evidence of a connective tissue attachment to laser microgrooved abutments: a canine study. Int J Periodontics Restorative Dent 2010;30(3):245–55.

Orentlicher G, Goldsmith D, Horowitz A. Applications of 3-dimensional virtual computerized tomography technology in oral and maxillofacial surgery: current therapy. J Oral Maxillofac Surg 2010;68(8):1933–59.

Ozan O, Turkyilmaz I, Ersoy AE, et al. Clinical accuracy of 3 different types of computed tomography-derived stereolithographic surgical guides in implant placement. J Oral Maxillofac Surg 2009;67(2):394–401.

Pecora GE, Ceccarelli R, Bonelli M, et al. Clinical evaluation of laser microtexturing for soft tissue and bone attachment to dental implants. Implant Dent 2009;18(1): 57–66.

Razavi T, Palmer RM, Davies J, et al. Accuracy of measuring the cortical bone thickness adjacent to dental implants using cone beam computed tomography. Clin Oral Implants Res 2010;21(7):718–25.

Rosenfeld A, Mandelaris G, Tardieu P. Prosthetically directed placement using computer software to insure precise placement and predictable prosthetic outcomes. Part 1: diagnostics, imaging, and collaborative accountability. Int J Periodontics Restorative Dent 2006;26:215–21.

Rosenfeld AL, Mandelaris GA, Tardieu PB. Prosthetically directed implant placement using computer software to ensure precise placement and predictable prosthetic outcomes. Part 2: rapid-prototype medical modeling and stereolithographic drilling guides requiring bone exposure. Int J Periodontics Restorative Dent 2006;26(4): 347–53.

Rosenfeld AL, Mandelaris GA, Tardieu PB. Prosthetically directed implant placement using computer software to ensure precise placement and predictable prosthetic outcomes. Part 3: stereolithographic drilling guides that do not require bone exposure and the immediate delivery of teeth. Int J Periodontics Restorative Dent 2006; 26(5):493–9.

Rothman, Stephen LG. Computerized tomography of the enhanced alveolar ridge. In: Anderson-Wiedenbeck C, editor. Dental applications of computerized tomography. Chicago: Quintessence Publishing; 1998. p. 87–112.

Sarment DP, Shammari K, Kazor CE. Stereolithographic surgical templates for placement of dental implants in complex cases. Int J Periodontics Restorative Dent 2003; 23:287–95.

Schulze RK, Berndt D, d'Hoedt B. On cone-beam computed tomography artifacts induced by titanium implants. Clin Oral Implants Res 2010;21(1):100–7.

Shapoff CA, Lahey B, Wasserlauf PA, et al. Radiographic analysis of crestal bone levels around Laser-Lok collar dental implants. Int J Periodontics Restorative Dent 2010;30(2):129–37.

tenBruggenkate CM, Krekeler G, Kraaijenhagen HA, et al. Hemorrhage of the floor of the mouth resulting from lingual perforation during implant placement: a clinical report. Int J Oral Maxillofac Implants 1993;8(3):329–34.

Thomas SL, Angelopoulos C. Contemporary dental and maxillofacial imaging. Dent Clin North Am 2008;52(4).

Uchida Y, Noguchi N, Goto M, et al. Measurement of anterior loop length for the mandibular canal and diameter of the mandibular incisive canal to avoid nerve damage when installing endosseous implants in the interforaminal region: a second attempt introducing cone beam computed tomography. J Oral Maxillofac Surg 2009;67(4):744–50.

Valente F, Schiroli G, Sbrenna A. Accuracy of computer-aided oral implant surgery: a clinical and radiographic study. Int J Oral Maxillofac Implants 2009;24(2):234–42.

Weiner S, Simon J, Ehrenberg DS, et al. The effects of laser microtextured collars upon crestal bone levels of dental implants. Implant Dent 2008;17(2):217–28.

Worthington P, Rubenstein J, Hatcher DC. The role of cone-beam computed tomography in the planning and placement of implants. J Am Dent Assoc 2010; 141(Suppl 3):19S–24S.

Oral Cancer Detection

Orville Palmer, MD, MPH, FRCSC[a],*, Roger Grannum, DDS[b,c]

KEYWORDS

• Oral cancer • Cancer prevention • Screening for oral cancer

In an average year close to 21,000 Americans will be diagnosed with oral or pharyngeal cancer. Cancer of the oral cavity includes the following subsites: lip (excluding skin of the lip), tongue, salivary glands, gum, mouth, pharynx, oropharynx, and hypopharynx. The disease will cause more than 6000 deaths. Of the newly diagnosed cases, slightly more than a half will be alive in 5 years. These statistics have not significantly changed in many years, even with the push for early detection and prevention. These figures place oral cancer ahead of many other cancers in terms of death toll. "Oral cancer accounts for 3% of all cancers in the United States, but it is the sixth most common cancer in males and the twelfth most common in females."[1]

The majority of Americans do not visit the dentist on a regular basis. Dental visits are usually left until the patient is suffering symptoms. Oral cancer is especially dangerous because in its early stages it is relatively painless. These facts account for the high death rate associated with oral cancer. It is usually discovered late in its development with an associated poor prognosis. Approximately 94% of all oral cancers are squamous cell carcinomas. Less common oral cancers include mucoepidermoid carcinoma, adenoid cystic carcinoma and, rarely, malignant melanoma. According to the Oral Cancer Foundation, approximately $3.2 billion is spent in the United States each year on treatment of head and neck cancers.

DEMOGRAPHICS

As one would expect, squamous cell carcinoma behaves like most other carcinomas in that it becomes more prevalent with increased age. To fully understand the published statistics in the literature, the reader must first determine which reference points are being used. In some literature the statistics are based solely on intraoral disease and do not include any disease of the vermillion region. The contrary is apparent in many other articles, where all areas of the mouth are included in the definition. Neville

---

The authors have nothing to disclose.
[a] Division of Otolaryngology, Head and Neck Surgery, Department of Surgery, Harlem Hospital Center, 506 Lenox Avenue, New York, NY 10037, USA
[b] Private Practice of Oral and Maxillofacial Surgery, Woodhull Medical Center, 760 Broadway, Brooklyn, NY 11206, USA
[c] Department of Dentistry, Woodhull Medical and Mental Health Center, 760 Broadway, Brooklyn, NY 11206, USA
* Corresponding author.
E-mail address: odp3@columbia.edu

Dent Clin N Am 55 (2011) 537–548
doi:10.1016/j.cden.2011.02.009
0011-8532/11/$ – see front matter © 2011 Elsevier Inc. All rights reserved.

and colleagues[1] conclude that in the United States the incidence of intraoral cancer is highest in white males older than 65 years. For middle-aged males the highest incidence occurs in African American males. According to all sources, the rate of oral cancer continues to increase in the African American community; by contrast the rates are decreasing for non-blacks. A good reference for the epidemiology of the disease is the United States Government Surveillance Epidemiology and End Results Report (SEER).[2] Females of all ethnicities and races in the United States have a lower incidence of the disease according to the National Cancer Institute. However, within this group African American females have the highest incidence and mortality rates, just like their male counterparts.

We now live in a global society so we should be somewhat familiar with global statistics. Whites and blacks are still more likely to suffer the effects of this disease and, consistent with what is found in the United States, males more so than females. One very interesting fact put forward by the National Cancer Institute is that Filipinos are the only race in whom the incidence of oral cancer is the same for both males and females.

ETIOLOGY

Most literature concedes that oral cancer has a high correlation with a person's lifestyle. There are multiple extrinsic agents associated with oral cancer. Tobacco use of all types, whether it be pipes, cigars, cigarettes, or smokeless tobacco, must also be included as one of the major causes. Betel nut chewing, practiced in parts of Asia, also has a high association. Over a lifetime people who chew these nuts, which come from the areca palm, have an 8% chance of contracting oral cancer. The next major association is alcohol consumption and abuse. It is not widely thought that alcohol by itself is a major inducing agent. However, in conjunction with tobacco use it is thought to have a potentiating effect. According to Kuriakose and Sharan,[3] the risk for development of oral cancer is 3 to 9 times greater in people who drink or smoke and up to 100 times greater in people who drink and smoke heavily.

Iron deficiency is also associated with an increased risk of squamous cell carcinoma of the esophagus, oropharynx, and posterior mouth. Patients with Plummer-Vinson and Paterson-Kelly syndromes are at highest risk. Vitamin A deficiency has also been shown to place individuals at risk for oral cancer. Research has shown that people whose diets are lacking fruits and vegetables are more susceptible to the disease. Blood levels of retinol and the amounts of dietary β-carotene ingested are inversely proportional to the risk of contracting oral squamous cell carcinoma and leukoplakia.[1]

A thorough knowledge of the causative agents of cancer will help in the prevention and early detection of the disease. Because most people contract the disease after age of 40, some of the literature places age as a risk factor. "The age of diagnosed patients may indicate a time component in the biochemical or biophysical processes of aging cells that allows malignant transformation, or perhaps, immune system competence diminishes with age."[4]

New research has shown that there are biologic risk factors as well. Tumor-producing viruses are thought to play a role in the development of oral squamous carcinoma. Human papillomavirus 16 (HPV 16) has been definitively implicated in oral cancers, particularly those that occur in the posterior oral cavity and oropharynx. HPV 16 and HPV 18 are the primary biologic agents associated with cervical cancer. These cancer-associated types of HPV cause dysplastic tissue growths that usually appear flat and are nearly invisible. Dysplastic tissue is the presence of abnormal cells on the surface of the skin. Dysplasia is not cancer, but is a tissue change often seen prior to invasive malignancy. These biologic factors are not thought to follow the same mechanism as the extrinsic factors. HPV-related disease appears to occur on the tonsillar area, the base of the tongue, and the oropharynx, and non-HPV–positive tumors tend to involve the anterior tongue, floor of the mouth, the mucosa that covers the inside of the cheeks, and alveolar ridges. At the cellular level, the mouth is structurally very similar to the vagina and cervix. These organs have the same type of epithelial cells that are the targeted by HPV. The majority of oral cancers are of epithelial cells, primarily squamous cell carcinomas, not unlike the cancers that affect the cervix. It has been shown that smoking and drinking alcohol help promote HPV invasion, especially marijuana smoking.

HPV 16 tumors usually occur in a younger population than the tobacco and alcohol malignancies. Tobacco oral cancers occur most frequently in the fifth through the seventh decade of life, more so in white males and in nonsmokers. "The HPV positive group is the fastest growing segment of the oral cancer population."[4]

PREVENTION

The obvious method of preventing oral cancer would be to refrain from alcohol and tobacco use; however, it is not quite that simple. In a 2005 article in *JADA*, Cruz and colleagues[5] split prevention into two categories. Primary prevention, as they called it, consists of "avoidance of tobacco use and alcohol abuse, as well as appropriate intake of fruits and vegetables." Secondary prevention consists of regular oral head and neck examinations, and treatment of any premalignant conditions or in situ neoplasms.

In 2000 the Department of Health and Human Services published a report called *Healthy People 2000*, which consisted of several goals and guidelines to not only prevent but also to reduce oral cancer **Box 1**.[6]

As the goals were published back in 2000, they fail to address one of the major concerns of today, namely the transmission of the HPV virus. The transmission of HPV to the oral cavity through unprotected oral sex is becoming very prevalent.

It would seem, therefore, that education and health care promotion may hold the key to reducing the number of cases of oral cancer. With regard to cigarette smoking, great strides have been made in reducing the number of smokers in the United States. A similar government initiative will be required if the amount of alcohol consumed in this country is to be reduced. Regarding education, both physicians and dentists must also play their part. It is imperative that both disciplines stay up to date with the latest knowledge and technology pertinent to this matter. For physicians it is also imperative that if they are in any doubt they refer suspicious oral lesions to the dentists. All patients should undergo head and neck examinations yearly or every 6 months if they exhibit risk factors associated with the disease. Patients from lower socioeconomic brackets are more likely to visit a medical doctor than a dentist when they have symptoms that do not involve the teeth.

It is essential that health care providers understand the oral cancer examination procedure, and know the clinical appearance of oral precancerous and cancerous lesions, thus allowing them to routinely perform a systematic oral cancer examination for all their patients.

There have been no studies conducted in the United States to determine the impact of head and neck examinations and the early detection of cancer. Sensitivity and specificity tests have reported rates ranging from 58% to 99%. Many investigators have suggested that sensitivity will be improved when providers are better trained to recognize specific signs and symptoms of early cancer and pre-cancer. Furthermore, they suggest that if practitioners understand disease progression and regression, they will be more likely to detect disease in its early stages.

Box 1
Healthy People 2000 oral cancer objectives

Reverse the increase in cancer deaths to achieve a rate of no more than 130 per 100,000 people.

Increase complex carbohydrates and fiber-containing foods in the diets of adults to 5 or more daily servings for vegetables (including legumes) and fruits, and to 6 or more daily servings for grain products. Reduce cigarette smoking to a prevalence of no more than 15% among people aged 20 and older.

Reduce the initiation of cigarette smoking by children and youth so that no more than 15% have become regular cigarette smokers by age 20.

Reduce smokeless tobacco use by males aged 12 through 24 to a prevalence of no more than 4%.

Increase to at least 75% the proportion of primary care and oral health care providers who routinely advise cessation and provide assistance and follow-up for all of their tobacco-using patients.

Reduce the proportion of young people who have used alcohol, marijuana, and cocaine in the past month.

Reduce the proportion of high school seniors and college students engaging in recent occasions of heavy drinking of alcoholic beverages to no more than 28% of high school seniors and 32% of college students.

Reduce alcohol consumption by people aged 14 and older to an annual average of no more than 2 gallons of ethanol per person.

Increase to at least 75% the proportion of primary care providers who screen for alcohol and other drug use problems, and provide counseling and referral as needed.

Reduce deaths due to cancer of the oral cavity and pharynx to no more than 10.5 per 100,000 men aged 45 through 74 and 4.1 per 100,000 women aged 45 through 74.

Increase to at least 70% the proportion of people aged 35 and older using the oral health care system during each year.

Increase to at least 40% the proportion of people aged 50 and older visiting a primary care provider in the preceding year who have received oral, skin, and digital rectal examinations during one such visit.

Sensitivity is the proportion of truly diseased persons in the screened population who are identified as diseased by the screening test, that is, the probability of correctly diagnosing a case, or the true positive rate. Specificity is the proportion of truly non-diseased persons who are so identified by the screening test, that is, the probability of correctly identifying a nondiseased person with a screening test, or the true negative rate. (Definition from JM Last's *A Dictionary of Epidemiology*, Oxford Press, 1988.)

CHEMOPREVENTION

Chemoprevention is defined as the administration of agent(s) to block or reverse carcinogenesis.[3] With regard to oral cancer, the goal of chemoprevention has been to reverse any premalignant transformations and the prevention of second primary tumors. The agents associated with chemoprevention of oral cancer are retinoids, β-carotene, vitamin E, selenium, and cyclooxygenase-2 inhibitors. In 2003 the National Cancer Institute reported a negative result for the use of ketorolac in topical form for oral leukoplakia.

β-Carotene and the retinoids are the most commonly used antioxidant supplements for chemoprevention of oral cancer. The success rate of these agents is unreliable at best, but they still may be appropriate if there is recurrence after surgical excision. Patients with leukoplakia involving a large area of the oral mucosa might also be candidates for antioxidants, as might patients with extensive medical problems that increase their surgical risk.[4]

Retinoids are compounds consisting of natural forms or synthetic analogues, and are the most widely investigated agents for chemoprevention in oral cancer. Of the more than 1500 synthetic analogues of vitamin A, 13-*cis*-retinoic acid (13-cRA), also known as isotretinoin or Accutane, has generated the most interest. 13-cRA has been shown to cause temporary remission of oral leukoplakia, but it also causes side effects in a high percentage of patients.[4] A study done by Hong and colleagues[7] in which they looked at the role of high-dose retinoic acid in the treatment of leukoplakia found that 67% f the treatment group showed a response compared with only 10% of the control group. Other studies have shown that there may be a propensity for remission once the treatment has been stopped.

β-Carotene is a member of the carotenoids, which are highly pigmented (red, orange, yellow), fat-soluble compounds naturally present in many fruits, grains, oils, and vegetables (green plants, carrots, sweet potatoes, squash, spinach, apricots, and green peppers). α-, β-, and γ-carotene are considered provitamins because they can be converted to active vitamin A. β-Carotene supplements alone have been associated with clinical improvement; rates have ranged from 14.8% to 71%.[4] Unlike the retinoids, there have been no side effects reported in patients given β-carotene supplements. However, little is known about recurrence rates after treatment.

PRECANCEROUS LESIONS
Leukoplakia

Leukoplakia has several different variations, but in general is classified as a white plaque that does not rub off and cannot be clinically identified as anything else. The majority of cases of leukoplakia are merely responses to some kind of irritant in the form of hyperkeratosis, but in 25% to 30% of cases some form of dysplasia is present. Practitioners should be especially vigilant if it appears on the ventral tongue, floor of the mouth, or posterior pharynx (**Fig. 1**).

Some of the variations of leukoplakia include:

1. Proliferative verrucous leukoplakia (PVL): very rare but has a high potential for malignant transformation

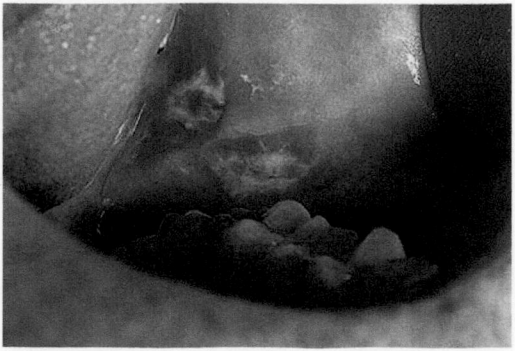

Fig. 1. Leukoplakia.

2. Granular leukoplakia: clinically the surface is not smooth and looks like small granules or nodules. It has a fairly high potential for malignant transformation
3. Smooth, thick leukoplakia has a smooth surface as its name portrays, but will be thick in appearance with low potential for malignant transformation
4. Smooth, thin leukoplakia, the opposite of the above with very little chance of malignant transformation.

Erythroplakia

An erythroplakia is a red lesion which, like leukoplakia, cannot be classified as another entity. Although it is less common than leukoplakia it has a far greater propensity for malignant transformation. The lesions are flat, macular, of velvety appearance, and may have white spots indicative of an area of keratosis (**Fig. 2**).

ORAL SUBMUCOUS FIBROSIS

This particular lesion is usually seen in people from India and South East Asia. It has a strong association with the chewing of betel quid, which as mentioned earlier comes from the areca nut. It is a chronic disease of the oral cavity, which manifests in inflammation and progressive fibrosis of the submucosal tissues (lamina propria and deeper connective tissues). As the condition progresses there can be rigidity and an eventual inability to open the mouth. This condition has an extremely high potential for malignant transformation (**Fig. 3**).

Lichen Planus

There is no real evidence in the literature to this point as to whether lichen planus undergoes malignant transformation or shows any signs of dysplasia. However, it is extremely difficult to differentiate lichen planus from epithelial dysplasia. Lichen planus is chronic and very common. It is believed that if as a practitioner one is unsure, a biopsy should be recommended (**Fig. 4**).

There are many other lesions that may appear in the oral cavity, but most have a very low potential for any malignant transformation. A biopsy should be considered for any mucosal lesion that persists for more than 14 days after all irritants have been eradicated.

Depending on the source, between 5% and 20% of dysplasias will become malignant, although expecting a greater probability of malignant change for dysplasias with a greater histologic degree of epithelial dysplasia seems intuitive. The tenet that the

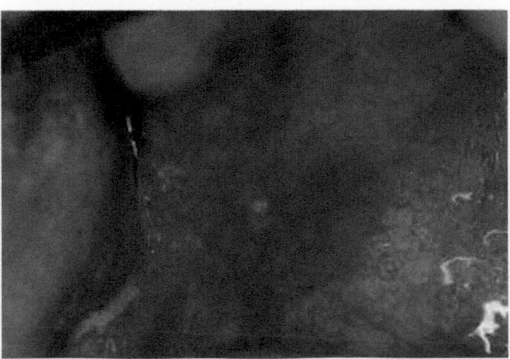

Fig. 2. Erythroplakia.

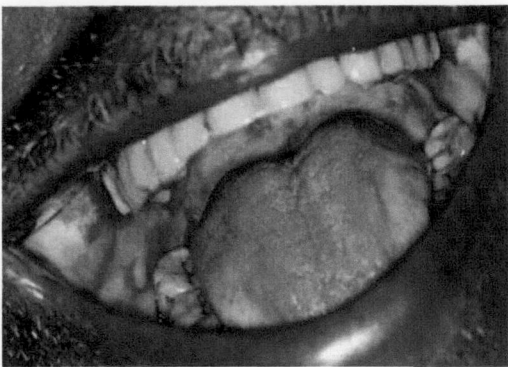

Fig. 3. Malignant transformation of erythroplakia.

greater the dysplasia, the greater the chance of malignant transformation has not been proved. However, certain manifestations have been associated with an increased risk of malignant transformation.

Curiously, according to DeJong and colleagues[8] if a patient has a premalignant lesion it is more likely to undergo malignant transformation if that person is a nonsmoker. Other factors that can lead to an increased risk of malignant transformation are any kind of erythroleukoplakia, multiple lesions, or if the lesion is located in a one of the aforementioned high-risk areas.

DETECTION

The recently introduced technologies are all aimed at early detection, and are simple enough for nonsurgeons to employ.

To date there is no consensus on oral cancer screening guidelines. Individual guidelines have been implemented by independent insurance companies, government agencies, and multiple medical and dental societies. The one thing missing is a consensus by all involved as to how medical and dental practitioners should screen patients effectively. **Table 1**, taken from the oral cancer foundation Web site,[4] demonstrates this fact.

It is in the best interest of all medical and dental practitioners to implement their own set of guidelines for the treatment of their patients. There are many early detection modalities on the market; some are more efficacious than others. A common-sense approach should be brought to the early detection of oral cancer.

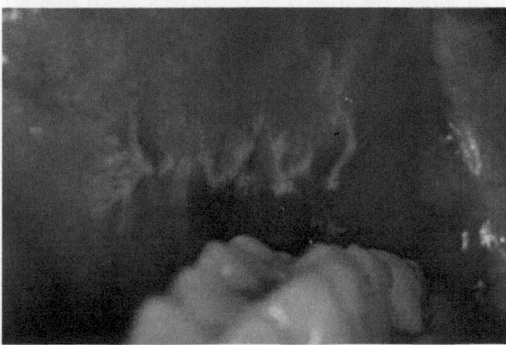

Fig. 4. Lichen planus.

Table 1
Differing recommendations by organization

Organization	Routine	High-Risk Group Only	Screening Recommendations
American Cancer Society	Yes	No	Examination for cancer of the oral region every 3 years for persons 21 years and older and annually for those 40 years and older
US Preventive Task Force	No	Yes	All patients should be counseled to discontinue the use of all forms of tobacco and to limit consumption of alcohol. Clinician should remain alert to signs and symptoms of oral cancer and premalignancy in persons who use tobacco or alcohol
Canadian Task Force	No	Yes	There is insufficient evidence to include or exclude screening for oral cancer from the periodic health examination in the general population. Only high-risk people warrant an annual oral examination by a physician or dentist

Data from www.oralcancerfoundation.org.

The first action to be undertaken should be that the government and private bodies should implement nationwide campaign to educate people on oral cancer, including risk factors, self detection, and awareness. This campaign should take the shape of those that educate people about breast cancer, colon cancer, and obesity. An educated population should theoretically be easier to treat.

Like breast cancer, the first step in early detection should begin at home in the form of self examination. Patients in high-risk groups should be encouraged to perform self examination at home on a regular basis between dental visits or doctor's visits.

Patients should be educated as to what to look for and how to perform such examinations. When a patient first visits a practitioner, a thorough history and physical (H&P) should be undertaken. This H&P should be meaningfully updated on subsequent visits. The H&P should obviously include questions on all the known risk factors.

A complete oral examination should be performed by dental and medical practitioners during visits. These examinations are extremely quick to perform and can be performed yearly. A study in Sri Lanka undertaken by Warnakulasuriya and colleagues[9] found that when paramedical providers were trained and employed in the detection of oral cancer and precancerous lesions they were able to screen significant numbers of patients, far more than medical and dental providers were able to screen. Once initial screening has taken place, a complete head and neck examination should be undertaken. A description of how to perform a head and neck examination can be found in dental text books or on the Internet. If no lesions are found, the patient can be placed on a 6-month or yearly recall depending on risk factors. If a suspect lesion is found then there are many ways to proceed. The first may be to watch the lesion, if it is small, for 2 weeks and see if it heals. If it does not heal then it should be investigated further. A basic rule of thumb can that be all lesions meeting the following criteria should be investigated[4]:

- A sore or lesion in the mouth that does not heal within 2 weeks
- A lump or thickening in the cheek

- A white or red patch on the gums, tongue, tonsil, or lining of the mouth
- A sore throat or a feeling that something is caught in the throat
- Difficulty chewing or swallowing
- Difficulty moving the jaw or tongue
- Numbness of the tongue or other area of the mouth
- Swelling of the jaw that causes dentures to fit poorly or become uncomfortable.

If the patient is in a dental office then dental radiographs should be thoroughly reviewed and evaluated. If the practitioner feels comfortable, the most reliable thing to do would be to perform an incisional biopsy and send it to a pathologist. It is essential that the practitioner take a deep enough sample for the pathologist to analyze. If the practitioner does not feel comfortable performing an incisional biopsy then he or she has several options. The patient can be referred to an oral and maxillofacial surgeon, who may be the most experienced in diagnosing oral cancer. The dentist also has the option to perform a noninvasive procedure, of which there are several. Brush cytology is probably the best known of the noninvasive procedures. Brush cytology Brush Biopsy (CDx Laboratories, Suffren, NY, USA) was first introduced back in 1999. It was initially intended to be used on lesions that showed a low level of suspicion for squamous cell carcinoma. As such, if a positive result was found the patient would then undergo a more formal incisional biopsy. Multiple studies have shown encouraging results for brush biopsy and the detection of precancerous lesions. The advantages to this procedure are that it can be done in the dentist's office, is not painful, and requires no anesthetic. A small bristled brush is rotated over the suspicious lesion several times or until pinpoint bleeding is attained. The sample is then transferred to a microscope slide, which is also provided in the kit. Once completed, the slide is sent to the laboratory to be read.

There is some very promising work being done by Weigum and colleagues,[10] which involves the use of nano-biochips to detect early precancerous oral lesions. After a conventional brush biopsy has been performed the samples are then sent to the laboratory, where specific biomarkers are then looked for. In their article the marker being looked for was the epidermal growth factor receptor. Several parameters were used to distinguish which specimens were positive or negative. The technology is still in its infancy, but appears to be extremely promising in the early detection of oral cancer.

SCREENING METHODS

Chemiluminescence was initially used by gynecologist for the early detection of cervical dysplasias. Like many other screening tests it has been adapted for use in the oral cavity, under the trade names ViziLite Plus (Zila Inc, Phoenix, AZ, USA) and Microlux/DL (AdDent Inc, Danbury, CT, USA).

The ideal screening is a noninvasive, inexpensive method with a high sensitivity and specificity, providing a reasonably high positive predictive value. It should also able to differentiate a benign from a precancerous or cancerous lesion. The methods for detection of precancerous and cancerous lesion comprise direct white light examination, chemiluminescence, or direct fluorescence visualization. The chemiluminescence method makes use of acetic acid and tolonium chloride, by themselves or in combination.

Conventional Screening

Conventional screening (CS) for oral lesions involves inspection and palpation under halogen or incandescent illumination. Neck examination looking at all 6 neck zones is involved as a part of this screening method. Meta-analysis performed by McIntosh and colleagues[11] using biopsy and histopathology as the gold standard shows a sensitivity and specificity of 0.85 and 0.97, respectively. The inherent problem with this method is that about 10% of the population have some form of oral mucosal abnormality. Most of these lesions are benign. CS does not accurately distinguish between a benign, malignant lesion and a premalignant lesion. CS cannot detect a premalignant lesion in a normal-appearing mucosa, which may lead to delay in diagnosis and ultimately poorer prognosis.

Acetic Acid

Acetic acid rinse as a detection method uses conventional acetic acid or, more recently, commercially available chemiluminescence kits containing a chemical mixture with acetic acid as its illumination source. Microlux/DL and ViziLite are the commonly known kits.

ViziLite contains 1% acetic acid, sodium benzoate, a base of propylene glycol and alcohol, with a raspberry flavor. The chemiluminescent ViziLite light stick comprises an inner fragile glass vial of hydrogen peroxide and an outer plastic capsule containing acetylsalicylic acid. When the capsule is flexed the inner glass ruptures, releasing the peroxide. The chemical reaction produces a blue-white light (wavelength 430–580 nm) lasting for 10 to 12 minutes. The mouth is first examined using CS at which point the size, morphology, and surface characteristics are noted. The mouth is rinsed with 30 mL of the acetic acid solution. The ViziLite capsule is then activated and placed in the ViziLite retractor. The oral cavity is then examined under dimmed lighting and photographed if any abnormal findings are noted. Sensitivity, specificity, and positive predictive value for this method are 1.0, 0.18, and 0.2, respectively in a study done by McIntosh and colleagues,[11] and 1.0, 0.14, and 0.8 in a study by Ram and Siar.[12] Therefore, the usefulness of this method seems to be user dependent.

The Microlux/DL kit provides similar findings after the mouth is examined using CS. In this method the mouth is the examined before and after a 60-second 1% acetic acid rinse, using the standard LED headlight with overhead lights dimmed. Abnormal areas are photographed and biopsied. The sensitivity, specificity, and positive predictive value are 0.78, 0.71, and 0.37, respectively.

Both the ViziLite and Microlux/DL methods are poor discriminators between benign and malignant tumors as well as being poor discriminators of underlying pathology, and add little more to CS findings for new emerging lesions.

Tolonium Chloride

Tolonium chloride represents another chemiluminescent diagnostic tool. Tolonium chloride solution is used by itself or mixed with 10 mL of 1% acetic acid and 4.19 mL absolute alcohol. This is a quick, inexpensive test used as an oral rinse or to paint a suspicious lesion. It is a blue dye that selectively stains the acidic component of tissue with which it comes into contact, namely DNA and RNA. It has been used around the world as a method of early detection for oral cancer. However, in the United States it has not been approved by the Food and Drug Administration for that purpose.

Tolonium chloride has been used in the past for detection of carcinoma in situ and invasive carcinoma. It has also found use in postsurgical tumor recurrence, carving out a surgical field for biopsy or resection in tumors of the bronchus, cervix, larynx, and oral cavity. In a meta-analysis performed by Rosenberg and Cretin[13] looking at 12 studies ranging from 12 to 1190 subjects, the sensitivities range from 0.86 to 1.0 with the average being 0.97, while the specificities range from 0.7 to 1.0 with the average being 0.91. The positive predictive value averages about 15%, meaning that of all the cases tested positive on testing, only 15% are positive on definitive histopathology on biopsy.

Linegan and colleagues[14,15] determined multiple problems with the studies conducted with toluidine blue:

- No studies performed in primary care environment
- Data from studies in secondary care are not necessarily applicable to the general population
- No randomized controlled trials
- Some studies only include carcinomas or dysplasia, and some include both
- Histologic diagnosis is rarely used as gold standard
- Methods vary: single rinse, double rinse, or painting
- Confusion over inclusion of equivocal (pale) staining as positive or negative.

Direct Fluorescence Visualization

There have been multiple studies conducted on the efficacy of these reflective tissue fluorescence systems as an adjunct for oral cancer detection. Lingen and colleagues[14] make a valid criticism of all the studies: that there is no comparison with the diagnostic gold standard, which is the scalpel biopsy.

Ever since it was discovered that tissue fluorescence could be used for cancer detection, there has been great interest in the areas of fluorescence imaging and spectroscopy. In fluorescence spectroscopy, tissues are exposed to various excitation wavelengths; subsequently, differences between normal and abnormal tissues can be identified. Fluorescence imaging involves the exposure of tissue to specific wavelengths of light, which results in the autofluorescence of cellular fluorophores. The fluorophores are changed by cellular alterations, meaning that the way the light is scattered and absorbed will be altered; this leads to color changes that can be seen. Consequently fluorescence imaging and spectroscopy are good at distinguishing between normal and malignant tissue. However, based on the mechanism of each technique, imaging is far more feasible as a screening tool in the oral cavity.

The VELscope (LED Dental Inc, White Rock, BC, Canada) is being marketed as an oral cancer screening tool. The VELscope allows for direct visualization of the oral cavity. A blue light is emitted from the unit and when it meets normal oral mucosa there is a light green autofluorescence, which can only be viewed through the handpiece that is attached to the device. Abnormal tissue will autofluoresce to a lesser degree, appearing dark when viewed through the scope. This coloration is quite easy to recognize because the surrounding mucosa will have the light green appearance. Lane and colleagues[16] investigated the ability of the VELscope to identify precancerous or cancer lesions. These investigators found that the VELscope showed a sensitivity of 0.98 and a specificity of 1.00 for distinguishing between dysplasias and cancers. Comparisons were made with the gold standard scalpel biopsy and histology findings. One important point is that all the lesions could be seen with the naked eye. It still remains to be seen how good the device would be in the detection of lesions invisible to naked eye. Data on the VELscope as a screening tool is still forthcoming.

SUMMARY

Although the oral cavity is relatively accessible to examination, malignant processes tend to present late and with poor prognosis. To improve tumor outcome, early detection and treatment are essential. Many screening tools are available, but their clinical usefulness has not been scientifically proved. At present, available screening tools may help in visualizing an existing lesion or its borders, but they add little in discriminating between a premalignant, malignant, or inflammatory process. Good history taking and examination still seem to be our most cost-effective tools.

REFERENCES

1. Neville B, Damm D, Allen C, et al. Oral and maxillofacial pathology. Philadelphia; London; New York; St Louis; Sydney; Toronto: W.B. Saunders Company; 2002. p. 356–9.
2. U.S. National Cancer Institute. National Cancer Institute. Surveillance Epidemiology and End Results. (SEER). Available at: http://seer.cancer.gov. Accessed June 22, 2010.
3. Kuriakose M, Sharan R. Oral cancer prevention. Oral Maxillofac Surg Clin North Am 2006;18:493–511.
4. Available at: www.oralcancerfoundation.org. Accessed June 22, 2010.
5. Cruz G, Ostroff J, Kumar J, et al. Preventing and detecting: oral health care providers' readiness to provide health behavior counseling and oral cancer examinations. J Am Dent Assoc 2005;136:594–601.
6. Department of Health and Human Services. Healthy people 2000. Rockville (MD): US Department of Health and Human Services, Public Health Service; 1991. DHHS publication no. (PHS) 91-50212.
7. Hong W, Endicott J, Itri L, et al. 13-cis retinoic acid in the treatment of oral leukoplakia. N Engl J Med 1986;315:1501–5.
8. DeJong WF, Albrecht M, Banoczy J, et al. Epithelial dysplasia in oral lichen planus. Int J Oral Maxillofac Surg 1984;13:221–5.
9. Warnakulasuriya KA, Ekanayake AN, Sivayoham S, et al. Utilization of primary health care workers for early detection of oral cancer and precancer cases in Sri Lanka. Bull World Health Organ 1984;62(2):243–50.
10. Weigum S, Floriano P, Reddind S, et al. Nano-Bio chip sensor platform for examination of oral exfoliative cytology. Cancer Prev Res (Phila) 2010;3(4):518–28.
11. McIntosh L, McCullough M, Farah CS. The assessment of diffused light illumination and acetic acid rinse (Microlux/DLTM) in the visualisation of oral mucosal lesions. Oral Oncol 2009;45:227–31.
12. Ram S, Siar CH. Chemiluminescence as a diagnostic aid in the detection of oral cancer and potentially malignant epithelial lesions. Int J Oral Maxillofac Surg 2005;34:521–7.
13. Rosenberg D, Cretin S. Use of meta-analysis to evaluate tolonium chloride in oral cancer screening. Oral Surg Oral Med Oral Pathol 1989;67(5):621–7.
14. Lingen M, Kalmar J, Karrison T, et al. Critical evaluation of diagnostic aids for the detection of oral cancer. Oral Oncol 2008;44(1):10–22.
15. Zhang L, Williams M, Poh CF, et al. Toluidine blue staining identifies high risk primary oral premalignant lesions with poor outcome. Cancer Res 2005;65(17): 8017–21.
16. Lane P, Gilhuly T, Whitehead P, et al. Simple device for the direct visualization of oral-cavity tissue fluorescence. J Biomed Opt 2006;11(2):024006.

Office Computer Systems for the Dental Office

Frances E. Sam, DDS[a], Andrea M. Bonnick, DDS[b,c],*

KEYWORDS

• Dental office • Software • Computers • Chartless • EHR

Traditionally, the practicing dentist has had to act as bookkeeper, accountant, marketing and promotions expert, and in countless other capacities in addition to clinician. The profession has always had its innate challenges if any measure of success was to be achieved. Of course, delegating some of these responsibilities to competent team members has helped to relieve the impossible load of the average practitioner. However, disorganized and frenzied team dynamics can add to the overall stresses.

Over the years, the pressures associated with dentistry have been well documented.[1] Practice management has been consistently identified as a major factor.[2] Fortunately, impressive technological advances have alleviated much of the strain that running a flourishing practice can create. The fields of dental informatics and information technology have since presented us with options to assuage management concerns and, more recently, clinical issues.

Over the past 25 years, the growing field of dental informatics has played a significant role in the evolution of dentistry. Succinctly stated, "Dental informatics is the application of computer and information sciences to improve dental practice, research, education and management."[3(p61)] Intersection of this field with that of information technology has affected us in a variety of ways. For example, it has resulted in the extensive database MEDLINE, clinical simulation programs, and distance learning.[4] It has also resulted in the array of dental office computer systems that are now in use. There exists a plethora of hardware and software that today's practitioner can customize to the needs of any type of practice.

The authors have nothing to disclose.
a Department of Oral and Maxillofacial Surgery, Howard University College of Dentistry, 600 West Street, NW, Room 424, Washington, DC 20059, USA
b Oral and Maxillofacial Surgery Program, Department of Oral and Maxillofacial Surgery, Howard University Hospital, 2041 Georgia Avenue, NW, Washington, DC 20060, USA
c Department of Dentistry, Howard University Hospital, 2041 Georgia Avenue, NW, Washington, DC, USA
* Corresponding author. Department of Oral and Maxillofacial Surgery, Howard University Hospital, 2041 Georgia Avenue, NW, Washington, DC 20060.
E-mail address: abonnick@howard.edu

Dent Clin N Am 55 (2011) 549–557
doi:10.1016/j.cden.2011.02.010
0011-8532/11/$ – see front matter © 2011 Elsevier Inc. All rights reserved.

As in the past, there remains a relatively slow acceptance for computers to take on increasing responsibility. Many practitioners own software but use it in a limited capacity. The associated expenses and time-consuming training may act as deterrents for many. However, dentistry, as all other professions, finds itself in the tide of the new digital world. It is estimated that approximately a third of practitioners currently have computers within their operatories. Because computers have become a part of everyday life, it is expected that we shall see further integration into what is considered mainstream practice.

HISTORY OF COMPUTERS AND DENTISTRY

Over the past 4 decades, we have witnessed the integration of computers into various functions of the dental office. The emergence, however, had to overcome initial resistance. The cost of computer analysis was deemed "bad for productivity"[5(p659)] and that "computers should be reserved for more challenging tasks."[5(p660)] Employees were considered far more efficient than the unfamiliar processing units.

Granted, the relative expense of the option was high compared with what it would cost now. Extravagant costs prohibited small practices from purchasing their own units. Acquiring computer data would have been a considerable expense. Fortunately, the appearance of the microchip in the early 1980s soon made computers for the household and small businesses a possibility.[6] However, the heavy reliance on human labor was indicative of a traditional mindset in which computers were considered unnecessary for "simple" tasks.

During the 1980s, a growing interest in technology for the dental office developed. Practitioners realized how the incorporation of computers could lighten the load of busy practices while affecting productivity in substantial ways. They acted as centralized databases mainly used by front desk personnel. Administrative tasks such as compiling production reports, patient recalls, and accessing transaction information no longer encumbered overworked staff.[7]

As popularity was gained, traditional use of the computers grew to include additional bookkeeping and accounting duties, handling of insurance claims, and patient scheduling. During the mid to late 1980s, promotion and marketing efforts had become a prevalent part of the dental community. Software companies became conscious of the marketing aspect of dental practices. Subsequently, letter-writing functions and demographic analyses were featured as part of their offerings.[6]

In 1984, only 11% of dentists reported having computers in their offices.[8] By 1991, 48% of dentists had computers in their offices.[9] The dental world had been firmly infiltrated. Within the following 10 years, the number rose to 85%.[10]

During that decade, technology started to include clinical features in addition to data and financial management functions. Areas such as periodontal charting, voice activation, and imaging capabilities were actively being explored; however, these features were largely independent of each other. A divide existed between practice management software and clinical technology.[6] Perhaps this was because, despite the innovations in clinical applications, the overwhelming majority of dentists were still using computers mainly for administrative tasks.[10,11] However, the concept of a fully functioning intraoffice network was budding. Major innovations were about to further redefine the manner in which dentistry was practiced.

CONTEMPORARY USE OF OFFICE COMPUTER SYSTEMS

In the mid 1990s, the appearance of the intraoral camera resulted in computer monitors moving into the operatory. This enabled the practitioner to inspect subtleties not visible to the naked eye, and it also introduced the opportunity for enhancement of patient education.[6,12] Although options such as treatment planning and charting were also available, they were likely to be run by programs different from the practice management programs. As a result, practitioners were not taking full advantage of these new developments.

Unlike the stand-alone offerings of the 1990s, today's software choices have successfully combined administrative functions along with clinical features, thereby augmenting the role of chairside computers. By 2003, approximately 25% of dentists were using computers at chairside.[13] Currently, some of the most popular systems include Dentrix (Henry Schein, Inc, Melville, NY, USA), Eaglesoft (Patterson Dental, St Paul, MN, USA), and Softdent (Kodak Dental Systems, Atlanta, GA, USA). All offer similar basic functions but each offers its own unique features (Table 1).

In an ideal situation, updates to medical history can be reviewed at a glance. Relevant clinical information can then be documented in real time by voice recognition and radiographs can be viewed instantaneously. The patient can then be educated on any number of issues. Subsequently, an electronic signature may be obtained for consent, if necessary, by use of a writing tablet. After delivering treatment, future appointments can be scheduled in accordance with the established treatment plan before the patient departs the chair. Billing matters can be addressed by the front desk before the patient leaves, as personnel would have immediate access to data already entered into the system.

Conventionally, these data are usually stored on a dedicated server and protected by numerous security measures. In addition, companies usually offer off-site backup of information as part of their packages. Presently, Curve Dental (Orem, UT, USA) offers a completely Web-based practice management system, meaning that it runs independent of servers. The user requires only a browser and an Internet connection. It is also offered on a subscription basis. This presents yet another interesting option in the abundance of quality software that currently exists.

The judicious practitioner must make the decision as to what is appropriate for a particular practice. What may be suitable for one office may not be necessary in another. Note that in addition to purchasing the practice management software, a compatible image management software and digital imaging system would also be necessary for the chartless office, which is in the early stages of adoption by practitioners.

Chartless offices appear to be an emerging trend for 2 reasons. One reason is the growing interest in "green" practices. The reduction of paper waste, as well as chemical waste associated with conventional x-ray methods, can ultimately decrease operating costs while positively affecting the environment. The second reason has to do with upcoming changes in the health care system.

WHAT THE FUTURE HOLDS

Further reliance on technology is inevitable, as the structure of health care will drastically change by 2015.[14] The American Recovery and Reinvestment Act of 2009 has set forth a 5-year timeline for hospitals and other eligible health care professionals to adopt health care information technology (HIT).

The Office of the National Coordinator for Health Information Technology (ONCHIT), a staff division of the Department of Health and Human Services, is responsible for developing a nationwide health information network (NHIN). This interconnectivity is expected to increase efficiency, reduce the astronomic costs of health care, and improve clinical outcomes.

Table 1
Comparison of dental office computer systems

	Dentrix (Henry Schein)	Eaglesoft (Patterson Dental)	Softdent (Kodak)	Easy Dental (Henry Schein)	Practice Works (Kodak)	Curve (Curve Dental)
Operating systems	Windows	Windows	Windows	Windows	Windows	Windows or Mac
Treatment planning	●	●	●	●	●	●
Charting	●	●	●	●	●	●
Insurance & e-claims	●	●	●	●	●	●
Patient recall	●	●	●	●	●	●
Scheduling	●	●	●	●	●	●
Voice recognition	●	●	●			
Mobile applications	●		●			●
Additional features	Guru patient education	Caesy patient education Touch screen options	Customized patient ed Touch screen options	Guru patient education		Web based Subscription based
Current users	30,000+	25,000+	30,000+	24,000+	12,000+	<1000

Through this electronic network, health care providers will be able to access the electronic heath records (EHR) of patients. This includes comprehensive medical histories, laboratory results, pharmaceutical information, vision records, and so forth. The American Dental Association is currently working on the creation and implementation of the dental component of the EHR. This undoubtedly sets the tone for the future of dental practice.

Previous studies indicate that 1% to 2% of dental practices in the United States run as truly chartless offices.[13,14] However, the industry currently appears to be averaging 35% with regard to offices that have computers within the operatory (Laci L. Phillips, Aztec, NM, personal communication, August 2010). This suggests that the potential to be chartless exists. The hesitation to convert is reflected in the health care industry at large.[15]

A survey conducted by the *New England Journal of Medicine* showed that only 1.5% of hospitals had made the transition to comprehensive EHRs.[16] A 2008 study revealed that 4% of physicians surveyed had extensive EHR systems and 13% had a basic system.[17] For both groups, cost was cited as the major hindrance to implementation. That, along with the overwhelming choices a dental practitioner must make regarding software, may explain the gradual acceptance in the field of dentistry.

In addition to government mandates, the expectations of patients will also dictate the way we will practice in years to come. As it stands, the popularity of personal health records (PHR) is rising. With this application, patients have the ability to create and maintain their own health records online. Two types exist: stand-alone and integrated PHRs.[18] The integrated version allows for interconnectivity between the physician's EHR and the patient's PHR. Significant patient populations are already actively using this technology.

Although we have glimpses of the near future, we are unable to predict the exact course of events. Our once 1-dimensional view of technology's place in dentistry has expanded to affect every aspect of practicing, from accounting to treatment to patient education. We have transitioned from an isolated use of computers to viable office networks. In the next few years, we will be completely interconnected with a massive health network (**Fig. 1**). How the individual practice management systems will integrate with a national network remains to be seen.[19] A considerable adjustment period for the entire health community should be expected by all members.

Information gathering and communication patterns will continue to evolve as technology proceeds to the next level. Regardless of the trajectory we embark on, our association with technology should consistently result in increased efficiency, an improved patient experience, and cost-effectiveness for the practice.

INHERENT BENEFITS

Dental office computer systems promote efficiency when properly implemented. Instead of physically having to pull charts and search for information, all records can be pulled up at a glance. Because many tasks can be automated, such as recall

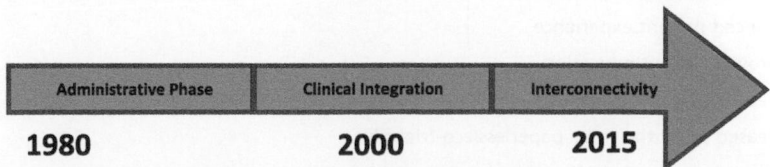

Fig. 1. The role of dental office computer systems over time.

and appointment reminders, this enables personnel to attend to other pressing matters. Invariably, increased efficiency and organization will reduce the amount of stress and anxiety experienced by all members of the dental team.[20]

Generally speaking, the overall patient experience should be enhanced with the addition of office computer systems. The efficiency of the system results in extra time, which translates to greater productivity of the team. Even if that productivity is simply having an extra 5 minutes to interact with patients, it strengthens relationships, which encourages patients to return. Patients evaluate their experiences on far more than the dental work received. They appreciate being treated as individuals, not cases.[21] Modern technology is often blamed as the cause of impersonal interactions. In this regard, technology used effectively can help to improve interpersonal connections.

In addition, technology can be used for patient education. Oftentimes, patients are unable to visualize what is relayed to them verbally. They are not familiar with dental terminology and dentists are not always the strongest communicators. Visual imagery can greatly improve patient comprehension and, subsequently, patient satisfaction.[22,23]

Many of the available programs have highly sophisticated patient education modules. With the support of visual aids, patients become better equipped to make informed decisions regarding their oral health. Patients often judge practitioners on how effectively they relay information.[24] Options such as Kodak's education module and Henry Schein's Guru[25] offer customized patient information through interactive programs.

Incorporation of current technology also sends a subconscious message of competence to the patient. Patients like to see that their health professionals are progressive. They may feel more confident that they are receiving quality care. When they have innovative experiences, they are likely to carry that information to others. All practitioners know that word of mouth is a significant practice builder.

Last, dental office computer systems are sizable investments and this may discourage hesitant practitioners from upgrading existing systems. However, on closer examination, such systems turn out to be highly cost effective in the long term.

Expenses associated with paper charts, filing systems and cabinets, and off-site storage are eliminated. Paper communications to colleagues, patients, and insurance companies can be reduced. The associated mailing charges significantly decrease. With the use of digital imaging systems, there are no more costs for film, mounts, and processing chemicals. In addition, time gained with increased efficiency also adds to the economic benefits, which can add up to tens of thousands of dollars per year (**Box 1**).[26]

Box 1
Advantages of office computer systems

- Increased efficiency
- Increased productivity
- Enhanced patient experience
- Improved patient education
- Increased cost-effectiveness
- Increased potential to be paperless/eco-friendly
- Improved progressive office appearance

Box 2
Current challenges of office computer systems

- Steep learning curve
- User interfaces
- Initial expense
- Voice recognition software
- Infection control

A WORK IN PROGRESS

All aforementioned advantages of office computer systems depend heavily on the proficiency of the users. When surveyed, 26% of individuals using practice management programs found nothing they disliked about the systems.[13] One area in which people expressed concern was in ease of use. Although many of the software functions are intuitive in nature, operator proficiency is not instantaneous. Initially, a significant amount of time may be spent on training because the learning curve for application of these systems is undoubtedly steep.

This presents a serious challenge to offices wishing to adapt to contemporary methods. Although appropriate training and technical support can help alleviate this problem, focus on user interfaces is of importance. Continuous improvements in software design will greatly help this particular challenge.[27]

Another concern revealed was that of infection control.[13] Entry of clinical data cannot be performed by individuals wearing personal protective equipment (PPE) so as not to contaminate any entry devices. Most of the data entry was found to be performed by hygienists and assistants.

The use of voice recognition software can help alleviate this problem. However, difficulty in successfully using these programs has been off-putting for many users.[28,29] Although the concept of voice recognition is straightforward, it requires some effort on the part of the practitioner.

"Training" of the software is necessary for the program to effectively identify the speech patterns of the individual user.[30] Therefore, different profiles would have to be created for each user of the program. Over time, this aspect of speech recognition software has greatly improved, resulting in progressively less training time being required. As practitioners find this application becoming easier to implement, it will greatly facilitate the process of creating electronic health records while maintaining infection control standards (**Box 2**).

SUMMARY

Over the past 3 decades, we have seen the computerization of dental offices come to light. From peripheral duties to complete integration, the future of dentistry has been irrevocably changed. The reality is that the world at large is changing rapidly and, as all other professions, we have to change with it. The initial discomforts of transition should not stand in the way of progression. If the technology exists that allows us to improve patient care, then as professionals we should be eager to embrace it.[31]

For those who resist the evolution of the modern dental practice, growth will be impeded as more patients will come to expect what technology has to offer. With the accessibility of the Internet, patients will become even more discriminating in their choice of practitioners. Resistance to contemporary schemes implies that all methods a practitioner uses will be outdated. Whether or not that is true is irrelevant. In the eyes of well-informed patients, traditionally acceptable methods may begin to appear less than standard when compared with more modern systems.

As it stands, health care will reach a milestone by 2015. The concept of interconnectivity was brought forth during the last administration, but we are now in the midst of actively manifesting that vision. Over the next few years, making a series of intelligent choices will help the conversion to electronic health records be a less arduous process.

To willingly remain unfamiliar with current technology in the dental world is to operate counter to the direction the profession is moving. Each practitioner must decide what aspects of technology are appropriate for an individual practice, but the larger picture must be kept in mind. We will not be operating as isolated entities as in the past. Interconnectivity and interoperability will be key characteristics of tomorrow's health care system. Gradual inclusion of appropriate software and hardware will allow dedicated dental teams to adapt favorably and ultimately connect them with the health community at large.

Much is to be gained by all parties with the acceptance of technology in practice. Thirty years ago it was written that "The computer is everywhere today, but its use in dentistry lags noticeably behind other fields...."[32(p226)] Fortunately, we can choose otherwise. Total integration of dental office computer systems is simply the way of the future.

REFERENCES

1. Rada RE, Johnson-Leong C. Stress, burnout, anxiety and depression among dentists. J Am Dent Assoc 2004;135(6):788–94.
2. Bourassa M, Baylard JF. Stress situations in dental practice. J Can Dent Assoc 1994;60(1):65–7, 70–1.
3. Eisner J. The future of dental informatics. Eur J Dent Educ 1999;3(Suppl 1):61–9.
4. Schleyer T, Spallek H. Dental informatics: a cornerstone for dental practice. J Am Dent Assoc 2001;132(5):605–13.
5. O'Connor JT. In-office data analysis without a computer. J Am Dent Assoc 1980; 101(4):655–60.
6. Snyder TL. Integrating technology into dental practices. J Am Dent Assoc 1995; 126(2):171–8.
7. Ricks M. A computer helped humanize my office. Dent Manage 1980;20(3): 18–24.
8. Kiser A, Nash K. Computers in dentistry on the rise. J Am Dent Assoc 1992; 123(2):106–7.
9. American Dental Association. 1992 survey of dental practice. Chicago: American Dental Association; 1991.
10. American Dental Association. 2000 survey of current issues in dentistry. Dentists' computer use. Chicago: American Dental Association; 2001.
11. Flores-Mir C, Palmer NG, Northcott HC, et al. Computer and Internet usage by Canadian dentists. J Can Dent Assoc 2006;72(3):145.
12. Johnson LA. A systematic evaluation of intraoral cameras. J Calif Dent Assoc 1994;22(11):34–42, 44–7.
13. Schleyer TK, Thyvalikakath T, Spallek H, et al. Clinical computing in general dentistry. J Am Med Inform Assoc 2006;13(3):344–52.
14. DiGangi P. Chartless future for everyone closer than you think. Dent Econ 2009; 99(3). Available at: http://www.dentaleconomics.com/index/display/article-display/

357580/articles/dental-economics/volume-99/issue-3/features/chartless-future-for-everyone-closer-than-you-think.html. Accessed February 15, 2011.

15. Bigalke JT. Filling the healthcare IT gap by 2015. Healthc Financ Manage 2009; 63(6):38–40.
16. Jha AK, DesRoches CM, Campbell EG, et al. Use of electronic health records in U.S. hospitals. N Engl J Med 2009;360(16):1628–38.
17. DesRoches CM, Campbell EG, Rao SR. Electronic health records in ambulatory care—a national survey of physicians. N Engl J Med 2008;359:50–60.
18. Tang PC, Lee TH. Your doctor's office or the Internet? Two paths to personal health records. N Engl J Med 2009;360(13):1276–8.
19. Schleyer TK. Should dentistry be part of the National Health Information Infrastructure? J Am Dent Assoc 2004;135(12):1687–95.
20. Technology makes dental practice more efficient. Dent Abstr 2005;50(3):134.
21. Yamalik N. Dentist-patient relationship and quality care. 3. Communication. Int Dent J 2005;55(4):254–6.
22. Hu J, Yu H, Shao J, et al. An evaluation of the dental 3D multimedia system on dentist–patient interactions: a report from China. Int J Med Inf 2008;77(10):670–8.
23. Cooper BR. Patient education software: technology in the dental office. Dent Assist 2007;76(3):16–7.
24. Lahti S, Tuutti H, Hausen H, et al. Dentist and patient opinions about the ideal dentist and patient—developing a compact questionnaire. Community Dent Oral Epidemiol 1992;20(4):229–34.
25. Acharya A, Wali T, Rauch J. GURU: Patient education software. J Dent Educ 2009;73(1):137–9.
26. Dykstra BA. The economics of the digital dental record: can you afford not to make the switch? Dent Econ 2009;99(9). Available at: http://www.dentaleconomics.com/index/display/article-display/369534/articles/dental-economics/volume-99/issue-9/features/the-economics-of-the-digital-dental-record-can-you-afford-not-to-make-the-switch.html. Accessed February 15, 2011.
27. Thyvalikakath T, Schleyer TK, Monaco V. Heuristic evaluation of clinical functions in four practice management systems. J Am Dent Assoc 2007;138(2):209–18.
28. Yuhaniak-Irwin J, Schleyer T. A preliminary comparison of speech recognition functionality in dental practice management systems. AMIA Annu Symp Proc 2008;988.
29. Yuhaniak-Irwin J, Fernando S, Schleyer T, et al. Speech recognition in dental software systems: features and functionality. Stud Health Technol Inform 2007;129(Pt 2):1127–31.
30. Glenn T. Speech recognition technology for physicians. Physicians News Digest 2005. Available at: http://www.physiciansnews.com/business/505glenn.html. Accessed February 15, 2011.
31. Ganz CH. Advanced clinical technology—clinical tool or expensive toy? J Can Dent Assoc 1995;61(10):857–60, 863–5.
32. Crandell CE. Use of computers in dental office management. Int Dent J 1980; 3(3):226–33.

The Use of CAD/CAM in Dentistry

Gary Davidowitz, DDS[a,b,*], Philip G. Kotick, DDS[b,c]

KEYWORDS

- CAD/CAM • CEREC • E4D • iTero • Lava COS
- Dental laboratory

Computer-aided design (CAD) and computer-aided manufacturing (CAM) have become an increasingly popular part of dentistry over the past 25 years.[1] The technology, which is used in both the dental laboratory and the dental office, can be applied to inlays, onlays, veneers, crowns, fixed partial dentures, implant abutments, and even full-mouth reconstruction. CAD/CAM is also being used in orthodontics.

CAD/CAM technology was developed to solve 3 challenges. The first challenge was to ensure adequate strength of the restoration, especially for posterior teeth. The second challenge was to create restorations with a natural appearance. The third challenge was to make tooth restoration easier, faster, and more accurate. In some cases, CAD/CAM technology provides patients with same-day restorations.

Dentists and laboratories have a wide variety of ways in which they can work with the new technology. For example, dentists can take a digital impression and send it to a laboratory for fabrication of the restorations or they can do their own computer-aided design and milling in-house.

When laboratories receive a digital impression, they can create a stone model from the data and either continue with traditional fabrication or rescan the model for milling. Alternatively, the laboratory can do all of the design work directly on the computer based on the images received.

This article discusses the history of CAD/CAM in dentistry and gives an overview of how it works. It also provides information on the advantages and disadvantages, describes the main products available, discusses how to incorporate the new technology into your practice, and addresses future applications.

[a] International Advanced Aesthetic Dentistry Program, NYU College of Dentistry, 345 East 24th Street, New York, NY 10010, USA
[b] Department of Cariology and Comprehensive Care, NYU College of Dentistry, 345 East 24th Street, New York, NY 10010, USA
[c] International Comprehensive Dentistry Program, NYU College of Dentistry, 345 East 24th Street, New York, NY 10010, USA
* Corresponding author. Department of Cariology and Comprehensive Care, NYU College of Dentistry, 345 East 24th Street, New York, NY 10010.
E-mail address: gd33@nyu.edu

Dent Clin N Am 55 (2011) 559–570
doi:10.1016/j.cden.2011.02.011
0011-8532/11/$ – see front matter © 2011 Elsevier Inc. All rights reserved.

dental.theclinics.com

HISTORY OF DENTAL CAD/CAM

Computer-aided design and manufacturing were developed in the 1960s for use in the aircraft and automotive industries,[2] and were first applied to dentistry a decade later.

Some of the most important figures in dental CAD/CAM development are Drs François Duret of France, Werner Mörmann of Switzerland, Dianne Rekow of the United States, and Matts Andersson of Sweden.

Dr Duret was the first person to develop a dental CAD/CAM device, making crowns based on an optical impression of the abutment tooth and using a numerically controlled milling machine as early as 1971.[3] He produced the first dental CAD/CAM restoration in 1983[4] and demonstrated his system at the French Dental Association's international congress in November 1985 by creating a posterior crown restoration for his wife in less than an hour.[5] Dr Duret later developed the Sopha system.

Dr Mörmann was the developer of the first commercial CAD/CAM system. He consulted with Dr Marco Brandestini, an electrical engineer, who came up with the idea of using optics to scan the teeth. By 1985, the team had performed the first chairside inlay using a combination of their optical scanner and milling device. They called the device CEREC, an acronym for computer-assisted ceramic reconstruction.[6]

Dr Rekow worked on a dental CAD/CAM system in the mid-1980s with colleagues at the University of Minnesota. This system was designed to acquire data using photographs and a high-resolution scanner, and to mill restorations using a 5-axis machine.[7]

Dr Andersson developed the Procera (now known as NobelProcera, Nobel Biocare, Zurich, Switzerland) method of manufacturing high-precision dental crowns in 1983.[8] He was also the first person to use CAD/CAM for composite veneered restorations.[9]

Early technology permitted the creation of inlays, onlays, veneers, and crowns. More recently, CAD/CAM systems have been able to provide fixed partial dentures and implant abutments.

Another use of CAD/CAM is in orthodontics. One example of this is Invisalign (Align Technology, Inc, Santa Clara, CA, USA), a treatment that uses multiple clear, removable appliances designed and manufactured via CAD/CAM to straighten teeth.

CAD/CAM systems are becoming increasingly popular in dental offices. More than 30,000 dentists around the world own scanning and milling machines; 10,000 of these are in the United States and Canada. Worldwide, more than 15 million CEREC restorations alone have been completed.[10]

OVERVIEW OF CAD/CAM

In brief, in-office dental CAD/CAM systems consist of a handheld scanner, a cart that houses a personal computer together with a monitor, and a milling machine.

The scanner head is placed intraorally above the tooth preparation and the resulting data appear on the monitor as 2-dimensional (2-D) or 3-dimensional (3-D) images. Design work is done on the monitor and the instructions are sent to a computer-assisted processing machine for milling.

Restorations are milled from prefabricated blocks of porcelain. Options include feldspathic, leucite, or lithium disilicate materials as well as blocks of composite.[11] After the restoration is examined and approved, it is polished and inserted using conventional bonding techniques.

Results with in-office milling machines appear to be as good as those from laboratory milling machines. A systematic review of 16 articles that comprised 1957 restorations found no significant differences in 5-year survival rates between chairside CEREC restorations (90.2% to 93.8%) and Celay laboratory restorations (82.1%).[12]

ADVANTAGES AND DISADVANTAGES OF CAD/CAM

The use of CAD/CAM technology for dental restorations has numerous advantages over traditional techniques. These advantages include speed, ease of use, and quality.

Digital scans have the potential to be faster and easier than conventional impressions because casts, wax-ups, investing, casting, and firing are eliminated.[13] According to Sirona, half-arch impressions with the most recent version of CEREC take 40 seconds and full-arch impressions take 2 minutes.[14] CAD/CAM also makes design and fabrication faster; a full-contour crown takes just 6 minutes to mill.[15]

Having a milling machine on site means that patients can receive their permanent restoration the same day they come in, without making a second appointment. Patients no longer need to have provisional restorations, which take time to fabricate and fit.[13] If anesthetics are needed, they only need to be administered once.

The quality of CAD/CAM restorations is extremely high because measurements and fabrication are so precise. In a study of 117 subjects by Henkel,[16] each subject had 2 crowns made. One crown was made based on physical impressions using standard trays and impression material and another was made based on electronic impressions. Without knowing which one was which, dentists chose the crown based on the electronic impression 68% of the time.

Perhaps this difference in the finished product should not be surprising, given the wide variation in quality of traditional impressions. Writing in a 2005 article, Christensen[17] stated that he had seen impressions sent to laboratories in which more than 50% of the preparation margins were not discernible. Traditional impressions suffer from problems, such as bubbles and tears in the impression material, cords or other debris embedded in the impression material, and missing teeth.[17]

CAD/CAM restorations have a natural appearance because the ceramic blocks have a translucent quality that emulates enamel, and they are available in a wide range of shades.[13] Ceramic wears well in the mouth, even when used for posterior teeth; because it is no more abrasive than conventional and hybrid posterior composite resins, it causes minimal wear to the opposing teeth.[13]

Finally, quality is consistent because prefabricated ceramic blocks are free from internal defects and the computer program is designed to produce shapes that will stand up to wear.

Savings in time and labor have the potential to reduce costs, and the promise of faster, high-quality restorations should appeal to patients and patients are also happy to avoid the need for gag-inducing impressions.

Another benefit is that all the scans can be stored on the computer; whereas, standard stone models take up space and can chip or break if stored improperly.[18]

Still, CAD/CAM systems have disadvantages. The initial cost of the equipment and software is high, and the practitioner needs to spend time and money on training.[13] Dentists without a large enough volume of restorations will have a difficult time making their investment pay off.

Just as with conventional impressions, in taking an optical scan the dentist needs to obtain an accurate recording of the tooth in need of restoration. The scan needs to emphasize the finish line and precisely duplicate the surrounding and occlusal teeth. Digital scanning requires the same type of soft-tissue management, retraction, moisture control, and hemostasis that is so important for conventional impressions.

Digital impression systems may not save time as they are currently used because of the need for multiple steps. For example, dentists who use certain scanners must first send the images for a cleanup process, which is followed by setting of the margins by a dental technician. The images next go to the clinician's dental laboratory for review and then back for model milling. Finally, the models and dies are then sent to the clinician's dental laboratory for fabrication of the restoration.[16]

OFFICE-BASED DEVICES

Four products are presently available for digital impressions in the dental office: CEREC AC (Sirona, Charlotte, NC, USA), E4D Dentist (D4D Technologies, Richardson, TX, USA), iTero (Cadent, Carlstadt, NJ, USA), and Lava COS (3M ESPE, St Paul, MN, USA). Taking digital impressions allows dentists to do away with selecting trays, mixing materials and waiting for them to set, cleaning up the mess from the impressions, disinfecting the impressions, and shipping the impressions to a laboratory.

The CEREC and E4D devices can be combined with in-office design and milling; whereas, the iTero and Lava COS devices are reserved for image acquisition only. In-office milling allows same-day restorations.

The CEREC System

CEREC, introduced in 1987, was the first dental system to combine digital scanning with a milling unit. The system allows dentists to provide restorations made from commercially available ceramic blocks in a single visit.

The earliest models produced inlays and onlays only.[6] The newest model, known as CEREC AC powered by BlueCam (Sirona, Charlotte, NC, USA) and introduced in 2009,[19] also has the ability to take half-arch or full-arch impressions and create crowns, veneers, and bridges.

The current acquisition system employs intense blue light from blue light-emitting diodes (LEDs). The camera projects blue light onto the teeth, which reflects it back at a slightly different angle. This method of visualization is referred to as *active triangulation*.

To use the system, the entire tooth preparation to be scanned is coated with a layer of special titanium dioxide powder, which makes translucent areas of the teeth opaque and permits the camera to register all of the tissues. Several optical impressions are then taken from an occlusal orientation, being sure to obtain images of the tooth to be restored as well as the adjacent and opposing teeth. The scanner is able to focus automatically.

After the impression is complete, a 3-D rendering of the tooth to be restored appears on the monitor. The dentist is able to mark where the die should begin and end based on this image. The software program then generates a proposed restoration based on comparisons to the surrounding teeth, which can then be altered or fine tuned as needed.

After the design is approved, the milling process can begin. A block of ceramic or composite material in the correct color is simply inserted into the milling unit.[15]

Alternatively, the dentist can obtain a digital impression and send the data to a dental laboratory. The laboratory can then design and mill the restoration using CAD/CAM technology. They can also use the digital image to fabricate a hard resin model based on the data and proceed to fabricate the restoration in the conventional manner.

The E4D Dentist System

The E4D Dentist system, which made its debut in 2008, is presently the only other system besides CEREC that permits same-day in-office restorations.[18] Dentists can purchase the design center and laser scanner alone, or also purchase the milling unit.

This system includes a laser scanner, called the IntraOral Digitizer, along with a design center and milling unit. The scanner is small, so patients do not need to open their mouth as wide (**Fig. 1**).

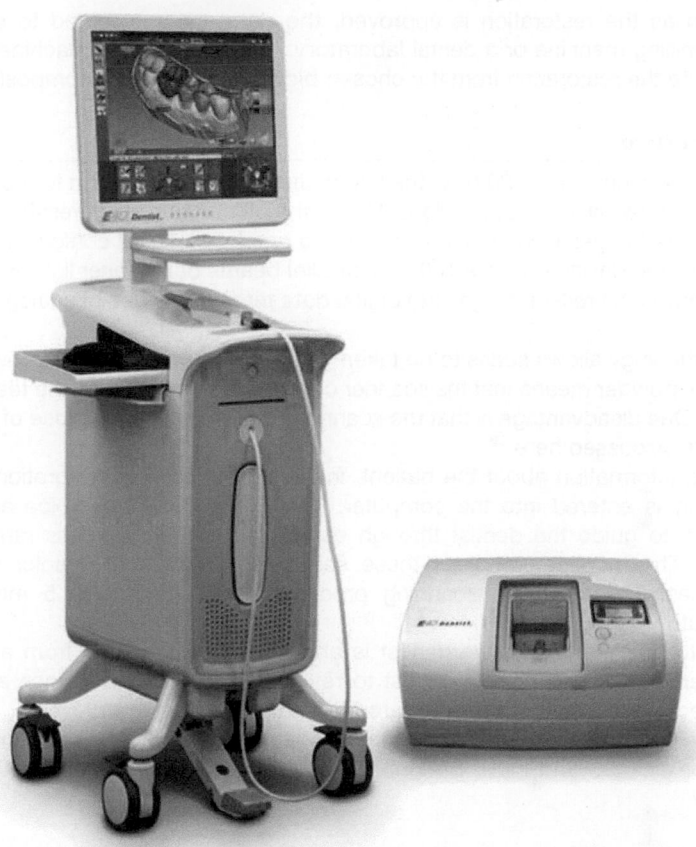

Fig. 1. E4D. (*Courtesy of* D4D Technologies.)

The E4D system requires the use of powder in some but not all cases. To use the system, the restoration site is prepared as it is for a traditional impression. The scanner is placed near the target tooth, and has 2 rubber feet that hold it a specific distance from the area being scanned.

Looking at a computer monitor, the image of the target tooth is centered on the screen. A foot pedal is then released, which activates the image capture using software called ICEverything (D4D Technologies, Richardson, TX, USA). The software on the screen then prompts the dentist to adjust the scanner for the next image. As each picture is taken, the software gradually creates a 3-D image. The image can then be viewed from any angle to confirm that the scan is complete.

Instead of scanning the opposing arch, an occlusal registration is created with an impression material and is placed atop the target tooth. The scanner captures the combination of registration material and uncovered teeth, using this information to design restorations of the correct heights.

The design system automatically detects the finish lines and marks them on the screen. After the dentist approves these markings, the computer proposes a restoration model for the target tooth. Currently, one advantage of E4D is that the designer can work on up to 16 restorations at once.

As soon as the restoration is approved, the data are transmitted to either the in-house milling machine or a dental laboratory. The office milling machine will then manufacture the restoration from the chosen blocks of ceramic or composite.

The Cadent iTero

Cadent introduced iTero in 2007 as the first digital impression system for conventionally manufactured crowns and bridges. Unlike the other 3 digital impression systems, which acquire images using triangulation, iTero employs parallel confocal imaging.[20] Specifically, the device projects 100,000 parallel beams of red laser light at the teeth and transforms the reflected light into digital data through the use of analog-to-digital converters.[21]

This technology allows scans to be taken without coating the teeth in powder. The absence of powder means that the scanner can be rested directly on the teeth during scanning. One disadvantage is that the scanner head is larger than those of the other 3 scanners discussed here.[18]

To start, information about the patient, including the type of restoration and the tooth color, is entered into the computer. The system provides voice and visual commands to guide the dentist through each scan; a typical series ranges from 15 to 30. The monitor combines these scans to provide a 3-D color model of both arches. The complete scanning process takes about 3 to 5 minutes for a full mouth.

During the review phase, the dentist is able to review the scan from any angle. A digital articulator permits the dentist to review the occlusal clearance and make any needed modifications to the prepared teeth or opposing arch.

After the scan is approved, a dedicated wireless connection transmits the scan to Cadent for cleanup and initial design. The file then gets transmitted to the dental laboratory.

The Lava Chairside Oral Scanner

The Lava Chairside Oral Scanner (COS) was launched in February 2008.[18] The system includes a mobile cart, a touch screen display, and a scanner with a camera at the end (**Fig. 2**).

The camera, which contains 192 LEDs and 22 lens systems, employs active wavefront sampling to capture images at video rate.

After preparing the tooth and retracting the gingival tissue, the dentist dries the arch and gives it a light dusting of titanium dioxide powder. Just enough powder is used to permit the scanner to identify reference points.

The scan is obtained by moving the wand first over the occlusal surfaces, then over the buccal surfaces, and finally over the lingual sufaces. An additional scan is taken of the occlusal surfaces.

The monitor image, which appears instantly, can be rotated and magnified to ensure that all areas have been scanned properly and no holes appear. The dentist also has the ability to switch between 3-D and 2-D images. Finally, the system is compatible with 3-D glasses for a true 3-D experience.

After signing off on the scans, the data is sent wirelessly to the laboratory, where the die is cut and the margin marked digitally. Then the data go to 3M, where a technician reviews and synthesizes the images before creating a stone model. This stone model is then sent to the laboratory.

The Lava COS can be used to make any type of crown or bridge, not just Lava crowns and bridges.

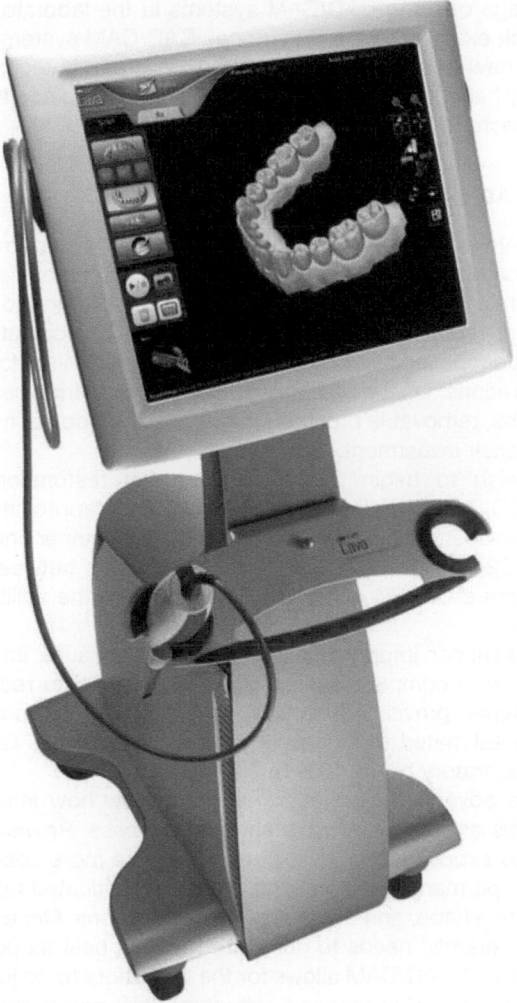

Fig. 2. Lava COS. (*Courtesy of* 3M ESPE.)

LABORATORIES

Laboratories are increasingly using CAD/CAM to create restorations. CAD/CAM technology is the only way to create zirconia copings because the design program is able to adjust precisely for the shrinkage caused by sintering.

A common way for laboratories to use CAD/CAM is for the laboratory to scan the stone model with a digital scanner. After waxing up the model, a second scan is done. The design program combines the 2 images digitally to determine the form of the restoration.

The best known of these systems is InLab, CEREC's laboratory-based designing and milling system. This system is able to fabricate 3-unit bridge frames and automatic virtual occlusal adjustments. The system is able to mill zirconia cores or full-ceramic restorations using materials, such as IPS Empress or IPS e.max (both from Ivoclar Vivadent, Amherst, NY, USA).

A major advantage of using CAD/CAM systems in the laboratory is that the final restoration can look exactly like the provisional. CAD/CAM systems also shorten the learning curve for new dental technicians, although a dental technician still finishes each restoration by hand. CAD/CAM technology does not replace the need for skilled dental laboratory technicians.

INCORPORATING CAD/CAM INTO YOUR PRACTICE

The age of CAD/CAM in dentistry has clearly arrived. Now it is up to individual dentists to decide how much of the new technology they want in their office and how quickly. Some dentists wish to have the latest technology and are willing to spend the money to have it. However, another point to consider is patient population. Dentists with younger, more affluent patients may be able to charge a premium for the convenience of same-day restorations. On the other hand, those whose practices consist primarily of direct restorations, removable prosthodontics, and periodontal treatments may not be able to recoup their investment.

Dentists who wish to begin providing same-day restorations can purchase a complete CEREC AC or E4D system at a cost of approximately $90,000 to $112,000.[22] A lower-cost option is to purchase a digital scanner only; prices for these range from about $24,000 to $41,000.[22] Each scan costs between $16 and $35.[22] Dentists who choose a CEREC AC or E4D scanner have the ability to add a milling unit at a later date.

Using a digital scanner improves patient comfort because impressions can be uncomfortable. Using a complete system has the potential to reduce costs related to impression material, provisional crowns, time in the office, and laboratory bills. Dr Parag Kachalia estimated that dentists who switch to office CAD/CAM systems can reduce their laboratory bill by 60% to 70%.[22]

Dentists who do advanced aesthetic treatment know how important provisional veneers and crowns are to the overall treatment success. Provisionals are used to not only protect the exposed tooth tissues and to give a more cosmetic appearance during the time the permanent restorations are being fabricated but also to allow for a trial run of the size, shape, and contour of the restorations. Once these parameters are accepted, the ceramist needs to duplicate them as best as possible in the final restorations. The use of CAD/CAM allows for the laboratory to do just that in an exact way. The laboratory technician makes 2 virtual models; one of the provisionals and one of the final impression of the prepared teeth. They virtually superimpose the provisionals over the prepared teeth. The veneers are then milled in that precise shape, with the ceramist cutting back a small portion to allow for layering and detail work (**Figs. 3–7**).

Using CAD/CAM technology in this way allows the ceramist to duplicate the emergence profile, incisal edge position, contours, and exact dimensions of the provisional veneers.

THE FUTURE OF CAD/CAM

Over the next decade, as prices come down and dentists become more comfortable with the new technology, we can expect to see increased use of CAD/CAM in dentistry. Same-day restorations will become more popular and will likely expand to fixed partial and removable dentures. One area for improvement would be representation of jaw movement using CAD/CAM; current design software only captures shapes.

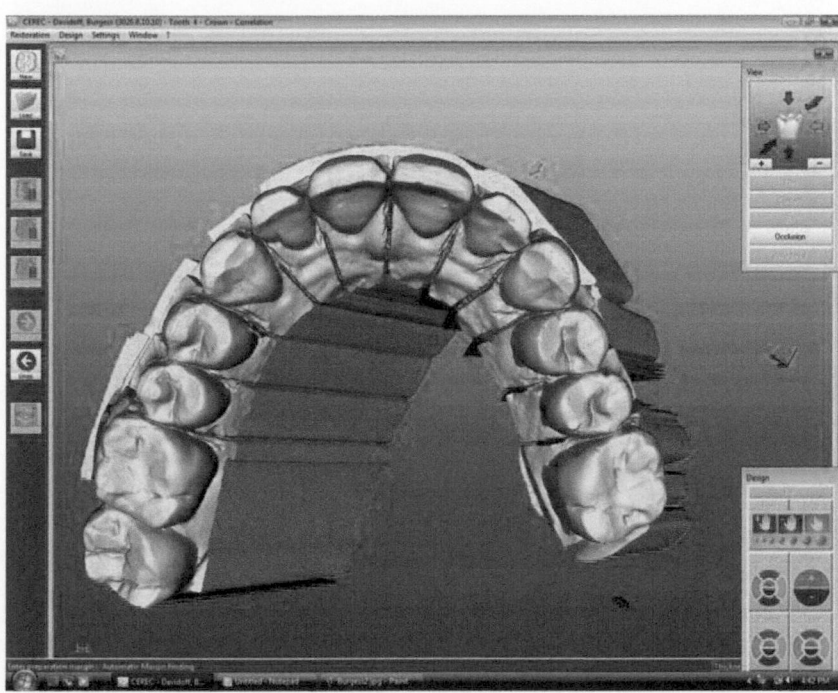

Fig. 3. Virtual cutting of the dies. (*Courtesy of* Jon Brooks, MDT, Smile-Vision.)

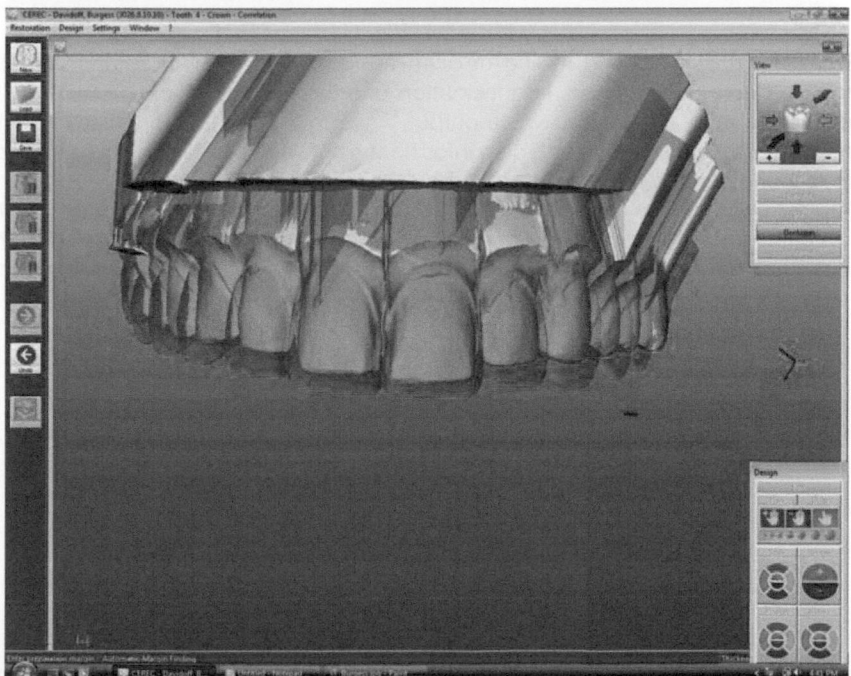

Fig. 4. Overlay of provisional virtual model over final virtual model. Note that the teeth were being lengthened by about 2 to 3 mm. (*Courtesy of* Jon Brooks, MDT, Smile-Vision.)

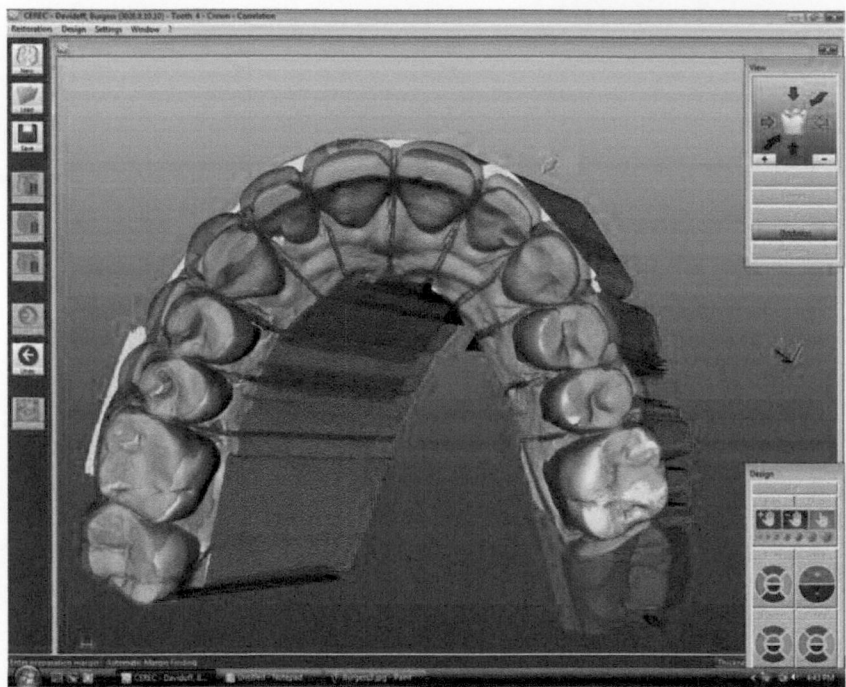

Fig. 5. Labial overlay of models. Note how emergence profile can exactly mimic the provisionals. (*Courtesy of* Jon Brooks, MDT, Smile-Vision.)

Scanning, designing, and milling devices are expected to become increasingly simple and convenient to use. In anticipation of future advances, the CEREC AC is prepared for voice control and voice output.[15] Improvements in technology should avoid some of the back-and-forth data information between the dentist, the manufacturer, and the dental laboratory.

Another potential use of dental CAD/CAM could be in third-world countries where laboratories and skilled ceramists might not be readily available.[5] CAD/CAM technology could allow technicians to do much of the work and restorations could be created on the spot.

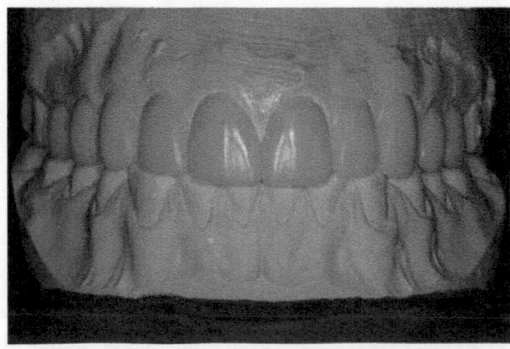

Fig. 6. Wax-up for provisionals. (*Courtesy of* Jon Brooks, MDT, Smile-Vision.)

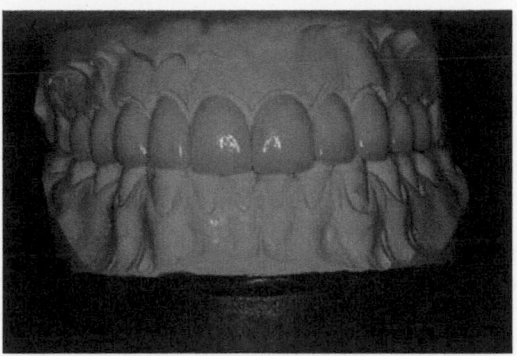

Fig. 7. Final restorations on model. (*Courtesy of* Jon Brooks, MDT, Smile-Vision.)

SUMMARY

Using CAD/CAM technology in the dental office and laboratory may have seemed like science fiction 20 years ago, but today it is reality. We now have the ability to create inlays, onlays, veneers, crowns, fixed partial dentures, implant abutments, and full-mouth reconstruction using CAD/CAM.

CAD/CAM units are still expensive to purchase and use. But as prices come down and more health care providers embrace the technology, we can expect digital scanners and computer-assisted design and manufacturing to become standard in dentistry.

ACKNOWLEDGMENTS

Devon Schuyler, MA, ELS assisted in the preparation of this manuscript.

REFERENCES

1. Duret F, Blouin JL, Duret B. CAD-CAM in dentistry. J Am Dent Assoc 1988;117(6): 715–20.
2. American Machinist. The CAD/CAM hall of fame, 1998; Available at: http://www. Americanmachinist.Com/304/Issue/Article/False/9168/Issue. Accessed August 13, 2010.
3. Duret F, Preston JD. CAD/CAM imaging in dentistry. Curr Opin Dent 1991;1(2): 150–4.
4. Priest G. Virtual-designed and computer-milled implant abutments. J Oral Maxillofac Surg 2005;63(9 Suppl 2):22–32.
5. Preston JD, Duret F. CAD/CAM in dentistry. Oral Health 1997;87(3):17–20, 23–4, 26–7.
6. Mormann WH. The evolution of the CEREC system. J Am Dent Assoc 2006; 137(Suppl):7s–13s.
7. Rekow D. Computer-aided design and manufacturing in dentistry: a review of the state of the art. J Prosthet Dent 1987;58(4):512–6.
8. History of Nobel Biocare. Nobel Biocare. Available at: http://Corporate.Nobelbiocare. Com/En/Our-Company/History-And-Innovations/Default.Aspx?V=1. Accessed August 10, 2010.
9. Andersson M, Carlsson L, Persson M, Bergman B. Accuracy of machine milling and spark erosion with a CAD/CAM system. J Prosthet Dent 1996;76(2):187–93.

10. FAQS. Answers you need for the results you desire. Sirona; 2008. Available at: http://www.Cereconline.Com/Cerec/Faqs.Html. Accessed February 15, 2011.

11. Materials–options and partners. Available at: http://www.Cereconlin.Com/Cerec/Materials.Html. Sirona; 2008. Accessed August 6, 2010.

12. Wittneben JG, Wright RF, Weber HP, Gallucci GO. A systematic review of the clinical performance of CAD/CAM single-tooth restorations. Int J Prosthodont 2009; 22(5):466–71.

13. Mormann WH, Brandestini M, Lutz F, Barbakow F. Chairside computer-aided direct ceramic inlays. Quintessence Int 1989;20(5):329–39.

14. The CEREC Acquisition Center powered by Bluecam. Available at: http://www. cereconlin.com/cerec/acquisition-center.html. Sirona; 2008. Accessed August 6, 2010.

15. CEREC AC: CAD/CAM for everyone [pamphlet]. Charlotte (NC): Sirona.

16. Henkel GL. A comparison of fixed prostheses generated from conventional vs digitally scanned dental impressions. Compend Contin Educ Dent 2007;28(8): 422–4, 426–8, 430–1.

17. Christensen GJ. The state of fixed prosthodontic impressions: room for improvement. J Am Dent Assoc 2005;136(3):343–6.

18. Birnbaum N, Aaronson HB, Stevens C, et al. 3D digital scanners: a high-tech approach to more accurate dental impressions. Inside Dentistry 2009;5(4).

19. Sirona introduces CEREC AC powered By Bluecam [press release]. Charlotte (NC): Sirona; 2009.

20. Cadent Itero. Creating the perfect byte [pamphlet]. Carlstadt (NJ): Cadent; 2008.

21. Lava Chairside Oral Scanner C.O.S [pamphlet]. St Paul (MN): 3M ESPE; 2009. 70-2009-3999-2.

22. Kachalia PR, Geissberger MJ. Dentistry a la carte: in-office CAD/CAM technology. J Calif Dent Assoc 2010;38(5):323–30.

Technological Advances in Nontraditional Orthodontics

Andrea M. Bonnick, DDS[a,b,c],*, Mark Nalbandian, DDS[d],
Marianne S. Siewe, DDS, MS[d]

KEYWORDS

- Self-ligation • Lingual braces • Invisalign • SureSmile
- Cone beam computed tomography • Miniscrews
- Distraction osteogenesis • Bioengineering

Technology boldly tells step aside, lead, or follow. Orthodontics has taken a lead driven by the increasing numbers of adult population seeking care that is esthetic, efficient, and at a reasonable cost.

Most of the recently introduced technologies to current orthodontic therapy for both children and adults are geared toward reduced orthodontic time, minimal postoperative pain, and enhanced periodontium.

SELF-LIGATING BRACKETS

These are 4-walled rectangular brackets that contain a large lumen and are passively ligated with extremely low-force archwires with specific expanded arch forms used in a sequential series during treatment. The aim of self-ligation is to stay within the lowest force necessary at every phase of treatment. This helps to elicit optimum tooth movement through enhanced physiologic response of the periodontal ligament and surrounding supportive hard and soft histologic structures.[1] Examples of self-ligation systems are

The authors have nothing to disclose.

[a] Department of Oral and Maxillofacial Surgery, Howard University Hospital, Howard University College of Dentistry, 2041 Georgia Avenue Northwest, Washington, DC 20060, USA

[b] Oral and Maxillofacial Surgery Program, Howard University Hospital, 2041 Georgia Avenue Northwest, Washington, DC 20060, USA

[c] Department of Dentistry, Howard University Hospital, 2041 Georgia Avenue Northwest, Washington, DC 20060, USA

[d] Department of Orthodontics, Howard University College of Dentistry, 600W Street, Northwest, Washington, DC 20059, USA

* Corresponding author. Department of Oral and Maxillofacial Surgery, Howard University Hospital, Howard University College of Dentistry, 2041 Georgia Avenue Northwest, Washington, DC 20060.

E-mail address: abonnick@howard.edu

Dent Clin N Am 55 (2011) 571–584
doi:10.1016/j.cden.2011.02.012
0011-8532/11/$ – see front matter © 2011 Elsevier Inc. All rights reserved.

Damon (Ormco Corporation, Glendora, CA, USA), Speed (Stride Industries, ON, Canada), SmartClip by 3M Unitek (Monrovia, CA, USA) (**Fig. 1**). When self-ligating brackets have a wire that pulls through them, they produce less friction than conventional brackets. Questions that should be answered by this system are

Does this low friction lead to a reduced treatment time and faster tooth movement? Do self-ligating appliances save chair time compared with elastomeric ligation, and are they more hygienic?[2]

According to Hamilton and colleagues,[3] the overall treatment time is no different between self-ligating brackets and conventional preadjusted appliances. However, further prospective studies are needed to prove the effectiveness of the self-ligation system in treatment time. Turpin[2] points out that in vivo studies would be a better measure of self-ligation appliance than current in vitro studies. However, the results of in vitro studies have provided information that could remain useful as long as they are considered with care. Turnbull and Birnie[4] showed that self-ligation is twice as fast to change archwires than conventional twin brackets and Alastik (3M Unitek, Monrovia, CA, USA), saving as much as 3 seconds per bracket and, therefore, reduces chair time. In addition, there is less need for chairside assistance, which can also save valuable time and reduce cost. A more recent report by Ong and colleagues[5] has shown that self-ligating brackets are no more efficient than conventional ligated brackets in anterior alignment or passive extraction space closure during the first 20 weeks of treatment in extraction cases.

A study by Pellegrini and colleagues[6] demonstrated that self-ligating appliances (brackets) promote less retention of bacteria, including streptococci, when compared with conventional appliances that use elastomeric ligatures. Concerning the periodontal status of mandibular anterior teeth in patients with conventional versus self-ligating brackets, a study by Pandis and colleagues[7] showed that the self-ligating

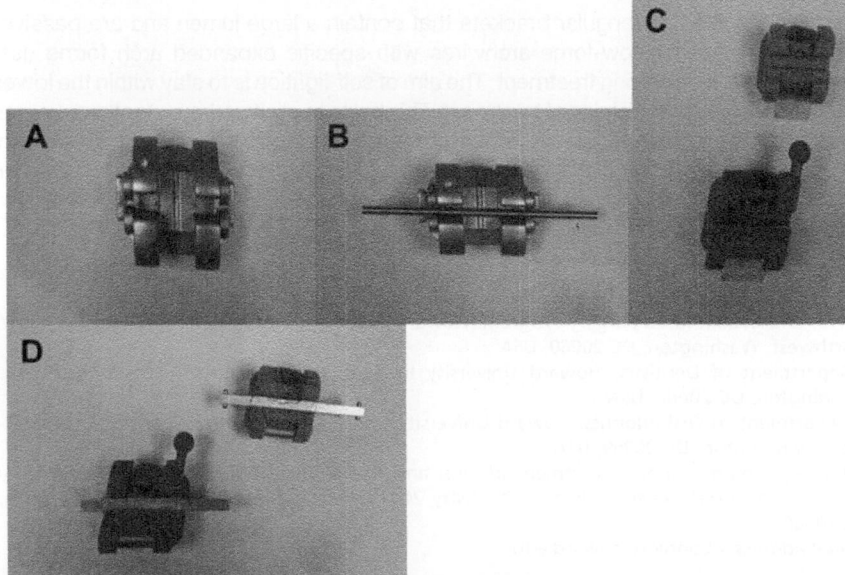

Fig. 1. Self-ligating bracket models without wire and with wire models: (*A, B*) SmartClip and (*C, D*) Damon brackets.

brackets had no advantage over the conventional brackets with respect to the status of the periodontal tissues of the mandibular anterior teeth.

LINGUAL ORTHODONTICS

This concept was initiated after Fujita and Kurz developed lingual brackets in the 1970s and 1980s.[8] Not all patients are candidates for lingual orthodontic techniques, and this is especially true for patients with expected low discomfort tolerance.[9] However, the development of indirect bonding techniques, the accuracy of bracket placement, the new metal alloys for archwires, and the wire bending methods simplified with the concept of the straight wire technique have contributed significantly to the reduction of patient discomfort and improved cooperation. In treatment with lingual orthodontics, patients should be carefully selected and diagnosed because some are more amenable than others. In patient selection, Echarri[9] categorizes favorable cases based on the following: Class I skeletal pattern, mesocephalic or mild brachycephalic, patient ability to open the mouth adequately and extend the neck, mild incisor crowding with anterior deep bite, long uniform lingual tooth surface with no restoration on it, good gingival and periodontal health, as well as the patient's keen compliance. Diagnostic considerations for lingual orthodontics should take into account esthetic factors; good periodontal and gingival health; dental considerations emphasizing on crowns, bridges, and restorations that are unfavorable; dentoalveolar discrepancy; vertical considerations; anteroposterior discrepancy; and preprosthetic cases.[9]

Lingual orthodontics has developed, and its future depends on 3 important issues: (1) advances in technology related to appliance design and laboratory protocols, (2) increasing the adult population seeking orthodontic treatment and the patient-driven demand for more esthetic acceptable appliances, and (3) a change in public and professional attitudes to lingual orthodontics in a more acceptable way.[10]

INVISALIGN

Invisalign, first introduced by Align Technology, Inc (Santa Clara, CA, USA) in 1997, is a technique that uses a series of customized transparent, removable aligners, which are designed and created using advanced computer technology, to orthodontically straighten teeth.[11] A high-quality set of pretreatment records, including photographs and radiographs, as well as polyvinyl siloxane impressions and a bite registration are taken and sent to Align Technology. These models are then digitized and are made available online in a 3-dimensional (3D) format so that the orthodontist can formulate a virtual prospective treatment plan using Align Technology's software known as ClinCheck.[12] This software allows the orthodontist to see a 3D representation of their treatment plan. Aligners are made and delivered to the orthodontist; on average, 20 to 30 aligners per arch are needed, with each set being replaced every 2 weeks. On average, case completion requires 12 months.[11]

Align Technology has made great advances in the Invisalign product since its inception. In addition to Invisalign Full, its foundation product, there are several other customizable options available now. Invisalign Express is a shorter-duration product that is ideal for treating minor crowding cases and for preparing the mouth for restorative dentistry.[11] Invisalign Teen addresses the unique considerations of treating adolescent patients, including compliance issues, as well as growth and development concerns.[11] Invisalign Assist, the company's customer service division, provides practitioners with product support to closely monitor the progress of cases, an ideal option for novice Invisalign users and for treating esthesis-centered cases.[11]

Invisalign also has developed various attachments, which have addressed some of the concerns voiced about the product in the past, including extrusion attachments that allow for more controlled and predictable extrusions of the upper and lower anteriors. Rotation attachments now allow for improved rotation of upper and lower canines, and velocity attachments produce more controlled movements of both the crown and root. Power ridges allow for optimal lingual root torque on upper incisors, without having to bond attachments.[11] Improvements in the ClinCheck software allow for interproximal reduction to be completed in the later stages of treatment, when the teeth are more aligned and thus are easier to access.[11]

There are many considerations to be made when deciding whether to use Invisalign or conventional braces; however, with the continued improvements seen with Invisalign technology, it has become a feasible and common treatment option.

SURESMILE

SureSmile, a product of OraMetrix (Richardson, TX, USA), is an orthodontic digital system that uses 3D imaging technology and computer software to facilitate diagnosis, treatment planning, and fabrication of customized orthodontic appliances.[13] Brackets are first bonded to the teeth as with conventional braces and are leveled with a straight wire.[14]

A 3D image is then created with brackets in place 3 to 6 months later using the OraScanner, a handheld light-based imaging device, which takes pictures of all surfaces of the teeth.[14] Cone beam computed tomography (CBCT) can be used alongside the OraScanner for an even more accurate representation of the orientation of the teeth, roots, and adjacent structures.[14] The resulting images are viewed using the therapeutic model, SureSmile software, that allows the operator to view the dentition from various perspectives and to consider several treatment alternatives by moving the teeth and extracting the teeth, along with other options.[15] Once the treatment plan has been formulated, the SureSmile Digital Lab sends a set-up model to the practitioner for approval before archwire customization begins.[15] The SureSmile archwire is created using robotics that precisely shapes the wire according to the specifications outlined in the set-up model and as confirmed/approved by the orthodontist.[15] Copper Ni-Ti (nickel-titanium) metal is used during the robotic customization process to create a shape memory alloy that permanently retains the wire-bending specifications.[15]

The ability to diagnose, plan treatment, and simulate the results of various treatment options, along with the extreme precision produced in the robotic-driven archwire bending process, improves orthodontic treatment in several critical areas.[15] The 3D models allow for detailed planning so that the teeth move the shortest distance to their target position, and the robotic wire bending greatly reduces errors that can be introduced to the archwire.[15] In fact, a study evaluating the efficiency and effectiveness of SureSmile showed that the process results in a lower mean ABO OGS (American Board of Orthodontics Objective Grading System) score and reduced treatment time as compared with conventional braces.[16] This technology improves the reproducibility, efficiency, and quality of orthodontic treatment.[13]

CONE BEAM COMPUTED TOMOGRAPHY

CBCT is an imaging modality originally developed for angiography and later used in radiation therapy planning in mammography and later intraoperatively in otolaryngologic surgery.[17] Although CBCT scanners have been around for more than 25 years, it was not until 2001 that the US Food and Drug Administration approved the first commercial system for oral and maxillofacial imaging. Some of the necessary technological advances that made the application of these scanners in the orthodontic office possible include:

1. The development of compact, cost-efficient, flat-panel digital detectors
2. The development of cost-efficient computers with the processing power to reconstruct the scans (a typical scan can range in size from 99–250 MB of data and include >500 slices[18])
3. The fabrication of highly efficient radiograph tubes
4. The development of machines that can scan limited field of views (FOVs).

The method of image data acquisition for a CBCT scanner involves a single rotation of an x-ray tube and a rectangular or round 2-dimensional detector. The fan beam CT scanners used in most hospital settings make use of a thin broad fan-shaped x-ray beam to acquire axial slices that are integrated yielding volumetric data (**Fig. 2**).

The advantages of the CBCT include greater efficiency in radiograph use, lower cost of the equipment, and quicker data acquisition that affects patient comfort. Furthermore, using CBCT, measurements made in any plane are usually precise, given that the voxels (the 3D equivalent of a pixel) are isotropic.

Although CBCT has various uses in dentistry, some of its benefits in orthodontics include:

- A 3D rendering of the craniofacial structures without distortion or magnification. Cross-sectional views can be taken without the interference of other structures

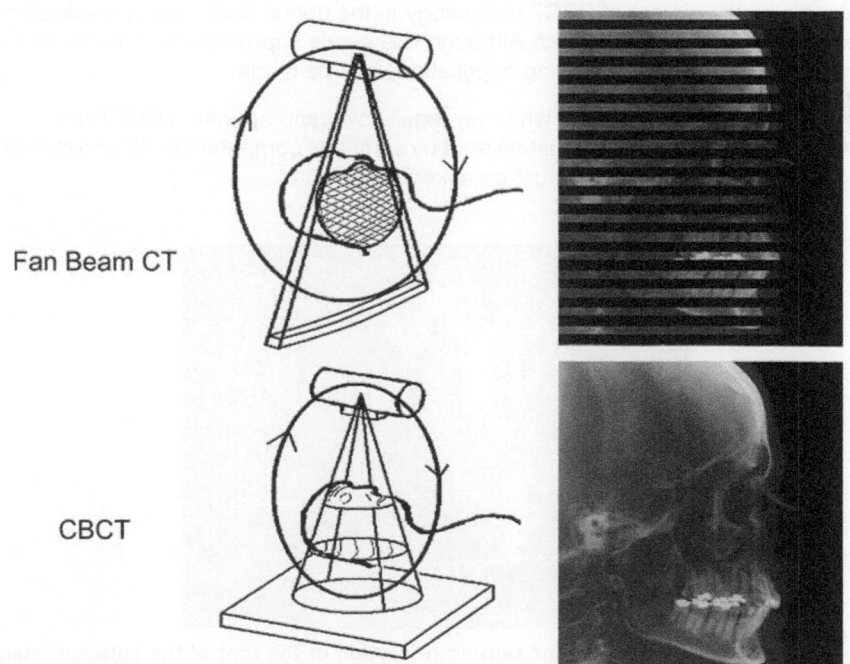

Fan Beam CT

CBCT

Fig. 2. Illustration of the difference between fan beam CT and CBCT technology. (*Adapted from* Farman AG, Scarfe WC. The basics of maxillofacial cone beam computed tomography. Semin Orthod 2009;15:4; with permission.)

superimposed on them (for this same reason, certain landmarks on a lateral cephalometric projection may not be visible or difficult to locate based on definition, ie, location of porion)

- Detection of affected teeth, their axial inclination, and proximity to total structures/other teeth can be better visualized (**Fig. 3**)
- Measurement of the airway is much more accurate than with 2D lateral cephalography
- Treatment planning for orthodontic miniscrews is made simpler. Evaluations of root proximity, bone thickness, and adjacent vital structures can be performed
- Assisting in creating physical biomodels in the treatment of patients with craniofacial syndromes
- An improved ability to detect occult pathologic condition (**Fig. 4**).

Although CBCT provides many benefits to the field of orthodontics, it is a radiologic survey and as such, should be prescribed only when the need is evident. Furthermore, effective radiation doses from a CBCT can be many times that of the conventional panoramic and lateral cephalometric radiography, which exposes the patient to 7.5 to 25.4 µSv.[19] When this value is compared with the effective dose from a CBCT radiographic survey, which exposes the patient to anywhere from 58.9 to 1025.4 µSv, depending on things such as the type of beam and filtration and the size of the selected FOV,[19] it becomes evident as to why this diagnostic tool must be used sparingly. Furthermore, the average natural background radiation in the United States is approximately 3000 µSv.[19] White and Pae[20] provide a useful algorithm (not included) to assist in the decision-making process when selecting radiographs for the orthodontic patient.

Along with the advent of CBCT technology in the dental field, several medicolegal questions have also been raised. Although it is nearly impossible to summarize this topic in 1 paragraph, the following suggestions can be made:

- Verify with state law as to who may legally own and operate a CBCT unit
- All of the image volume must be read by someone competent to do so (often this means that a radiologist must be asked to do so)

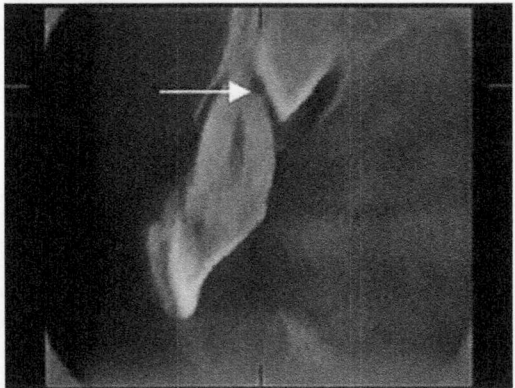

Fig. 3. An affected maxillary canine causing resorption of the root of the adjacent lateral incisor (*arrow*). (*Adapted from* Alqerban A, Jacobs R, Souza PC, et al. In-vitro comparison of 2 cone-beam computed tomography systems and panoramic imaging for detecting simulated canine impaction-induced external root resorption in maxillary lateral incisors. Am J Orthod Dentofacial Orthop 2009;136:764.e7; with permission.)

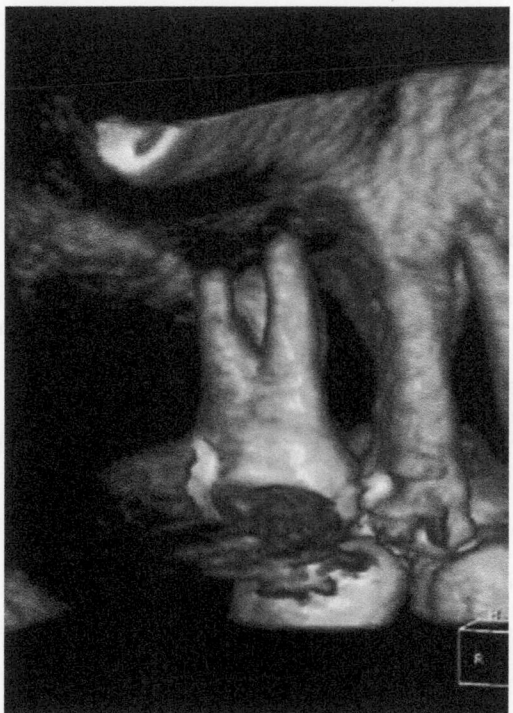

Fig. 4. The differential diagnosis of this "floating tooth" in the maxilla includes (1) localized severe periodontal bone loss, (2) Langerhans cell histiocytosis, and (3) a malignancy. (*Adapted from* Miles DA. Interpreting the cone beam data volume for occult pathology. Semin Orthod 2009;15:75; with permission.)

- When a radiologist is consulted, the dentist must make sure that the radiologist is licensed in the state in which the referring doctor practices. If the dentist consults with an out-of-state radiologist, the dentist must make sure the radiologist carries malpractice coverage that will cover him/her for out-of-state practice.[21]

In conclusion, the introduction of CBCT to the field of dentistry has proved CBCT to be a wonderful tool with great promise; however, the use of this technology must be exercised by competent individuals to maximize its benefits to patients and to avoid any foreseeable pitfalls.

MINISCREWS

Over the past few decades, the profession of orthodontics has witnessed an increase in the number of adult patients seeking treatment.[22] Unlike most adolescent patients, many adult patients present with missing teeth and/or teeth with reduced periodontal support. Traditional forms of anchorage may not be possible in such patients or even may not be accepted, as in the case of a headgear, which may be objectionable because of its impact on esthetics. With the advent of temporary anchorage devices (TADs), a biomechanically difficult or impossible situation may become easier to manage. A TAD is defined as a device fixed to bone with the purpose of reinforcing dental anchorage or eliminating the need for dental anchorage. The device is removed after it has fulfilled its purpose. Based on this definition, dental implants (endosseous implants) do not qualify as a TAD because they are not removed after obtaining the desired tooth movement. Examples of TADs (also called miniscrews or microscrews) are shown in **Fig. 5**.

Most orthodontic miniscrews range in diameter from 1.2 to 2.0 mm and are between 4 and 10 mm in length.[23] The dimensions of a selected miniscrew must be taken into consideration during its placement to avoid vital structures. Possible consequences of improper TAD placement include[24]:

- Damage to tooth roots or the periodontal ligament
- Damage to nerves (of concern is the greater palatine nerve in the palate and the inferior alveolar and mental nerves in the mandibular buccal region)
- Soft tissue emphysema caused by the use of an air syringe during device placement
- Nasal cavity and maxillary sinus perforation
- Miniscrew slippage/fracture
- Tissue overgrowth/infection (periimplantitis), usually occurs when the miniscrew is placed in alveolar mucosa.

The following guidelines, when followed, help minimize the potential complications associated with miniscrew placement and maximize the chances of attaining initial stability of the miniscrew:

- The use of radiographs to properly select the location of miniscrew placement
- Thorough knowledge of regional anatomy
- Use of pilot holes in the retromolar region or for TADs to be placed in the symphysis
- Placement of TADs in attached gingiva, where possible

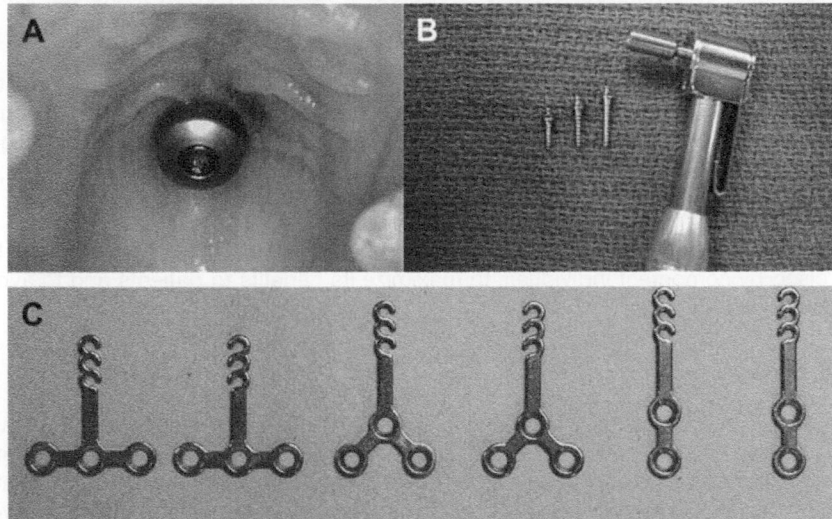

Fig. 5. (*A*) The Straumann Orthosystem palatal implant (Institut Strausmann AG, Basel, Switzerland). (*B*) Button-top TADs (Rocky Mountain Orthodontics, Denver, CO, USA) in 6, 8, and 10 mm and contra-angle driver. (*C*) Titanium bone plates for skeletal anchorage. (*Adapted from* Crismani AG, Bernhart T, Bantleon HP, et al. Palatal implants: the Straumann Orthosystem. Semin Orthod 2005;11:19; with permission; and Sugawara J, Nishimura M. Minibone plates: the skeletal anchorage system. Semin Orthod 2005;11:48; with permission.)

- Keeping the path of insertion unchanged throughout the placement
- Using an angle of insertion of 60° to 70°[25]
- Controlled insertion of the TAD using minimal pressure
- Minimizing torsional stress via wiggling of the hand driver off the miniscrew when insertion is completed. This process is done by first disassembling the driver handle from the shaft then the shaft from the miniscrew
- Instructing the patient on proper home care, including the use of chlorhexidine rinses.

Possible sites for miniscrew placement in the maxilla include the infrazygomatic crest, palate, infranasal spine (anterior nasal spine), retromolar area, and alveolar process.[22] In the mandible, miniscrews may be placed in the retromolar area, symphysis, and alveolar process.[22] When placing TADs in the alveolar process, it has been advocated that there be at least 3 mm of interradicular space for safe placement.[26] Furthermore, angulation of the miniscrew during placement can reduce the chance of root damage and increase the surface area that traverses the cortical bone and thereby enhancing primary stability of the miniscrew. Lee and colleagues[23] have demonstrated areas within both arches where the interradicular space is greater than 3 mm (**Fig. 6**).

It should be noted that these values are averages from a sample and each patient should be treated on an individual basis. Factors to take into consideration are curved/dilacerated teeth and crowded dentitions. Once placed, miniscrews may be loaded immediately (because primary cortical stability is the most important factor in their retention) because immediate loading stimulates bone adaptation.[27] However, immediate loading results in a minute amount of screw movement, which should be

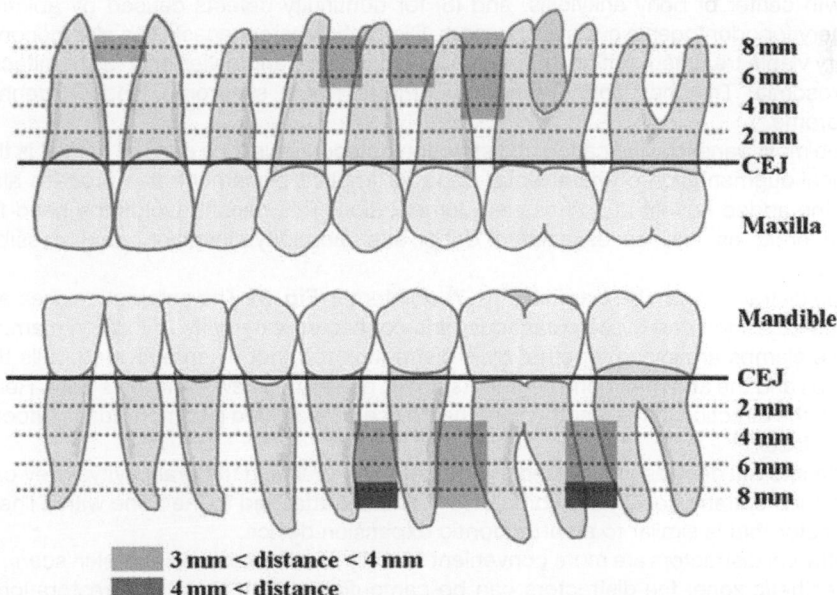

Fig. 6. Locations where the interradicular space is greater than 3 mm. CEJ, cemento-enamel junction. (*Adapted from* Lee KJ, Joo E, Lee JS, et al. Computed tomography analysis of tooth-bearing alveolar bone for orthodontic miniscrew placement. Am J Orthod Dentofacial Orthop 2009;135:491; with permission.)

taken into consideration during screw placement to ensure it is at a safe distance from vital structures.[27]

Orthodontic miniscrews have a broad range of applications. A few situations in which they have proved to be effective include molar uprighting, molar intrusion, molar protraction, molar distalization, nonsurgical treatment of open bites, and the correction of occlusal cants. By possessing a sound knowledge of the regional anatomy and following sound principles, TADs can be used to maximize their potential benefits and minimize complications.

DISTRACTION OSTEOGENESIS

Distraction osteogenesis was first described by Codvilla in 1905 after using the technique to elongate the femur. The technique of osteodistraction, sometimes referred to as callostasis, was pioneered by Ilizarov and evolved from the procedures of osteotomy, bone segment fixation, and skeletal traction. Craniofacial distraction osteogenesis was first introduced to clinical application by McCarthy, and since then, multiple modifications and clinical applications have been reported in the literature.[28]

Distraction osteogenesis is a technique of growing new bone (bone regeneration and osteosynthesis) between the surfaces of bone segments that are gradually separated by mechanical stretching or incremental traction of the preexisting bone tissue.

Distraction osteogenesis is indicated (1) for the lengthening of alveolar bone accompanied by proportionate stretching of adjacent soft tissue in preparation for implant placement, (2) for the correction of transverse discrepancies, (3) as a treatment option for the management of mandibular and midface hypoplasia in adults and children, (4) as an alternative surgical option for obstructive sleep apnea, (5) for acquired mandibular retrognathia secondary to trauma of the condylar complex leading to the loss of growth center or bony ankylosis, and (6) for continuity defects caused by ablative surgery for odontogenic cysts and tumors. Distraction osteogenesis has also become a very viable treatment option for congenital craniofacial anomalies such as hemifacial microsomia, Treacher Collins syndrome, Pierre Robin syndrome, and Goldenhar syndrome.

The most beneficial indication of distraction osteogenesis for a general dentist is the vertical augmentation of the alveolar bone for implant placement; this process also has the added benefit of soft tissue augmentation. This benefit avoids the need for bone graft, as well as associated donor-site morbidity, infection, and possible scarring.

The distractors can be external (**Fig. 7**) or internal (**Fig. 8**). The external devices are attached to the bone by percutaneous pins connected externally to fixation clamps. These clamps are joined together by a distraction rod that when activated pulls the clamps and the attached bone segments apart, generating new bone in its path. Relative to the direction of the lengthening, the devices are divided into monofocal, bifocal, and trifocal.[29]

The internal devices are located subcutaneously or within the oral cavity. They can be placed extramucosally or submucosally and are attached to the bone with a linear distractor that is similar to an orthodontic expansion device.

Intraoral distractors are more convenient socially and leave no residual skin scars. In the esthetic zone, the distractors can be camouflaged with temporary restorations. The surgical procedure can be performed under sedation or general anesthesia. A limited vestibular incision is made, and a full-thickness mucoperiosteal flap is developed, the osteotomy is outlined, and the segments are separated by chisels. It is important to avoid overzealous stripping of the periosteum to preserve the blood

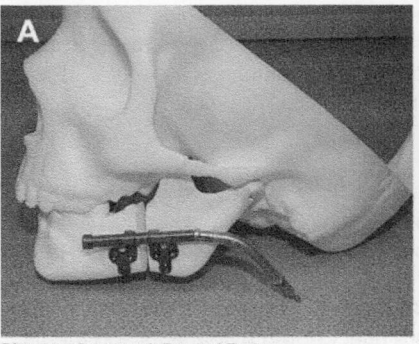
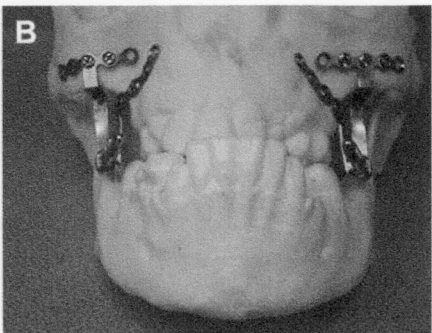

Distraction Osteogenesis Extraoral Device

Fig. 7. (*A, B*) Extraoral distractors.

supply of the bone. Clinically, distraction osteogenesis consists of 5 sequential periods: osteotomy, latency, distraction, consolidation, and remodeling.

Latency is the time required for reparative callus formation between the osteotomized bone segments. A period of 3 to 7 days is required depending on the age of the patient. Distraction activation is the period when traction force is applied to the segments. A rate of 1.0 mm/d is considered optimal, less than 1.0 mm/d can lead to premature ossification, and 2.0 mm/d causes fibrous connective tissue formation leading to delayed bone healing.[30] The period of consolidation starts when the desired expansion is achieved and lasts for 8 to 12 weeks. The ability of the distractor to maintain the stability of the newly formed bone is important for regeneration by direct osteogenesis. Unstable devices with unstable bone segments lead to increased endochondral bone formation and decreased bone regeneration. Remodeling begins after the distractor device is removed and continues up to 1 year.

Complications are reported as both mechanical and surgical. Common reports are fracture of the transport segment, breakage of the distractor, and control of vector forces for optimal outcome.[31]

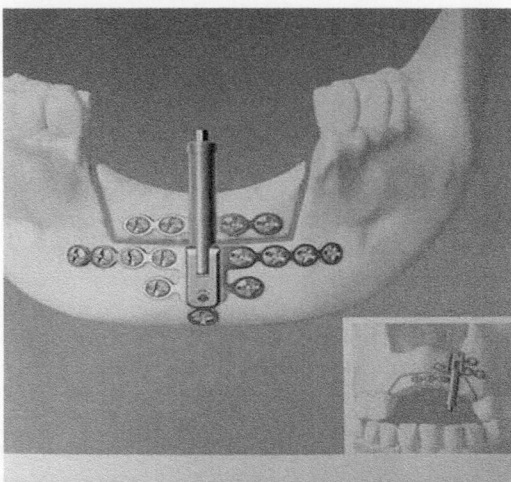

Fig. 8. Intraoral maxillary and mandibular alveolar distraction devices. (*Courtesy of* Synthes CMF; with permission.)

The application of distraction osteogenesis offers excellent solutions for surgical orthodontics, the management of developmental anomalies of the craniofacial skeleton, alveolar augmentation for rehabilitation of the edentulous patient, and reconstruction of continuity defects without donor-site morbidity.

PIEZOCISION

It is described as a minimally invasive, periodontally accelerated, orthodontic tooth movement procedure.[32] It was designed because of the growing number of adult patients seeking orthodontic treatment and their recurring request for a faster treatment approach. Early surgical techniques developed to accelerate tooth movement have been found to be quite invasive and were unaccepted by patients and the dental community. Dibard and colleagues[32] have developed a minimally invasive technique that combines piezoelectric incisions and microincisions with selective tunneling that helps to produce hard and soft tissue grafting. This technique is an orthodontic-guided procedure that is designed for orthodontic purposes but performed by a periodontist. Therefore, it is very versatile and requires a team approach for treatment. It is indicated for patients with Class II and deep bite, anterior and posterior dental crossbite, moderate to severe crowding, soft tissue deficiency, thin or recessive gingiva, and a need for bone or connective tissue grafts. The new approach has led to reduced orthodontic treatment time, minimal postoperation discomfort, great patient acceptance, and enhanced or stronger periodontium.[32]

Histochemical studies have shown that piezocision is less invasive and less traumatic than corticotomy procedures, and bone can regenerate in up to 8 weeks. However, one problem associated with it is that it can create gingival defect.

BIOENGINEERING

Bioengineering is considered a collaborative field, combining principles of engineering with those of the life sciences. Stem cells and regenerative medicine have a profound impact on the practice of orthodontics and dentistry. For a cell to be defined as a stem cell, 2 conditions must be met. First, it must possess the ability to self-replicate, and second, it must be able to differentiate into at least 2 different cell types. Stem cells may be derived from one of many sources. They may be embryonic stem cells (referring to the inner cell mass of the blastocyst during embryonic development), umbilical cord stem cells, amniotic fluid stem cells, or adult stem cells.[33] The adult stem cells may be further divided into bone marrow–derived mesenchymal stem cells (MSCs), tooth-derived stem cells, adipose-derived stem cells, and induced pluripotent stem cells (somatic cells that have been coaxed to act as embryonic stem cells).[33] To date, tooth-derived stem cells have been isolated from dental pulp, deciduous teeth, and the periodontium.[34]

The current benchmark for adult stem cells is the bone marrow–derived MSCs. They are presently being evaluated for potential contributions in cartilage defects in arthritis, bone defects, adipose tissue grafts in plastic and reconstructive surgery, cardiac infarcts, diabetes, liver disease, and neurologic regeneration such as in the treatment in Parkinson disease.[33] Among the craniofacial tissues that have been engineered using stem cells, there have been several recent milestones that should be of interest to orthodontists and the dental profession. Alhadlaq and Mao[35] have successfully engineered a mandibular condyle using rat MSCs that is similar in shape to that of humans. Further achievements include the engineering of distinct elements of the periodontium, craniofacial bone, cranial sutures, and adipose tissue.[34] Several researchers have successfully developed a tooth crown with distinct layers resembling the enamel, dentin, and pulp.[33]

Tooth-derived stem cells have the potential to solve many problems faced today in both dentistry and medicine. This potential coupled with the relative ease of acquiring tooth-derived stem cells, via extractions of noninfected primary or permanent teeth (either wisdom teeth or healthy teeth extraction for orthodontic reasons), make dental stem cells an attractive option. Future trends need to emphasize methods for preservation of tooth-derived stem cells, promotion of research in the multifaceted field of biomedical engineering, and its incorporation into the curriculums of dental schools and postdoctoral orthodontic residencies.

ACKNOWLEDGMENTS

The authors would like to acknowledge Davina Bailey, Dental Student, Howard University College of Dentistry.

REFERENCES

1. Bach RM. Self-ligation is not a scientific concept. Am J Orthod Dentofacial Orthop 2009;136:758.
2. Turpin DL. In vivo studies offer best measure of self-ligation. Am J Orthod Dentofacial Orthop 2009;135:141–2.
3. Hamilton R, Goonewardene MS, Murray K. Comparison of active self-ligating brackets and conventional pre-adjusted brackets. Aust Orthod J 2008;24:102–9.
4. Turnbull NR, Birnie DJ. Treatment efficiency of conventional versus self-ligating brackets: the effects of archwire size and material. Am J Orthod Dentofacial Orthop 2007;131:395–9.
5. Ong E, Mc Callum H, Griffin MP, et al. Efficiency of self-ligating vs conventionally ligated brackets during initial alignment. Am J Orthod Dentofacial Orthop 2010; 138(2):138–9.
6. Pellegrini P, Sauerwein R, Finlayson T, et al. Plaque retention by self-ligating vs elastomeric orthodontic brackets: quantitative comparison of oral bacteria and detection with adenosine triphosphate-driven bioluminescence. Am J Orthod Dentofacial Orthop 2009;135:426.e1–9.
7. Pandis N, Polychronoupoulou A, Eliades T. Self-ligating vs conventional brackets in the treatment of mandibular anterior crowding: a prospective clinical trial of treatment duration and dental effects. Am J Orthod Dentofacial Orthop 2007; 132:208–15.
8. Kyung Hee-Moon. The use of microimplants in lingual orthodontic treatment. Semin Orthod 2006;12:186–90.
9. Echarri P. Lingual orthodontics: patient selection and diagnostic considerations. Semin Orthod 2006;12:160–6.
10. Stuart McCrostie H. Lingual orthodontics: the future. Semin Orthod 2006;12: 211–4.
11. Align Technology. Invisalign. Available at: www.invisalign.com/. Accessed August 1, 2010.
12. Joffe L. Current products and practice Invisalign: early experiences. J Orthod 2003;30:348–52.
13. Muller-Hartwich R, Prager TM. SureSmile—CAD/CAM system for orthodontic treatment planning, simulation and fabrication of customized archwires. Int J Comput Dent 2007;10(1):53–62.

14. OraMetrix. SureSmile. Available at: www.suresmile.com. Accessed August 1, 2010.
15. Mah J, Sachdeva R. Computer-assisted orthodontic treatment: the SureSmile process. Am J Orthod Dentofacial Orthop 2001;120:85–7.
16. Saxe AK, Louie LJ, Mah J. Efficiency and effectiveness of SureSmile. World J Orthod 2010;11(1):16–22.
17. Farman AG, Scarfe WC. The basics of maxillofacial cone beam computed tomography. Semin Orthod 2009;15:2–13.
18. Miles DA. Interpreting the cone beam data volume for occult pathology. Semin Orthod 2009;15:70–6.
19. Brooks SL. CBCT dosimetry: orthodontic considerations. Semin Orthod 2009;15: 14–8.
20. White SC, Pae EK. Patient image selection criteria for cone beam computed tomography imaging. Semin Orthod 2009;15:19–28.
21. Friedland B. Medicolegal issues related to cone beam CT. Semin Orthod 2009; 15:77–84.
22. Melsen B, Verna C. Miniscrew implants: the Aarhus Anchorage System. Semin Orthod 2005;11:24–31.
23. Lee KJ, Joo E, Lee JS, et al. Computed tomography analysis of tooth-bearing alveolar bone for orthodontic miniscrew placement. Am J Orthod Dentofacial Orthop 2009;135:486–94.
24. Kravitz N, Kusnoto B. Risks and complications of orthodontic miniscrews. Am J Orthod Dentofacial Orthop 2007;131:S43–51.
25. Wilmes B, Su YY, Drescher D. Insertion angle impact on primary stability of orthodontic mini- implants. Angle Orthod 2008;78:1065–70.
26. Schnelle MA, Beck FM, Jaynes RM, et al. A radiographic evaluation of the availability of bone for the placement of miniscrews. Angle Orthod 2004;74:832–7.
27. Chen Y, Kang ST, Bae SM, et al. Clinical and histological analysis of the stability of microimplants with immediate orthodontic loading in dogs. Am J Orthod Dentofacial Orthop 2009;136:260–7, 28.
28. Samchukov ML, Cope JB, Cherkashin AM. Craniofacial distraction osteogenesis. St Louis (MO): Mosby; 2001.
29. Van Sickels J, Casmedes P, Weil T. Long term stability of maxillary and mandibular osteotomies with rigid internal fixation (principles of internal fixation using the AO/ASIF technique). In: Greenberg A, Prein J, editors. Craniomaxillofacial reconstructive and corrective bone surgery. New York: Springer; 2006. p. 648–50.
30. Batal H, Cottrell D. Alveolar distraction osteogenesis for implant site development. Oral Maxillofac Surg Clin North Am 2004;16(1):91–109, vii.
31. Samchukov ML, Cope JB, Cherkashin AM. The effect of saggital orientation of the distractor on the biomechanics of mandibular lengthening. J Oral Maxillofac Surg 1999;57(10):1214–21.
32. Dibard S, Sebaoun JD, Surmenian J. Piezocision: a minimally invasive, periodontally accelerated orthodontic tooth movement procedure. Compend Contin Educ Dent 2009;30(6):342–4, 346, 348–50.
33. Mao JJ. Stem cell and the future of dental care. N Y State Dent J 2008;74(2):20–4.
34. Mao JJ, Giannobile WV, Helms JA, et al. Craniofacial engineering by stem cells. J Dent Res 2006;85(11):966–79.
35. Alhadlaq A, Mao JJ. Tissue-engineered neogenesis of human-shaped mandibular condyle from rat mesenchymal stem cells. J Dent Res 2003;82(12):951–6.

Lasers and Radiofrequency Devices in Dentistry

James Green, DMD*, Adam Weiss, DDS, Avichai Stern, DDS

KEYWORDS

• Lasers • Radiofrequency devices • Implants • Oral surgery

Advances in technology are increasing and changing the ways that patients experience dental treatment. Technology helps to decrease treatment time and makes the treatment more comfortable for the patient. One technological advance is the use of lasers in dentistry. Lasers are providing more efficient, more comfortable, and more predictable outcomes for patients. Lasers are used in all aspects of dentistry, including operative, periodontal, endodontic, orthodontic, and oral and maxillofacial surgery. Lasers are used for soft and hard tissue procedures in the treatment of pathologic conditions and for esthetic procedures. This article discusses how lasers work and their application in the various specialties within dentistry.

PHYSICS OF LASERS AND THEIR INTERACTIONS WITH TISSUES

It is important to understand the physics of lasers before using them in surgical procedures. Lasers transfer energy to an electron and then that energy is emitted as laser energy when the atom returns to its lower energy state. This is based on Einstein's quantum theory of radiation hypothesis. The basis of this theory is that electrons are usually in a low-energy orbit close to the atomic nucleus and that these electrons can move to a higher energy state by absorbing external energy. When the electrons return to their original lower energy state, or orbit level, this absorbed energy is released spontaneously as light or photons. Therefore, a laser is an emission of energy accomplished by transferring energy to the electron of an atom. The low-energy electron is excited by a photon striking the atom; an electron absorbs this energy and sends the electron into an outer electron ring. This moves the electron further away from the nucleus of the atom. The further away the electron is from the atom, the more unstable it becomes. The electron in this higher energy and more unstable state wants to become more stable by returning to its ground state.[1] As the electron returns to this original ground state, it releases electromagnetic energy by spontaneous emission of photons or light. The

Oral and Maxillofacial Surgery, The Brooklyn Hospital Center, 121 Dekalb Avenue, Brooklyn, NY 11201, USA
* Corresponding author.
E-mail address: jrgreen4@gmail.com

Dent Clin N Am 55 (2011) 585–597
doi:10.1016/j.cden.2011.02.017
0011-8532/11/$ – see front matter © 2011 Elsevier Inc. All rights reserved.

energy in the laser beam is generated by using an electrical, chemical, or optical source to begin the emission of photons from the atom.

A laser is a device that controls the way that energized atoms release photons. The word "laser" is an acronym that stands for light amplification by stimulated emission of radiation. To produce this beam of light lasers use several components. These components consist of an energy source, an active medium, and a resonant chamber. Most energy sources for lasers are electrical. This energy source flows through the laser medium and excites the electrons to a higher energy state. Lasers in dentistry usually are made up of one of three commonly used mediums. These include the Nd:YAG laser, CO_2 laser, and dye laser. The Nd:YAG laser is composed of neodymium ions and crystal of yttrium-aluminum-garnet. The CO_2 laser is a gas laser incorporating carbon dioxide, nitrogen, and helium. Dye lasers are liquid lasers with fluorescent organic dyes injected into a tube.[2] The last component is the resonant chamber, which contains the laser medium and reflective mirrors. There is usually one highly reflective and one partially reflective mirror. These mirrors permit the laser light to exit.[3] Usually, there are intense flashes of electrical discharge that pump this medium and create a large collection of atoms with higher energy electrons. This pumping phenomenon is created by atoms absorbing energy, going to a higher state, and decaying and releasing this energy. This released energy is then absorbed by other atoms, causing these atoms to enter a higher energy state. The atoms are excited to a level that is two to three times greater than their ground state. This leads to population inversion, which is when there are more atoms in the excited state than in the lower energy ground state. As more and more atoms reach the higher energy state they spontaneously decay and release photons to travel within the laser chamber. Pumping continues to maintain the population inversion within the resonant chamber. Eventually, enough photons are released to produce a beam of coherent light that is reflected by the mirrors, giving rise to a laser beam.[4]

Lasers are different from normal light. A laser light has three distinguishing properties. The first is that the light released is monochromatic. The laser contains one specific wavelength of light. The laser is usually characterized by this wavelength and the wavelength is determined by the amount of energy released when the electron drops down to its ground state. The wavelength and absorption of the laser determines the laser's interaction with the tissue. The second property is that the laser is coherent or organized. The photons move with all the others and launch in unison. The third property is that the light is directional. The laser has a very tight beam and is concentrated. This allows the laser to remain coherent and not scatter over a long distance as opposed to a light bulb that allows light to go in all directions. The photon emitted has a very specific wavelength that depends on the state of the electron's energy when the photon is released. The wavelength of the laser determines the degree of scattering, tissue penetration, and the amount of energy absorbed by the tissues.[2] If there is more scattering, less energy is transmitted to the tissue. A laser with minimal scatter is more precise and delivered to a single spot on the tissue, allowing it to be used to cut the tissue. A laser with more scatter is better suited for coagulation of the tissue. Another factor that determines the laser's effect on the tissue is the exposure time. Exposure time is the amount of time the laser is directed at the target tissue.[2] The exposure time can be either continuous, pulsated, or other modes. Continuous mode delivers a constant laser beam to the tissue over a period specified by the operator. Pulsated delivery modifies the delivery of higher laser energy for shorter periods. The pulsation rate is usually measured in pulses per second. This pulsation prevents deeper tissue penetration and minimizes heat buildup. Superpulsation is a type of pulsing used to minimize adjacent tissue damage by using a high peak power pulse at a much shorter width. This is useful for procedures such as skin resurfacing.[5]

The current lasers are the Nd:YAG, CO_2, erbium:YAG, and argon ion. The ND:YAG is a solid state laser; the wavelengths of the laser beam are between 1064 and 1320 nm. This laser is minimally absorbed and is able to penetrate tissue to depths of up to 10 mm. This laser causes a great amount of tissue damage when compared with the CO_2 laser. The Nd:YAG is used for coagulation of angiomas, arthroscopic surgery of the temporomandibular joint (TMJ), and vascular tumor resections.[2] The CO_2 laser uses a gas medium primarily composed of CO_2. This laser produces wavelengths around 10,600 nm.[2] It is an excellent laser due to its properties of minimal scatter, rapid soft tissue vaporization, excellent water absorption, and negligible damage to surrounding tissue. Due to these properties, the CO_2 laser is able to focus precisely onto its target tissue and can be used as a scalpel type of laser. It also produces a hemostatic cutting because vessels below 0.5 mm are coagulated. The erbium:YAG laser produces a wavelength of around 2940 nm and it has very good energy absorption by water. This laser has a limited depth of penetration and causes less damage to adjacent tissue resulting in less erythema, edema, and pain. These properties make it excellent for intraoral and skin resurfacing procedures. This laser is also capable of cutting both bone and enamel, allowing it to be used in crown elongation, tooth exposure, implant uncovering procedures, and operative dentistry. The argon ion laser has a wavelength of around 488 to nm making it a low wavelength laser. It is primarily used for photocoagulation of small vessels.

ORAL AND MAXILLOFACIAL SURGERY
Snoring or Mild Sleep Apnea

Sleep apnea has become an increasing prevalent disorder in the population as obesity has risen. There is a variety of treatments for sleep apnea ranging from conservative therapy to surgical therapy depending on the documented severity. Several surgical treatments have shown success in treating sleep apnea. Some of these surgical treatments use lasers. The benefits of the laser in these procedures include excellent hemostasis, decreased postoperative pain and scarring, and the ease of use in the posterior airway. Currently, there are two commonly performed procedures for snoring and mild sleep apnea: laser-assisted uvulopalatoplasty (LAUPP) and laser-assisted uvulopalatopharyngoplasty (LA-UPPP).[6] The LAUPP procedure has been used by some surgeons for almost 10 years and is considered an effective method to treat socially unacceptable snoring.[7] The LAUPP has the advantage of being able to be done in the office under intravenous sedation and with local anesthesia. The goal of this procedure is to resect the uvula, soft palate, and tonsils. One must be careful in during resection of the soft palate because if too much is resected, this can lead to a compromise of palatal closure and velopharyngeal competence.[8]

Recently, several surgeons have changed their technique from LAUPP to LA-UPPP, basically performing UPPP with a laser instead of a scalpel. The goal of this procedure is to increase the posterior airway space and eliminate the need for multiple procedures. This surgical technique provides similar results to UPPP but has the advantages of being bloodless, having lower morbidity, and being more controllable. This procedure is usually performed in the operating room and can be done simultaneously with other procedures such as hyoid or genial advancements. The goal of the LA-UPPP is to remove the uvula, soft palate, and anterior and posterior tonsillar pillars, and then suture the lateral pharyngeal tissue providing increased airway dilation.[8]

Several postoperative complications have been documented, including bleeding, velopharyngeal insufficiency, airway compromise, infection, and scarring.[9]

SKIN REJUVENATION

Cosmetics have become increasingly popular in recent decades. People want to look younger and more attractive. With this rising trend has come an increase in the demand for skin rejuvenation procedures. Lasers have been used effectively for this purpose. Lasers are used for the revision of facial scars, treatment of aging, sun-related skin damage, and pathologic conditions of the face. The use of lasers for skin rejuvenations is often done without anesthesia, although pretreatment with a topical anesthetic is used by some clinicians. There is no need for wound closure, suction, or evacuation of a laser plume. Patients often get this procedure done during lunch breaks because there is minimal to no posttreatment down time.

Photoaging is a common cosmetic defect that results from environmental UV exposure. This UV exposure can lead to dry, rough, and course skin along with squamous cell carcinoma, basal cell carcinoma, and melanoma. Many treatments are available for photoaging, including the use of lasers. Lasers are used for skin resurfacing procedures by producing a controlled wound stimulates new skin growth. The depth of treatment is usually through the epidermis and into a specific layer of the dermis. The treatments are usually divided into superficial, mid, and deep, depending on what layer of the dermis they penetrate. The superficial depth makes it to the stratum corneum and papillary dermis, middepth to the upper reticular dermis, and deep to the midreticular dermis. After the laser treatment, the new skin replaces the damaged epidermal layer and a tighter dermal layer. The dermal layer becomes tighter due to the shortening of the existing collagen and the production of new collagen.[10] Laser skin resurfacing is best used for the treatment of acne scars, actinic keratosis, shallow rhytids, irregular pigmentation, and fine wrinkles. Lasers that target water, such as CO_2 lasers, produce nonspecific heating of the upper dermis, with the goal of promoting new collagen production.[11] Laser resurfacing most commonly uses CO_2 lasers that are pulsed, although the CO_2 laser should not be used for the treatment of deep rhytids due to the possibility of suboptimal scarring and hypopigmentation. The CO_2 laser vaporizes the epidermis and causes collagen shrinkage of the dermis, which results in contraction of the dermis. The ability to change the settings of the laser, such as pulsation and delivery time, gives the clinician better control than the use of chemical peels.[12] Other than the CO_2 laser the erbium:yttrium-aluminum-garnet (Er:YAG) laser can be used for skin rejuvenation procedures of patients with dark skin color or pigmentation. The Er:YAG laser is better absorbed by water than the CO_2 laser and results in less thermal injury.

Newer techniques for facial rejuvenation with lasers have emerged including nonablative laser resurfacing. Nonablative facial rejuvenation is designed to reduce facial rhytids, improve skin texture, decrease pore size, and aims to achieve a younger, healthier appearance.[13] This type of resurfacing limits the epidermal damage and simultaneously applies selective energy to the dermis. The epidermis is spared due to selective cooling and leads to improved healing and less need for anesthesia. This technique can be used for all skin types and is best for the treatment of fine skin lines and shallow rhytids.

Patients may also have scars that they want eliminated or minimized. For scars that are hypertrophic in nature, lasers capable of a wavelength in the range of 585 nm are beneficial.[14] This is usually accomplished with pulse dye lasers. The laser produces new collagen and remodels the existing collagen. Simultaneously the fibroblast scar response is minimized. Usually this is not done in one sitting and requires multiple laser scar revision therapies. It has been shown that laser scar revision therapy is more successful when used with other treatments such as steroid injections.[15]

There are several contraindications and possible complications associated with skin resurfacing and scar revision procedures. The contraindications include the use of certain medications, skin type, recent facial procedures, and active medical or skin disorders. If the patient is currently taking retinoids, steroids, Dilantin, or d-penicillamine, then laser resurfacing is contraindicated.[16] Facial cosmetic procedures that have recently been performed such as face lifts, rhinoplasty, and brow lifts are contraindications. This is because these procedures disrupt the lymphatic drainage system and can lead to severe edema. Medical conditions that are contraindications include prior radiation treatment of the head and neck, psychiatric disorders such as body dysmorphic syndrome, and a history of keloid scar formation. If the patient has active skin disorders, including acne, psoriasis, rosacea, or verrucae infections, laser skin resurfacing procedures should be postponed. Smoking is a relative contraindication because it can delay healing.[16]

Most complications from laser resurfacing procedures arise from overaggressive treatment. Complications include persistent erythema, hypopigmentation, and hyperpigmentation. Hyperpigmentation is usually seen in darker skinned individuals such as Hispanics, Asians, and African Americans. Usually this resolves on its own over time but it can be treated with Retin-A, hydroquinone, and topical steroids. Hypopigmentation is due to overtreatment and destruction of melanocytes. This complication usually manifests as a late complication and is much more serious because it can be permanent. No specific treatment is available for hypopigmentation. Hypertrophic scarring is another possible complication that is usually caused by overaggressive treatment into the underlying deep dermal layers. It is usually seen in dark skin types and is best treated by prevention. If it does occur, treatment is the same as for other hypertrophic scars, including steroid injections, topical steroids, and compression dressings.[17]

Vascular lesions of the face are best treated with lasers because tissue does not have to be excised, which can result in scarring and cosmetic defects. Lasers that target the hemoglobin chromophore, such as pulsed dye lasers at 580 nm with short pulses, are the preferred treatment of vascular lesions, including hemangiomas, vascular malformations, port-wine stains, ectasias, and telangiectasias. It is thought that these lasers cause the release of inflammatory mediators by heating of the microvasculature while sparing the adjacent normal tissue. These mediators may stimulate fibroblasts, which results in new collagen production and remodeling.[18] Many of these smaller lesions, such as the ectasias, can be treated in one session, but the larger port-wine stains require multiple sessions.

IMPLANTS

Implantology is arguably the fasting growing field in dentistry. As lasers become more predictable, their use is increasing. The advantages of using lasers are that they provide hemostasis while cutting the tissue so the patient experiences less pain and edema. Bone osteotomies can also be performed with a laser. Lasers can be used to efficiently uncover implants and manage peri-implant soft-tissue defects and hyperplastic tissues. The CO_2 laser is reflected by titanium but may be absorbed by surrounding tissues. Therefore, one should protect adjacent teeth and soft tissues when performing laser surgery near implants.[19] The uncovering of implants at second-stage surgery can be achieved with the laser in focused mode. Laser uncovering allows for excellent hemostasis, minimal postoperative pain, and the limited need for local anesthesia.[20] Additionally, the reduction of hyperplastic peri-implant tissues can return them to a healthier, more hygienic state. This reduction can be accomplished by lasing surrounding hyperplastic tissues while maintaining the laser tip parallel to the long axis of the implant in a similar fashion to the uncovering technique. Periodontal and periimplant gingival grafting has also been performed effectively with the CO_2 laser.[21] Also, the authors have found a supraperiosteal vestibuloplasty dissection can be done to prepare the recipient site with the laser in focus in intermittent mode or continuous mode.

Lasers can also be used in the sinus lift procedure. The procedure can be done by making the lateral osteotomy with a decreased incidence of sinus membrane perforation. The yttrium-scandium-gallium-garnet (YSGG) laser is the optimal choice for not cutting the sinus membrane.[22] The YSGG laser can also be used to make the osteotomy for a ramal or symphyseal block graft. Bone grafts done with lasers have been demonstrated to decrease the amount of bone necrosis from the donor site and the osteotomy cuts are narrower, resulting in less postoperative pain and edema.[23]

Periimplantitis is a complication of implants that is difficult to treat. This complication results in progressive loss of bone surrounding the implant and possible loss of the implant. It is believed that this is caused by bacteria contamination. It has been treated by antimicrobial therapy in an attempt to decontaminate the implant and surrounding tissues. The expectation is that decontaminating the surrounding tissue promotes regeneration of bone. It is difficult to accomplish mechanical debridement with curettes and ultrasonic scalers without damaging the implant. Lasers, specifically diode lasers, can decontaminate the implant and peri-implant tissue. First, toluidine blue is applied to sensitize the bacterial cell membrane to the laser light. Next, the laser is set at 905 nm and applied for 1 minute.[24] The CO_2 laser can also treat periimplantitis. The Nd:YAG should not be used to treat it because it can cause alteration to the implant itself.

GINGIVAL SURGERY

There are several different ways to remove gingival tissue, including a scalpel, electrosurgery, or a laser. Lasers have been used for gingival surgery with a high degree of precision and success. The use of the laser is ideal for gingival surgical procedures, given its excellent hemostasis, minimal scarring, and decreased postoperative pain. Electrosurgery provides excellent hemostasis during the removal of gingival tissue, but it can lead to the generation of excess heat. This excess heat can lead to irreversible recession of the gingival or damage to the underlying alveolar bone. This gingival recession can lead to exposure of margins, which can lead to decreased aesthetics especially in the anterior region.[25] If one is working in interproximal areas, an intermittent mode (20-millisecond pulses at 20 pulses per second) is recommended.[26] Diode lasers are optimal for gingival surgery due to their ability to be absorbed by gingival tissue and not by the adjacent tooth structure.[25]

Crown-lengthening procedures are commonly performed by the restorative dentist, periodontist, and oral and maxillofacial surgeon. Aesthetic crown lengthening is usually done with the use of a diode laser set at a wavelength of 810 nm. Diode lasers set at this wavelength are only absorbed by the gingival tissue and exhibit little or no affinity for hard tooth structure, metal alloys, composites, or porcelain. This advantage allows recontouring of the soft tissue around the tooth structures with little or no effect on the cementum or enamel. With this feature, no heat is conducted through the tooth, which prevents thermal pulpal injury. Before using the laser for crown lengthening or gingival recontouring procedures, a full periodontal examination must be performed.

The focus is on the biologic width, amount of attached gingival tissue, and the location of the crestal bone. It must be determined if the patient needs an osseous recontouring procedure with or without soft tissue contouring.

When performing the crown-lengthening or gingival-recontouring procedure, the diode laser tip contacts or is a few millimeters away from the gingival tissue. The gingival tissue is removed and recontoured along the tip of the laser with shallow tissue penetration. This leads to a slower but more controlled cutting of the soft tissue. The diode laser should be set in a pulsed mode to minimize thermal conduction to adjacent tissue and char formation. The laser should be used to create an external bevel providing optimal gingival contour and hemostasis.[25]

Periodontal disease is commonly treated with scaling and root planning (SRP) alone. Recently, the diode laser has been used in combination with SRP, decreasing postoperative pain associated with the procedure. In addition, the diode laser used at 810 nm and 0.8 W has decreased the number of microbial colony-forming units, including *Actinobacillus actinomycetemcomitans*. The diode laser also leads to faster wound healing when used with SRP. Overall, it appears that the diode laser can be used in the treatment of periodontitis by reducing the subgingival bacterial counts and pocket depths. However, there has been no evidence of the diode laser increasing the periodontal attachment levels.[27] Periodontal disease is thought to be an inflammatory response of the periodontal tissue to a bacterial infection of the periodontal pocket. The diode laser is not used to remove tissue but instead is used to decontaminate the periodontal pocket and reduce the number of bacteria within the pocket. It also decreases the number of exotoxins (ie, hyaluronidase and collagenase), which are considered responsible for periodontal tissue destruction.[27]

The technique of using the diode laser with SRP is performed by placing the tip of the laser into the pocket and moving it in a sweeping motion from anterior to posterior down to the base of the pocket. The laser uses a special optical fiber system that only allows the laser to exit at the tip and not from the side walls. The laser is inserted parallel to the root surface and one should be careful not to apply the laser directly on the root surface. The laser is focused on the tissue within the pocket causing a nonablative thermal event. This event causes a stimulatory effect on the gingival tissue and reduces the pocket depth while resulting in faster and less painful healing.[2]

In some cases, there are extreme areas of gingival overgrowth that necessitate treatment. In these circumstances, a combined approach has been described that involves scalpel excision of gross overgrowth followed by refinement and hemostasis with the laser. The advantages of using lasers over traditional scalpel incision include, but are not limited to, excellent hemostasis with no need for a dressing or splint and decreased postoperative pain. The main disadvantage is the potential for tooth damage when appropriate precautions are not taken.[28]

TREATMENT OF ORAL LESIONS

Treatment of various types of oral pathology also benefits from the use of laser treatment. As an example, common lesions such as herpetic lesions are successfully treated with lasers. Patients often find these lesions bothersome, affecting their quality of life. The irradiation from the ER:YAG laser can be used to facilitate an explosive process to cause the disruption of the virus such that it is no longer detectable. The herpetic vesicles are ruptured with minimal residual thermal damage and minimal pain, making anesthesia unnecessary.[29] Additionally, it has been documented that low-level laser therapy (LLLT) can be used in the latent period between attacks to lower the incidence of recurrence.[30]

In dentistry, LLLT has also been used as a treatment for other soft oral tissue lesions, and positive results have been seen in the healing of diseases such as exudative erythema multiforme, gingivitis, periodontitis, and different forms of oral ulcers.[31] In gingival tissues, LLLT has been shown to stimulate the DNA synthesis of myofibroblasts without any degenerative changes and transform fibroblasts into myofibroblasts, which may encourage wound healing.

Leukoplakia is a very common lesion often found on routine head and neck examinations. The identification and treatment of these lesions is very important as some of these lesions have premalignant potential. Ben-Bassat and colleagues[32] first described laser therapy for the treatment of oral leukoplakia in 1978. Since then, many studies have found laser therapy to be a safe and effective treatment. A variety of laser types have been used to treat oral leukoplakia, including the carbon dioxide (CO_2), Nd:YAG, argon, and potassium titanyl phosphate (KTP) lasers.[33] Advantages of using lasers to treat oral leukoplakia include the creation of a bloodless surgical field, leading to improved visualization and accuracy, reduced postoperative pain, and limited scarring and contraction.[34] However, the use of lasers does not come without disadvantages. The clinician cannot obtain samples for histologic analysis when ablative techniques are used. Also additional time-consuming safety measures need to be taken during the surgery. Lim and colleagues[35] demonstrated a statistically significant reduction in recurrence rates in those treated with KTP laser ablation compared with those treated with CO_2 laser ablation. These investigators felt that the KTP was more effective in preventing recurrence due to its greater tissue penetrance and greater effect on the surrounding tissues owing to the thermal scatter.

Aphthous ulcers are very common and very bothersome oral lesions. These lesions can be very painful, often in a disproportionate amount in relation to their size. Various topical steroids have been used for palliative treatment. Laser treatment of aphthous ulcers is an alternative to temporary palliative pharmacologic therapy. The laser provides relief of pain and inflammation, with normal wound healing of this uncomfortable and potentially recurrent oral lesion.[36]

Lasers can also be used for incisional and excisional soft tissue procedures. Laser excision of a labial or lingual frenum can be performed. The mucosa and underlying muscles are excised by the laser. The patient usually has less pain than traditional sharp dissection, but this procedure does take longer to heal. The laser is also used to excise benign lesions such as fibromas. This is done by done by applying the laser to the tissue in an elliptical manner adjacent to the fibroma. Another example of using a laser for benign lesions is to treat epulis fissuratum, mucoceles, and ranulas. To accomplish this, the CO_2 laser is used with a continuous mode of 4 to 10 W. The entire lesion is outlined and then undermined. The laser can be used for marsupialization of the ranula. If the laser is used, suturing is usually not needed after these procedures.[19]

TMJ Disorders

Laser therapy is also applied to the field of TMJ disorder (TMD). TMD can involve the masticatory musculature and the TMJ, or both. LLLT is effective in treatment of the muscular component of TMD. Based on the results of experimental studies and therapeutic evaluations, LLLT is suggested for the management of TMD through its analgesic, antiinflammatory, and biostimulating effects. It is thought that laser therapy is effective due to increased pain thresholds through the alteration of neural stimulation and firing pattern, and the inhibition of the medullary reflexes.[31] The effects of LLLTs are seen immediately as nerve cell membranes produce a local anesthetic-like effect and can last from days to weeks. Kulekcioglu and colleagues[37] recently investigated the effectiveness of LLLT in the treatment of TMD and compared treatment effects in myogenic and arthrogenic cases. They observed significant pain reduction in both treatment groups; and the number of tender points, maximal mouth opening, and lateral jaw motion were significantly improved in the active treatment group compared with the placebo group.

Lasers is also used in conjunction with arthroscopic surgery. The laser that is the most effective with this procedure is the holmium:YAG laser. This laser has good absorption and minimal thermal damage to the tissue within the TMJ. It is used in TMJ surgery for synovectomy, treatment of hypermobility with disc repositioning procedures, and release of anterior disk attachment for clicking and popping.[38] The laser is used to free adhesions that are within the joint, mobilizing the disk from the anterior attachments so the disk can be repositioned posteriorly within the joint. The repositioned disk is then stabilized with sutures. Adhesions can also limit mobility of the joint. The laser is used to help with lysis and lavage of adhesions found within the superior joint space. The laser is used to ablate the adhesions and then the joint is lavaged with normal saline.[39]

Hypermobility of the TMJ is characterized by subluxation of the condylar head anterior to the articular eminence, inability to reduce the joint, or severe pain when reducing the joint. The traditional treatment of this condition is eminectomy to allow the condyle to freely translate. Laser therapy is used to treat hypermobility by coagulation of the retrodiscal tissue. This coagulation stabilizes the disk in a new position and allows fibrosis. In traditional joint procedures, the patient begins physical therapy to increase joint motility. With laser treatment of hypermobility, the patient should be restricted from joint movement postoperatively. This prevents immediate subluxation of the joint. The patient is restricted for 3 months.[39]

Disk perforations are another example of TMJ disease that can be treated with arthroscopy and lasers instead of open-joint procedures. Before performing this procedure, the clinician should be sure there are no bony changes of the condylar head because bony changes on the articulating surface are a contraindication to disk repair. Disk perforations or tears that are treated by arthroscopy and lasers allow the clinician to preserve the disk and prevent the need for grafting and disk-replacement procedures. The Nd:YAG laser is commonly used for this procedure. The laser is used to recontour and smooth the torn fragments of the disk. After reducing and smoothing these fragments, the condyle should be able to function freely. Postoperatively, the patient should be given a splint, placed on a soft diet, and begin physical therapy.[39]

OPERATIVE DENTISTRY

Lasers are now being used in the field of operative dentistry as well. In 1989, it was demonstrated that the Er:YAG laser produced cavities in enamel and dentin without major adverse side effects.[40] The Er:YAG laser is used for removal of enamel, dentin, and nonmetallic restorations. Clinically, cavity preparation in enamel results in ablation craters with a white chalky appearance on the surface of the crater.[41] The Er:YAG laser causes an expansion of the hydroxyapatite by heating the water within the structure and leads to ablation of the crystal structure. When using this laser to remove tooth structure or decay it is not necessary to use local anesthetic because the friction and heat production with drilling is eliminated. Although lasers can remove enamel and dentin, their use is limited to smaller cavity preparations. Their use with more advanced preparations such as those done for indirect restorations is time-consuming and limited.[42]

Lasers are also being used for in office or power bleaching of teeth. The laser is used in conjunction with a hydrogen peroxide gel. The application of the laser raises the temperature of the hydrogen peroxide, leading to an accelerated chemical bleaching process.[2]

Lasers have been shown to be beneficial in the treatment of dentinal hypersensitivity. Many patients complain of sensitive teeth upon examination in the dental office. Laser treatment offers a possible treatment for these patients. A comparison of the desensitizing effects of an Er:YAG laser with those of a conventional desensitizing system on cervically exposed hypersensitive dentine[43] showed that desensitizing of hypersensitive dentin with an Er:YAG laser is effective, and the maintenance of a positive result is more prolonged than with other agents.

A diode laser can also be used to help aid the dentist in taking accurate impressions leading to an optimal prosthetic result. The diode laser can be used to expose subgingival finish lines and provide hemostasis, giving good moisture control. The alternative to exposing the subgingival margin has been to use retraction cord. The laser eliminates the need for the retraction cord and causes minimal adjacent soft tissue necrosis. The diode laser allows complete regeneration of this adjacent soft tissue with little or no recession of the gingiva. When using the laser for this purpose it is necessary to use a pulsed mode and air or water to cool the laser.

ORTHODONTICS

The diode laser is a great adjunctive tool for orthodontics. It can be used to treat gingival hyperplasia, aesthetic tissue recontouring with altered tooth eruption, and exposure of unerupted teeth. Most of these procedures can be done by the orthodontist with topical anesthesia alone. Oral hygiene is a constant problem for patients undergoing orthodontic treatment. Often, poor oral hygiene results in gingival hyperplasia as a result of inflammation of the tissue. The diode laser is used to debride this hyperplastic tissue. The laser is used to remove hyperplastic inflamed papillae and pseudopocketing, leading to an improvement in the overall gingival health.[44]

The diode laser is also used to remove soft tissue covering unerupted or partially erupted teeth. Delayed passive eruption can limit crown exposure, making it difficult for the orthodontist to place brackets. The laser is used to remove the soft tissue, exposing the crown and allowing proper orthodontic bracket placement. The laser is also used to expose unerupted teeth for orthodontic bracketing. The unerupted tooth is exposed with the diode laser, which provides excellent hemostasis and allows the tooth to be bracketed. By using the laser to expose the tooth, proper bracket placement is done, leading to proper orientation and alignment of the tooth. The laser is also used to perform crestal fiberotomies when treating rotated teeth and preventing relapse. The laser fiberotomies are quick and bloodless when compared with the use of a blade to perform the procedure.[44]

ENDODONTICS

Lasers are currently used in endodontics for the debridement of infected tissue and associated bacteria. It has been shown that the laser is capable of cleaning and sterilizing the root canal system. Takeda and colleagues[45] performed a study comparing the removal of the smear layer by traditionally used endodontic irrigants with lasers. The study showed that lasers are superior in their removal of microorganisms within the canal and in the removal of the smear layer surrounding the dentin when compared with chemical irrigants such as hypochlorite.[45] The laser is also beneficial due to its bactericidal effect and ability to sterilize the canal before obturation. The laser has several known benefits over traditional rotary instruments, including ease of use, decrease in separation of instruments, and decrease in number of endodontic failures.

SUMMARY

Lasers and radiofrequency devices have truly revolutionized the field of dentistry. Snoring and sleep apnea are very common issues that need to be addressed in the population along with the rise in obesity. Methods such as LAUPP have been developed as means of successfully treating sleep apnea. Demand for skin rejuvenation is also increasing in our society. Lasers provide a method of efficiently eradicating skin conditions such as acne and actinic keratosis in a controlled setting. Lasers also contribute to the rising field of implant dentistry. Lasers assist in sinus lifting, gingival manipulation surrounding the implant, and implant uncovering. Lasers are used for the creation of osteotomies to create bone grafts, which can be used to prepare sites for proper implant placement. Soft tissue lesions such as leukoplakia are also treated with lasers. Lasers are used to treat and even eradicate various forms of intraoral lesions. Clinicians should consider the use of lasers to treat certain types of TMD as well. Lasers are used in the field of operative dentistry, including the creation of cavity preparations, treatment of dentinal hypersensitivity, and bleaching of teeth. The field of orthodontics also benefits from the use of lasers. Lasers are used to manipulate gingival soft tissue to enhance and facilitate orthodontic treatment. Finally, lasers are used in endodontics for cleaning and sterilizing the root canal system.

REFERENCES

1. Guttenberg SA, Emery RW. Laser physics and tissue interaction. Oral Maxillofac Surg Clin North Am 2004;16:143–5.
2. Sosovicka M. Lasers in oral and maxillofacial surgery. Fonseca RJ. editor. Oral and maxillofacial surgery. St Louis (MO): Saunders/Elsevier; 2009. p. 237–58. Chapter 14.
3. Colt HG, Mathur PN. Basic principles of laser-tissue interactions. UpToDate version 14.3 2004:1–5.
4. Boulnois JL. Photophysical process in recent medical laser developments: a review. Lasers Med Sci 1986;1:47.
5. Hobbs ER, Bailin PL, Wheland RG, et al. Superpulsed lasers: minimizing thermal damage with short duration, high irradiance pulses. J Dermatol Surg Oncol 1987; 13:955–63.
6. Strauss A. Lasers in the management of snoring and mild sleep apnea. Oral Maxillofac Surg Clin North Am 2004;16:255–67.
7. Walker RP, Grigg-Damberger MM, Gopalsami C. Laser-assisted uvulopalatoplasty for the treatment of mild, moderate, and severe obstructive sleep apnea. Laryngoscope 1999;109:79–85.
8. Strauss RA. Lasers in the management of snoring and mild sleep apnea. Oral Maxillofac Surg 1993;51:784–9.
9. Fairbanks DN. Uvulopalatopharyngoplasty complications and avoidance strategies. Otolaryngol Head Neck Surg 1990;102:239–45.
10. Obagi ZE. Pre- and postlaser skin care. Oral Maxillofac Surg Clin North Am 2004; 16:181–7.
11. Goldberg D. Full face nonablative dermal remodeling with a 1320 nm Nd:YAG laser. Dermatol Surg 2000;26:915–8.
12. Niamtu J. Common complications of laser resurfacing and their treatment. Oral Maxillofac Surg Clin North Am 2000;12(4):579–92.
13. Boyden D. A brief overview of noninvasive lasers in cosmetic maxillofacial surgery. Oral Maxillofac Surg Clin North Am 2004;16:231–7.
14. Kilmer SL. Cutaneous lasers. Facial Plast Surg Clin North Am 2003;11:229–43.

15. Weinstein C. Ultrapulse carbon dioxide laser rejuvenation of facial wrinkles and scars. Am J Cosmet Surg 1997;14:3–10.
16. Fitzpatrick TB. The validity and practicality of sun reactive skin types I through VI. Arch Dermatol 1988;124:869–71.
17. Grover S, Apfelberg DB, Smoller B. Effects of varying density patterns and passes on depth of penetration in facial skin utilizing the carbon dioxide laser with automated scanner. Plast Reconstr Surg 1999;104:2247.
18. Bjerring P, Clement M, Heickendorff L, et al. Selective non-ablative wrinkle reduction by laser. J Cutan Laser Ther 2000;2:9–15.
19. Wlodawsky RN, Strauss RA. Intraoral laser surgery. Oral Maxillofac Surg Clin North Am 2004;16:149–63.
20. Arnabat-Dominguez J, Espana-Tost AJ, Berini-Ayates L, et al. Erbium:YAG laser application in the second phase of implant surgery: a pilot study in 20 patients. Int J Oral Maxillofac Implants 2003;18:104–12.
21. Barak S, Horowitz I, Katz J, et al. Thermal changes in endosseous root-form implants as a result of CO2 laser application: an in vitro and in vivo study. Int J Oral Maxillofac Implants 1998;13(5):666–71.
22. Kusek ER. Use of the YSGG laser in dental implant surgery: scientific rationale and case reports. Dent Today 2007;25:98–102.
23. Lee CY. Procurement of autogenous bone from the mandibular ramus with simultaneous third molar removal for bone grafting using the Er, Cr:YSGG laser: a preliminary report. J Oral Implantol 2005;31:32–8.
24. Romanos G. Point of care: is there a role for lasers in the treatment of peri-implantitis? J Can Dent Assoc 2005;71(2):117–8.
25. Lee EA. Laser-assisted gingival tissue procedures in esthetic dentistry. In: Tarnow DP, editor. Applications of 810 nm diode laser technology. A clinical forum. Mahwah (NJ): Montage Media; 2006. p. 2–6.
26. Israel M. Use of the CO2 laser in soft tissue and periodontal surgery. Pract Periodontics Aesthet Dent 1994;6(6):57–64.
27. Ciancio S. Wound healing of periodontal pockets using the diode laser: an interview. In: Tarnow DP, editor. Applications of 810 nm diode laser technology. A clinical forum. Mahwah (NJ): Montage Media; 2006. p. 14–7.
28. Roed-Petersen B. The potential use of CO2 laser gingivectomy for phenytoin-induced gingival hyperplasia in mentally retarded patients. J Clin Periodontol 1993;20(10):729–31.
29. Hughes PS, Hughes AP. Absence of human papillomavirus DNA in the plume of erbium:YAG laser-treated warts. J Am Acad Dermatol 1998;38:426–8.
30. Schindl A, Neumann R. Low-intensity laser therapy is an effective treatment for recurrent herpes simplex infection. Results from a randomized double-blind placebo-controlled study. J Invest Dermatol 1999;113:221–3.
31. Kahraman SA. Low-level laser therapy in oral and maxillofacial surgery. Oral Maxillofac Surg Clin North Am 2004;16:277–88.
32. Ben-Bassat M, Kaplan I, Shindel Y, et al. The CO2 laser in surgery of the tongue. Br J Plast Surg 1978;31:155.
33. Ishii J, Fujita K, Komori T. Laser surgery as a treatment for oral leukoplakia. Oral Oncol 2003;39:759.
34. Meltzer C. Surgical management of oral and mucosal dysplasias: the case for laser excision. J Oral Maxillofac Surg 2007;65:293.
35. Lim B, Smith A, Chandu A. Treatment of oral leukoplakia with carbon dioxide and potassium-titanyl-phosphate lasers: a comparison. J Oral Maxillofac Surg 2010; 68:597–601.

36. Colvard M, Kuo P. Managing aphthous ulcers: laser treatment applied. J Am Dent Assoc 1991;122(7):51–3.
37. Kulekcioglu S, Sivrioglu K, Ozcan O, et al. Effectiveness of low-level laser therapy in temporomandibular disorder. Scand J Rheumatol 2003;32:114–8.
38. McCain JP, de la Rua H. Principles and practice of operative arthroscopy of the human temporomandibular joint. J Oral Maxillofac Surg 1989;1:135–52.
39. Koslin M. Advanced arthroscopic surgery. Oral Maxillofac Surg Clin North Am 2006;18:329–43.
40. Husein A. Applications of lasers in dentistry: a review. Archives of Orofacial Sciences 2006;1:1–4.
41. Tokonabe H, Kouji R, Watanabe H, et al. Morphological changes of human teeth with Er:YAG laser irradiation. J Clin Laser Med Surg 1999;17(1):7–12.
42. Convissar RA. Lasers in general dentistry. Oral Maxillofac Surg Clin North Am 2004;16:165–79.
43. Schwarz F, Arweiler N, Georg T, et al. Desensitising effects of an Er: YAG laser on hypersensitive dentine, a controlled, prospective clinical study. J Clin Periodontol 2002;29:211–5.
44. Sarver DM. Use of the 810 nm diode laser: soft tissue management and orthodontic applications of innovative technology. In: Tarnow DP, editor. Applications of 810 nm diode laser technology. A clinical forum. Mahwah (NJ): Montage Media; 2006. p. 7–13.
45. Takeda FH, Harashima T, Kimura Y, et al. A comparative study of the removal of the smear layer by three endodontic irrigants and two types of lasers. Int Endod J 1999;32(1):32–9.

Treatment of Dentin Hypersensitivity

Richard D. Trushkowsky, DDS[a,*], Anabella Oquendo, DDS[b]

KEYWORDS

• Dentin hypersensitivity • Pulpal pain • Tubular occlusion
• Nerve activity

Dentin hypersensitivity is exemplified by brief, sharp, well-localized pain in response to thermal, evaporative, tactile, osmotic, or chemical stimuli that cannot be ascribed to any other form of dental defect or pathology. Pulpal pain is usually more prolonged, dull, aching, and poorly localized and usually lasts longer than the applied stimulus.[1] Up to 30% of adults have dentin hypersensitivity at some period of their lives.[2] Current techniques for treatment may be only transient in nature and results are not always predictable.[3] Two chief methods of treatment of dentin hypersensitivity are tubular occlusion and blockage of nerve activity.[4] A differential diagnosis needs to be accomplished before any treatment because many symptoms are common to a variety of causes.[5] Items to be considered: the pain—sharp, dull, or throbbing; how many teeth and their location; which part of the tooth elicits the pain; and the intensity of the pain. Clinical and radiographic examination is necessary to elucidate the cause. The following questions need to be asked: Can the pain be localized to one tooth or area of the tooth? Is the area sensitive to a moderate flow of air from an air water syringe? Is the tooth sensitive to percussion? Is there sensitivity to biting pressure or on release? What is the extent of the pain after the stimuli is removed? Do radiographs demonstrate caries or periapical pathology? Is the dentin exposed as a result of recession and are there any cracked cusps, open margins, or occlusal hyperfunction?[5]

MECHANISM

There are regional differences in dentin sensitivity.[6] Freshly exposed dentin in the coronal part of the tooth is more sensitive than cervical dentin. This may be due to the higher conduction velocity or structural differences in dentinal innervations and

The authors have nothing to disclose.
a Advanced Program for International Dentists in Aesthetic Dentistry, Department of Cariology and Comprehensive Care, New York University College of Dentistry, 345 East 24th Street, New York, NY 10010, USA
b Advanced Program for International Dentists in Interdisciplinary Dentistry, Department of Cariology and Comprehensive Care, New York University College of Dentistry, 345 East 24th Street, 421 First Avenue, New York, NY 10010, USA
* Corresponding author. 483 Jefferson Boulevard, Staten Island, NY 10312-2332.
E-mail address: ComposiDoc@aol.com

Dent Clin N Am 55 (2011) 599–608
doi:10.1016/j.cden.2011.02.013
0011-8532/11/$ – see front matter © 2011 Elsevier Inc. All rights reserved.

in the dentin structure itself. Hypersensitive dentin, however, is found most often in the cervical area. Chronic dentin exposure may affect mineralization and inflammatory reactions in the pulp.[6] The sensitivity of dentin has a direct correlation with the size and patency of the dentinal tubules. Absi and colleagues[7] discovered that hypersensitive teeth have an increased number of patent tubules and wider tubules than those of nonsensitive teeth. Even if the tubules are covered by a smear layer or pellicle, however, the teeth can be sensitive due to pulpal inflammation. Also, tubules that are patent at the surface may not be patent down to the pulp. Absi and colleagues demonstrated that the tubules may not be patent all the way. The tubules may be occluded by plaque, smeared dentin in the periphery, peritubular dentin, and closer to the pulp by secondary or reparative dentin. Intratubular is formed by a hypercalcified lining in the tubule that increases in width with age resulting in sclerotic dentin.[8] Weber[9] found physiologic sclerosis is greatest in the region equidistant from the dentin-enamel junction and the exterior of the pulp. Even when sclerotic dentin is present, less than 50% of the tubules are blocked.

The popular assumption has been that tubular occlusion is greater in areas of attrition or abrasion. Mendis and Darling[10] found, however, peritubular dentin to be only 20% thicker in these areas compared with areas than are not subject to attrition. In addition, increased peritubular dentin formation may not eradicate dentin permeability but only reduce it. The classic hydrodynamic theory[11–13] has proposed fluid movement in the tubules and increased nerve excitability as the mechanism eliciting dental sensitivity. A variety of stimuli can result in pressure change traverse the dentin, resulting in stimulation of intradental nerves. The reaction that occurs is proportional to the pressure and rate of fluid flow. Surprisingly, cold, which actually causes fluid movement away from the pulp, creates a swifter and more profound response than heat, which causes an inward flow. It is believed that pressure traverse the dentin results in activation of a mechanoreceptor response. The odontoblastic processes were thought to contribute to dentin sensitivity by a mechanism known as the odontoblast transducer mechanism. Because odontoblasts only protrude a short distance into the dentin tubules, however, they cannot contribute directly to stimulus transmission.

CAUSES

There are many varieties of potential causes for dentin sensitivity. There is no principal cause. The loss of enamel and removal of cementum from the root with exposure of dentin, however, is a major contributing factor. Causes also include gingival recession due to root prominence and thin overlying mucosa, dehiscences and fenestrations, frenum pulls, and orthodontic movement, which causes a root to be moved outside its alveolar housing.[14] Loss of enamel may be a consequence of attrition, erosion, abrasion, and abfraction. The loss of enamel, however, is usually a combination of two or more of these factors. Attrition is the wear that occurs when teeth are in direct contact and is usually associated with occlusal function. Excessive or parafunctional habits, such as bruxism, may result in extreme pathologic wear and increased sensitivity. Abrasion is the tooth wear caused by objects other than other teeth.[15] Toothbrush/toothpaste abrasion is an example. Toothbrushing by itself, however, has minimal effect on enamel and even with toothpaste the effect is minimal on both enamel and dentin. The combination of toothbrushing and erosive agents results in loss of tooth structure.[16,17] West and colleagues[18] found, however, that toothbrushing with toothpaste was able to erode or abrade dentin in various amounts and cause tubule opening. Brushing dentin that has a smear layer with silica-based toothpaste opened the most tubules. Abrasion may cause gingival recession and, as a result of the recession, the softer root surface is exposed.[5] Erosion is the loss of tooth structure by acids that are not of bacterial origin. Erosion can be caused by extrinsic or intrinsic acids. Intrinsic acid is a consequence of exposure to gastric acid (acid regurgitation or gastroesophogeal reflux disease) causing dissolution of teeth by the acid (periomolysis). Extrinsic acid can be a result of dietary or environmental factors. A variety of foods and drinks that may contain acid can contribute to the erosion by demineralization and chelation of calcium. Industrial erosion can occur by exposure to acid vapors produced in a battery factory and wine tasters. Swimmers are exposed to acid in pools maintained at a low pH of 2.7. The loss of tooth structure by erosion is an active process that consists of episodes of demineralization and remineralization.[19] Acidified fluoride gel demonstrated a protective effect against abrasion in eroded enamel[20] but fluoride does not seem to reduce dental erosion.[21] A variety of studies have indicated the possibility of iron reducing enamel demineralization,[22] but potential adverse problems, such as tooth staining, may prohibit its use. A recent study[19] demonstrated iron in a gel increased enamel resistance to acids and helped minimize dental erosion.

BLEACHING

The sensitivity that occurs with bleaching is a result of a reversible pulpitis that is caused by the flow of dentinal fluid from osmolarity changes in the pulp. These changes occur when the bleaching material rapidly penetrates enamel and dentin to the pulp. Hydrogen peroxide and urea penetrate through integral enamel, through the dentin, and into the pulp in 5 to 10 minutes.[20] Most often, the sensitivity is generalized, but many times a sharp shooting pain may occur. This can be from the peroxide penetrating into the pulp or mechanical pressure due to an ill-fitting tray or occlusion on the tray.[21] The estimates of tooth hypersensitivity caused by whitening are usually approximately 60% and the degree of discomfort can be minor to excruciating.[22] Sensitivity usually stops on conclusion of the bleaching treatment and sometimes during treatment. Unfortunately, the patients who exhibit unendurable pain during the procedure do not comply with treatment and a poor result is the consequence. The components of whitening gels are usually carbamide peroxide or hydrogen peroxide; glycerin or propylene glycol is the carrier; and carbapol is used as a polymer-thickening agent. Phosphoric or citric acid is often added in slight amounts to increase the acidity and improve shelf life. The carbamide peroxide breaks down in saliva into hydrogen peroxide and urea. Subsequently, the urea breaks down into ammonia and carbon dioxide. Hydrogen peroxide enters the tooth and forms oxygen and water. The oxygen oxidizes the pigment molecule present in the enamel and dentin and creates a bleached effect.

The three basic classifications of bleaching, which include in office, tray, and over the counter, all incur some degree of sensitivity. Usually higher concentrations of peroxide results in a greater degree of sensitivity.[23,24] The addition of low levels of potassium nitrate to tray bleaches has reduced but not eradicated sensitivity.[25]

PERIODONTAL TREATMENT

Periodontal treatment is sometimes needed to preserve the dentition by eliminating inflammation, regenerating missing periodontium, maintaining esthetics, and stopping the progression of the disease. Unfortunately, patient discomfort often occurs while undergoing periodontal treatment. Postoperative pain and dentin hypersensitivity are often occurrences. Some patients find both the nonsurgical and surgical treatment painful. It has been reported that periodontal therapy can be an important source of dentin hypersensitivity.[26] On conclusion of periodontal therapy, the gingival protective barrier is reduced as a result of the removal of tissue that covers the root surface. Scaling and root planing can remove 20 to 50 μm of cementum and expose the dentinal tubules to a variety of stimuli. von Troil and colleagues[27] found 50% of patients undergoing scaling and root planing had dentin hypersensitivity after treatment. Wallace and Bissada[28] felt that scaling and root planing did not produce hypersensitivity but periodontal surgery that resulted in extensive exposure of root surface did produce dentin hypersensitivity. Smokers also presented with increased pain level in dentin hypersensitivity.[29]

TREATMENT—SELF-APPLIED AND OFFICE SUPPLIED

Self-applied treatments to reduce sensitivity consist of materials that occlude dentinal tubules, coagulate or precipitate tubular fluids, encourage secondary dentin formation, or obstruct pulpal neural response. Desensitizing toothpastes that contain potassium salts, either nitrates or chlorides, are believed to act by depolarizing the nerve surrounding the odontoblastic process, resulting in interference of transmission. Usually it takes 2 weeks with twice-a-day usage to get a reduction in sensitivity. Instead of having patients brush with the toothpaste, the paste could be placed in a soft tray to increase contact time. Haywood and colleagues[30] recommended placing 5% potassium nitrate in bleaching trays to minimize sensitivity that may occur as a result of bleaching. Ten-minute to 30-minute applications seemed to assuage any sensitivity that may occur. Ideally, the desensitizing toothpaste should not have sodium lauryl sulfate because a large amount of this ingredient may cause tissue irritation.

LASER TREATMENT

Laser treatment has also been recommended for the treatment of dentin hypersensitivity. The treatment seems to be only transient, however, and the sensitivity returns in time. In order for a laser to actually alter the dentin surface, it has to melt and resolidify the surface. This effectively closes the dentinal tubules. This does not occur. It is felt that laser treatment reduces sensitivity by coagulation of protein and without altering the surface of the dentin.[31] Dicalcium phosphate-bioglass in combination with Nd:YAG laser treatment has sealed dentin tubules to a depth of 10 μm, and dicalcium phosphate-bioglass plus 30% phosphoric acid occluded exposed tubules up to 60 μm.[32]

FLUORIDE TREATMENT

Patients can apply stannous fluoride in a 0.4% gel or sodium fluoride in a 0.5% mouth rinse or a 1.1% gel. Fluorides reduce the permeability of dentin probably by precipitation of insoluble calcium fluoride inside the dentinal tubules and reduce sensitivity.[33] Gel-Kam Dentin Block (Colgate Oral Pharmaceuticals, New York, NY, USA) consists of 1.09% sodium fluoride, 0.4% stannous fluoride, and 0.14% hydrogen fluoride that can be applied in a tray.

PRO-ARGIN

In 2002, Kleinberg[34] developed a material to reduce sensitivity based on saliva's natural role in reducing sensitivity. Saliva usually allows calcium and phosphate ions to migrate to open dentin tubules and form a precipitate of salivary glycoproteins and calcium phosphate that occludes the tubules.[35] The material developed by Kleinberg consisted of arginine, which is an amino acid that has a positive charge at physiologic pH; bicarbonate as a pH buffer; and calcium carbonate, which provides a source of calcium. This material was able to plug and seal exposed dental tubules to decrease sensitivity. Confocal laser scanning microscopy has demonstrated the occlusion to be resistant to acid exposure and normal pulpal pressure.[36,37] Kleinberg[34] found that the application of arginine-calcium carbonate applied in a paste provided instantaneous relief that lasted for 28 days.[36] Atomic-force microscopy also demonstrated that the normal helical fine structure of intertubular dentin, normally present, was not discernible, due to a surface coating, and the tubules were closed.[36]

OXALATE

Pashley and Galloway[38] felt that using potassium oxalate resulted in calcium oxalate crystals, occluding the tubules (monopotassium-monohydrogen oxalate [Protect® Sensitizing Solution, Sunstar Americas, Guelph, ON, Canada]).[39] BisBlock (Bisco, Schaumburg, IL, USA) contains calcium oxalate crystals, and etching before placement allows the crystals to form deep in the tubules. Once a nonacidic adhesive has been applied (ie, One-Step or One-Step Plus, Bisco), it penetrates the oxalate crystals and entraps them within the adhesive during polymerization. This prevents dislodgement of the crystals and prepares for bonding. The use of potassium nitrate and oxalate desensitizers, however, may reduce bond strength with some adhesives.[40] In addition, Yiu and colleagues[41] found convective water fluxes through dentine may be reduced by applying BisBlock to acid-etched dentine before bonding with One-Step or Single Bond (3M ESPE, St Paul, MN, USA). Reducing adhesive permeability with the use of oxalate desensitizer, however, is not applicable to low-acidity adhesives, such as Opti-Bond Solo Plus (Kerr, Orange, CA, USA) and Prime & Bond NT (Dentsply Caulk, Milford, DE, USA).[41] D/Sense Crystal (Centrix, Shelton, CT, USA) is applied with a syringe and reacts with dentin to form a precipitate of microcrystals of calcium oxalate and potassium nitrate. Pain-Free Desensitizer (Parkell, Edgewood, NY, USA) is a copolymer emulsion consisting of liquid A: emulsion of polymethyl-methacrylate/polystyrene sulphonic acid coploymer and liquid B: 2% oxalic acid solution. The acid diffuses into the dentinal tubules and reacts with the intratubular dentin (peritubular) matrix and releases calcium ions. Calcium ions react with the oxalic acid to form calcium oxalate crystals. The emulsion of the copolymer then coalesces to form a complex mass with calcium oxalate. The dentinal tubules are then occluded by resin tags inside the tubules and on the surface. Super Seal (Phoenix Dental, Fenton, MI, USA) is a chelating agent that complexes with the calcium-rich zone of peritubular dentin to form a crystal plug in the tubule. Kolker and colleagues[42] found that dentin sensitivity was down 97.5% with use of Super Seal. Super Seal does not interfere with subsequent bonding; formation of a hybrid layer after periodontal surgery does not interfere with normal healing when a flap is repositioned.

CASEIN PHOSPHOPEPTIDE–AMORPHOUS CALCIUM PHOSPHATE

Recaldent (Cadbury Enterprises Pte Ltd, Parsippany, NJ, USA) (casein phosphopeptide–amorphous calcium phosphate [CPP-ACP]) is available as a crème (Tooth Mousse, GC Corporation, Tokyo, Japan). The peptides present in Recaldent become bound to the dentin surface and this causes a mineral deposit formation in the dentin surface resulting in decreased opening of the dentinal tubules. The recent introduction of Tooth Mousse Plus, which contains fluoride (900 ppm), provides the added benefit of fluoride to aid in remineralization and tubule occlusion.[43]

CALCIUM PHOSPHATE PRECIPITATION

Chiang and colleagues[44] found a mesoporous silica biomaterial containing nanosized calcium oxide particles mixed with 30% phosphoric acid can occlude dentinal tubules and considerably reduce dentin permeability even in the presence of pulpal pressure. When the supersaturated calcium and hydrogen phosphate ion containing nanosized calcium oxide particles paste is brushed on the surface, the ions diffuse into the dentinal tubules and form di-calcium phosphate dihydrate precipitation at a depth of 100 μm.[44]

CARBONATE HYDROXYAPATITE NANOCRYSTALS AND SODIUM FLUORIDE/POTASSIUM NITRATE DENTIFRICE

Most of the materials used to treat dentin hypersensitivity usually aim to reduce stimuli conduction and apatite dissolution rather than attempting to encourage mineralization by apatite crystallization and possibly by remineralization. When hydroxyapatite is dissolved or abraded it cannot suddenly remineralize because enamel posses no cells and dentin apposition occurs only in the direction of the pulp. Synthetic hydroxyapatite (carbonate hydroxyapatite) biomimetic nanocrystals, introduced recently, have demonstrated the ability to remineralize altered enamel surfaces and close dentinal tubules.[45] There is a progressive closing of the dentinal tubules in several minutes and subsequently a remineralized layer forms in a few hours.[45]

GLUTARALDEHYDE

Desensitizers, such as Calm-it (Dentsply Caulk), Gluma Desensitizer (Heraeus Kulzer, Armonk, NY, USA), and Glu/Sense (Centrix, Shelton, CT, USA), are based on aqueous glutaraldehyde, which occludes the tubules by cross-linking of dentinal proteins. The presence of hydroxyethyl methacrylate acts as a wetting agent[46] and glutaraldehyde reacts with the serum albumin in dentinal fluid, resulting in precipitation of the serum albumin. This reaction causes the polymerization of 2-hydroxyethyl methacrylate (HEMA) and blockage of dentinal tubules.[47] Tubular occlusion can be visualized at a depth of 200 μm.[48] Telio CS Desensitizer (Ivoclar Vivadent, Amherst, NY, USA) contains polyethylene glycol dimethacrylate (PEG-DMA) and glutaraldehyde. PEG-DMA acts to precipitate plasma proteins in the tubules and glutaraldehyde is a cross-linking agent that bonds to amine groups of protein and forms highly cross-linked, insoluble protein aggregates. PEG-DMA precipitates the protein and the glutaraldehyde forms covalent bonds to the proteins and the result is the formation of firm plugs of protein that seal the tubules.[49] Hemaseal & Cide (Advantage Dental Products, Lake Orion, MI, USA) contains HEMA and 4% chlorhexadine.

SEAL & PROTECT AND ADMIRA PROTECT

Seal & Protect (Dentsply Caulk) consists of methacrylate resins, dipentaerythritol penta acrylate monophosphate, nanofillers, triclosan (a broad-spectrum antibacterial agent), and acetone. Photoinitiators and stabilizers are also present. The area to be treated is isolated, rinsed, and blot dried. Seal & Protect is then applied in sufficient amounts to keep the area wet for 20 seconds. A gentle stream of compressed air is used to volatilize the acetone solvent and the material is light cured for 10 seconds. A second coat is then applied, dried, and light activated. Admira Protect (Voco, Briarcliff Manor, NY, USA) consists of acetone, bisphenol A glycidyl methacrylate

(BIS-GMA), acidic adhesive monomer, organically modified ceramics, HEMA, and urethane dimethacrylate with fluoride release. The material is applied to a slightly moist surface, air dried, and light cured and then a second application is applied and light cured for 10 seconds.

PREHYBRIDIZED DENTIN

Postcementation hypersensitivity may occur after a newly cemented restoration is placed. The symptoms are usually a short, sharp pain that occurs when a tooth is exposed to thermal or chemical stimuli. Usually, postcementation hypersensitivity may occur when a tooth that has recently been restored with a crown or inlay/onlay. The patient may exhibit short, sharp pain when the tooth is exposed to thermal or chemical stimuli.[50] There are causes that have to be considered resulting in dentin hypersensitivity: overheating, excessive drying of the dentin during preparation, bacterial infiltration due to possible microleakage, and tooth preparation that comes in close proximity to the pulp (within 0.5 mm).

Prehybridized dentin or immediate dentin sealing has been suggested to make the dentin less sensitive while a restoration is fabricated in the laboratory. Because a hybrid layer is created immediately after preparation, teeth treated with the immediate dentin sealing technique were better able to tolerate thermal and functional loads in comparison to teeth that were sealed when the restorations were placed.[51]

VARNISH

Glass ionomers have been shown to reduce root sensitivity immediately and long term.[52,53] There has been a recent introduction of Vanish XT Extended Contact Varnish (3M ESPE, St Paul, MN, USA) for root sensitivity. The liquid contains a methacrylate-modified polyalkenoic, HEMA, water, initiators (including camphorquinone), and calcium glycerophosphate. The paste contains HEMA, BIS-GMA, water, initiators, and fluoroaluminosilicate glass. Calcium glycerophosphate was also added to provide calcium and phosphate to the oral environment. In a study by Rusin and colleagues,[54] Vanish XT Extended Contact Varnish demonstrated excellent bonding and sealing ability on dentin with open tubules or smear-layer occluded tubules. The resin-modified glass ionomer infiltrated the smear layer with resin, penetrated the dentin tubules, and created resin tags, thereby demonstrating the potential to reduce sensitivity on exposed root dentin.[54] Vanish 5% Sodium Fluoride White Varnish contains 5% fluoride and tricalcium phosphate. The tricalcium phosphate is mechanical ball milled with fumaric acid producing a free phosphate and funtionalized calcium. The calcium is protected by the fumaric acid and only reacts with the fluoride when it is applied to the teeth. Vanish also contains a modified rosin that is white or tooth colored. Profluorid L (Voco) contains 5% sodium fluoride for high-solubility and short-term effect and 5% calcium fluoride for low-solubility and long-term effect (according to the manufacturer). Calcium cations aid in the remineralization process. Profluorid L also contains eugenol, which provides an analgesic effect but is also detrimental to bonding as eugenol destroys the initiator. Duraphat (Colgate Oral Pharmaceuticals) is a 5% sodium fluoride varnish applied in the office with a syringe-style applicator at approximately 0.3 to 0.5 mL of varnish to each tooth, and dental floss can be used to draw the varnish interproximally. Topical fluorides are believed to form a barrier by precipitating calcium fluoride on the exposed dentin surface and reduce dentin permeability. Ritter and colleagues[55] found a single application of topical fluoride varnish reduced dentin hypersensitivity for at least 24 weeks.

DISCUSSION

For a few patients, dentin hypersensitivity may represent only a minor inconvenience but for many the degree of discomfort and emotional anguish can be overwhelming.[56] The adult population is living longer and problems with gingival recession and erosion often increase.[57] In addition, the distress caused by the dentin sensitivity leads to modification of behavior, such as change in diet, cancelled dental appointments, and inadequate plaque control. This may lead to caries, gingival inflammation, and periodontal breakdown. Initially desensitizing toothpastes (usually containing a potassium salt), varnishes, high-fluoride level mouth rinses, and precipitants are used. If subsequent adhesive techniques are required, a restoring dentist has to be aware of any possible interference with bonding. A restoration or a connective tissue graft for areas of recession may have to be considered if pain persists. The least invasive technique that provides long-term relief should be selected.

REFERENCES

1. Porto IC, Andrade AK, Montes MA. Diagnosis and treatment of dentinal hypersensitivity. J Oral Sci 2009;51(3):323–32.
2. Addy M. Etiology and clinical implications of dentine hypersensitivity. Dent Clin North Am 1990;34:503–14.
3. Orchardson R, Gangarosa LP, Holland GR, et al. Dentine hypersensitivity—into the 21st century. Arch Oral Biol 1994;39(Suppl):113S–9S.
4. Pradeep AR, Sharma A. Comparison of clinical efficacy of a dentifrice containing calcium sodium phosphosilicate to a dentifrice containing potassium nitrate and to a placebo on dentinal hypersensitivity: a randomized clinical trial. J Periodontol 2010;81(8):1167–73.
5. Haywood VB. Dentin hypersensitivity: bleaching and restorative consideration for successful management. Int Dent J 2002;52:7–10.
6. Närhi M, Yamamoto H, Ngassapa D, et al. The neurophysiological basis and the role of inflammatory reactions in dentine hypersensitivity. Arch Oral Biol 1994;39(Suppl):23S–30S.
7. Absi EG, Addy M, Adams D. Dentine hypersensitivity. A study of the patency of dentinal tubules in sensitive and non-sensitive cervical dentine. J Clin Periodontol 1987;14(5):280–4.
8. Holland GR. Mophological features of dentine and pulp related to dentine sensitivity. Arch Oral Biol 1994;39(Suppl):3S–11S.
9. Weber YN. Human dentine sclerosis: a microradiographic survey. Arch Oral Biol 1974;19:163–9.
10. Mendis BR, Darling AI. Distribution with age and attrition of peritubular dentine in the crowns of human teeth. Arch Oral Biol 1979;24(2):131–9.
11. Gysi A. An attempt to explain the sensitiveness of dentin. Br J Dent Sci 1900;43:865–8.
12. Bränström MA. Hydrodynamic mechanism in the transmission of pain-producing stimuli through the dentin. In: Anderson DJ, editor. Sensory mechanisms in dentine. Oxford (UK): Pergamon Press; 1963. p. 73–9.
13. Bränström M. Sensivity of dentine. Oral Surg Oral Med Oral Pathol 1966;21:517–26.
14. Canadian Advisory Board on Dentin Hypersensitivity. Consensus-based recommendations for the diagnosis and management of dentin hypersensitivity. J Can Dent Assoc 2003;69:221–6.
15. Smith BG. Toothwear: aetiology and diagnosis. Dent Update 1989;16:204–12.

16. Absi EG, Addy M, Adams D. Dentin hypersensitivity-the effect of toothbrushing and dietary compounds on dentin in vitro: an SEM study. J Oral Rehabil 1992; 19(2):101–10.

17. Davis WB, Winter PJ. The effects of abrasion on enamel and dentine after exposure to dietary acids. Br Dent J 1980;148(11–12):253–6.

18. West NX, Hughs J, Addy M. Dentin hypersensitivity: the effects of brushing desensitizing tooth pastes, their solid and liquid phases and detergents on dentin and acrylic, studies in vitro. J Oral Rehabil 1998;25:885.

19. Bueno MG, Marsicano JA, Sales-Peres SH. Preventive effect of iron gel with or without fluoride on bovine enamel in vitro. Aust Dent J 2010;55(2):177–80.

20. Cooper JS, Morrissette DB, Gasior EJ, et al. Penetration of the pulp chamber by carbamide peroxide bleaching agents. J Endod 1992;18:315–7.

21. Haywood VB. Treating tooth sensitivity during whitening. Compend Contin Educ Dent 2005;26(Suppl 9):11–20.

22. Leonard RH Jr. Efficacy, longevity, side effects, and patient perceptions of night-guard vital bleaching. Compend Contin Educ Dent 1998;19(8):766–70.

23. Matis BA, Mousa HN, Cochran MA, et al. Clinical evaluation of bleaching agents of different concentrations. Quintessence Int 2000;31(5):303–10.

24. Krause F, Jepsen S, Braun A. Subjective intensities of pain and contentment with treatment outcomes during tray bleaching of vital teeth employing different carbamide peroxide concentrations. Quintessence Int 2008;39(3):203–9.

25. Browning WD, Chan DC, Myers ML, et al. Comparison of traditional and low sensitivity whiteners. Oper Dent 2008;33(4):379–85.

26. Canakçi CF, Canakçi V. Pain experienced by patient undergoing different periodontal therapies. J Am Dent Assoc 2007;138(12):1563–73.

27. von Troil B, Needlemen I, Sanz M. A systematic review of the prevalence of root sensitivity following periodontal therapy. J Clin Periodontol 2002;29(Suppl 3): 173–7.

28. Wallace JA, Bissada NF. Pulpal and root sensitivity rated to periodontal therapy. Oral Surg Oral Med Oral Pathol 1990;69(6):743–7.

29. Chabanski MB, Gillam DG, Bulman JS, et al. Clinical evaluation of cervical dentine sensitivity in a population of patients referred to a specialist periodontology department: a pilot study. J Oral Rehabil 1997;24(9):666–72.

30. Haywood VB, Caughman WF, Frasier KB, et al. Tray delivery of potassium nitrate-fluoride to reduce bleaching sensitivity. Quintessence Int 2001;32(2):105–9.

31. Goodis HE, White JM, Marshall SJ, et al. Measurement of fluid flow through laser-treated dentine. Arch Oral Biol 1994;9(Suppl):128S.

32. Kuo TC, Lee BS, Kang SH, et al. Cytotoxicity of DP-bioglass paste used for the treatment of dentin hypersensitivity. J Endod 2007;33:451–4.

33. Morris MF, Davis RD, Richardson BW. Clinical efficacy of two dentin desensitizing agents. Am J Dent 1999;12(2):72–6.

34. Kleinberg I. SensiStat. A new saliva-based composition for simple and effective treatment of dentinal sensitivity pain. Dent Today 2002;21(12):42–7.

35. Panagakos F, Schiff T, Guignon A. Dentin hypersensitivity: effective treatment with an in-office desensitizing paste containing 8% arginine and calcium carbonate. Am J Dent 2009;22(Spec No A):3A–7A.

36. Cummins D. Dentin hypersentivity: from diagnosis to a breakthrough therapy for everyday sensitivity relief. J Clin Dent 2009;20(1):1–9.

37. Petrou I, Heu R, Stanick M, et al. A breaththrough therapy for dentin hyperensivity: how dental products containing 8% arginine and calcium carbonate work to deliver effective relief of sensitive teeth. J Clin Dent 2009;20(1):23–31.

38. Pashley DH, Galloway SE. The effects of oxalate treatment on smear layer of ground surfaces of human dentine. Arch Oral Biol 1985;30:731–7.
39. Moncada G, Fernandez E, Deyer E, et al. In-vivo study of calcium oxalate as a root surface desensitizer. Presented at IADR/AADR/CADR 83rd General Session. Baltimore (MD), March 9–12, 2005.
40. Türkkahraman H, Adanir N. Effects of potassium nitrate and oxalate desensitizer agents on shear bond strengths of orthodontic brackets. Angle Orthod 2007; 77(6):1096–100.
41. Yiu CK, Hiraishi N, Chersoni S, et al. Single-bottle adhesives behave as permeable membranes after polymerisation. II. Differential permeability reduction with an oxalate desensitiser. J Dent 2006;34(2):106–16.
42. Kolker IL, Vargas MA, Armstrong SR, et al. Effect of desensitizing agents on dentin permeability. J Dent Res 2002;81:A63. [IADR abstract #0295].
43. Walsh LJ. The effects of GC Tooth Mousse on cervical dentinal sensitivity: a controlled clinical trial. International Dentistry South Africa 2010;12:4–12.
44. Chiang YC, Chen HJ, Liu HC, et al. A novel mesoporous biomaterial for treating dentin hypersensitivity. J Dent Res 2010;89(3):236–40.
45. Orsini G, Procaccini M, Manzoli L, et al. A double-blind randomized-controlled trial comparing the desensitizing efficacy of a new dentifrice containing carbonate/hydroxyapatite nanocrystals and a sodium fluoride/potassium nitrate dentifrice. J Clin Periodontol 2010;37(10):510–7.
46. Stewardson DA, Crisp RJ, McHugh S, et al. The Effectiveness of Systemp.desensitizer in the treatment of dentine hypersensitivity. Prim Dent Care 2004;11(3):71–6.
47. Qin C, Xu J, Zhang Y. Spectroscopic investigation of the function of aqueous 2-hydroxyethylmethacrylate/glutaraldehyde solution as a dentin desensitizer. Eur J Oral Sci 2006;114(4):354–9.
48. Schüpbach P, Lutz F, Finger W. Closing of dentinal tubules by Gluma desensitizer. Eur J Oral Sci 1997;105(5):414–21.
49. Ivoclar Vivadent Product Profile. Schaan (Principality of Liechtenstein), January 2010.
50. Hu J, Zhu Q. Effect of immediate dentin sealing on preventive treatment for post-cementation hypersensitivity. Int J Prosthodont 2010;23(1):49–52.
51. Magne P, Kim TH, Cascione D, et al. Immediate dentin sealing improves bond strength of indirect restorations. J Prosthet Dent 2005;94(6):511–9.
52. Hansen EK. Dentin hypersensitivity treated with a fluoride-containing varnish or a light-cured glass –ionomer liner. Scand J Dent Res 1992;100(6):305–9.
53. Tantbirojn D, Poolthong S, Leevailoj C, et al. Clinical evaluation of a resin-modified glass—ionomer liner for cervical dentin hypersensitivity treatment. Am J Dent 2006;19(1):56–60.
54. Rusin RP, Agee K, Suchko M, et al. Effect of a new desensitizing material on human dentin permeability. Dent Mater 2010;26(6):600–7.
55. Ritter AV, de L, Dias W, et al. Treating cervical dentin hypersensitivity with fluoride varnish: a randomized clinical study. J Am Dent Assoc 2006;137(7):1013–20.
56. Bissada NF. Symptomatology and clinical features of hypersensitive teeth. Arch Oral Biol 1994;39(Suppl):31S–2S.
57. Zero DT, Lussi A. Erosion-chemical and biological factors important to the dental practitioner. Int Dent J 2005;12(Suppl 1):285–90.

Current Treatments and Advances in Pain and Anxiety Management

David Huang, DDS*, Edmund Wun, DDS, Avichai Stern, DDS

KEYWORDS

- Pain and anxiety management • Pain and anxiety control
- Pain and anxiety types • Physiology of pain and anxiety
- Preoperative and postoperative mortality and morbidity

The current management of pain and anxiety continues to evolve much as it has throughout its history. Beyond advances in pharmacology and technology, changes in societal views have historically influenced how we address these conditions. Discussing how cultural views have shaped medical management may help in understanding the continued evolution of treatment. Historically, the management of pain has evolved through many different societal and medical influences. Meldrum[1] elaborates on how pain contributes to philosophic, political, and religious ideology and has defined the suffering of individuals throughout human history. As the oldest medical problem and the universal physical affliction of humankind, little of its physiology has been understood until very recently.

In the 17th century, European physicians treated pain most often with opium, particularly laudanum, which was a mixture of opium in sherry. Yet pain was often seen as a medical necessity or diagnostic aid. Pain was used to relieve evil spirits or to amputate diseased limbs. It was a valued sign of the patient's vitality and of the effectiveness of treatment. Physical suffering was inevitable; the meaning, rather than actual pain, was what mattered to the physician. Pain was also attributed to serving as a counterirritant to disease.

The necessity of pain was questioned in medical opinions of the 1800s. Although the skilled surgeon took pride in his ability to operate quickly, the utility of sedation for long procedures was readily apparent. Dr William T.G. Morton, an American dentist, demonstrated the use of ether in 1846 to perform a dental extraction. The advent of anesthesia created much medical and societal controversy. Debates began over the ethics of operating on an unconscious patient and that the relief from pain might

The authors have nothing to disclose.
Department of Dentistry/Oral Maxillofacial Surgery, The Brooklyn Hospital, 121 Dekalb Avenue Box 187, Brooklyn, NY 11201, USA
* Corresponding author.
E-mail address: ddsdavidhuang@yahoo.com

Dent Clin N Am 55 (2011) 609–618
doi:10.1016/j.cden.2011.02.014
0011-8532/11/$ – see front matter © 2011 Published by Elsevier Inc.

dental.theclinics.com

actually impede healing. Religious writers called anesthesia a violation of God's law.[2] It wasn't until 3 decade later that anesthesia gained widespread acceptance.

Today the treatment of pain has changed dramatically; yet pain and its management or lack thereof continues to be one of the main obstacles in establishing routine dental care. It is estimated that as many as 75%[3] of adults experience some degree of dental fear and that up to 10%[4] may possesses a dental phobia that prevents them from seeking treatment in all but the most dire of circumstances. Neglect and procrastination result in conditions necessitating surgical treatment leading to increased perioperative and postoperative pain, which reinforces the pattern of treatment avoidance.

Pain management is important from a public health perspective as well. The American Society for Pain shows that pain results in more than 50 million lost workdays each year, worth an estimated $100 billion in the United States.[5] Currently, approximately 20 million Americans experience jaw and lower facial pain (temporomandibular joint disorder [TMD/TMJ]) each year.[5] Furthermore, as the population ages, we can expect that rates of acute and chronic pain will increase in elderly individuals.

TYPES OF PAIN AND ANXIETY

The International Association for the Study of Pain defines pain as an unpleasant sensory and emotional experience associated with actual or potential tissue damage.[6] It is a subjective experience. Nocioception is defined as the neural processes of encoding and processing noxious stimuli.[7] It is one of the pathophysiologic processes that produces pain. Although we appreciate that pain very often has a physical cause, it also has a psychological component that by itself may produce pain via psychosomatic pathways.

Pain is classified into acute versus chronic pain, with further differentiation based on pathophysiology, etiology, and/or the affected area.[8] Acute pain is usually self-limiting and resolves within a few weeks.[8] It tends to be nocioceptive in nature as pertaining to a disease, injury, or other form of tissue damage. It commonly occurs in trauma, during the postoperative period, and in acute medical illnesses. Acute pain can be further classified into somatic and visceral pain. Somatic acute pain that arises in the superficial structures has a sharp or throbbing sensation. Somatic pain arising from deeper musculoskeletal sources tends to be a dull aching, less localized throb. Conversely visceral pain is from damage or disease of an internal organ or its surroundings. Visceral pain can be dull and diffuse in nature, sharp and localized, or referred based on the specific etiology.

Chronic pain describes a condition that last longer than a month to years.[8] Its nature is largely neuropathic, but has nocioceptive components. Neuropathic pain tends toward paroxysmal lancating episodes with residual burning and throbbing. It tends to be associated with a hyperpathic state. Most forms of chronic pain are associated with a musculoskeletal disorder, or peripheral or central lesions. Musculoskeletal pain is nocioceptive, whereas peripheral and central lesions are neuralgic in nature.

Anxiety is a state of worry and nervousness that occurs in a variety of mental disorders, usually accompanied by compulsive behavior or attacks of panic, a vague unpleasant emotion that is experienced in anticipation of some misfortune.[9] There are several different types of anxiety with differing treatments. Nonetheless, anxiety itself as it pertains to medical or surgical treatment is often a healthy, if not ideal response. Nonpsychiatric physicians need to be able to distinguish between normal anxiety and phobias. Conditions such as generalized anxiety disorder and posttraumatic stress disorder may necessitate psychiatric treatment as part of long-term care. A preliminary evaluation of anxiety involves evaluating the objective consequences of the patient's heightened state. For example, is the patient's anxiety leading to neglect of care or endangerment of the patient and medical staff? Are there functional and physical manifestations of stress that interfere with daily and long-term function? Anxiety that obstructs personal, social, or professional life or presents with physical signs and symptoms, such as chest pain or shortness of breath, or suicidal and homicidal thoughts requires further workup and should not be dismissed as a necessary complication of treatment.

PHYSIOLOGY OF PAIN AND ANXIETY

Physiologically, pain begins with the activation of the first-order nocioreceptor of unmyelinated c fibers and a-delta fibers.[8] These neurons synapse with second-order neurons in the dorsal horn of the spinal cord. Second-order neurons include afferent, interneuron, sympathetic, and reflex neurons. Afferent branches then cross the midline to the contralateral spinothalamic tract and ascend to the thalamus. In the thalamus, second-order synapse with third-order neurons then send axons to synapse in the anterior cingulate and post-central gyrus of the cerebral cortex. Within the cortex, pain is processed, localized, and associated with emotions. During nocior-eception, chemical mediators are released peripherally and in the dorsal horn. These neurotransmitters can modulate the sensation of pain. The main excitatory peptides are substance P (subP) and calcitonin gene–related peptide (CGRP), which increase sensitization of nocioreceptors.[8] Continued stimulation of these receptors results in modulation of pain. Peripheral nocioreceptors decrease their threshold, and increase their frequency of firing to the same stimuli with continued firing after the stimulus is removed. Prostaglandins resulting from tissue damage directly activate nociorecep-tors. SubP and CGRP also cause degranulation of mast cells, vasodilatation, and formation of leukotrienes, resulting in neurogenic inflammation.[8] Centrally, excitatory neuropathies result in sensitization of second-order neurons, receptor field expansion, and hyperexcitability of neurons.[8]

The initial stimuli for anxiety can be a physical challenge or a perceived threat. This threat may be conscious or subconscious and results in stimulation of the amygdala. The amygdala modulates the response by attaching emotional significance to the stimuli. Feelings of agitation and anger accompanying the stimuli aid in creating and maintaining a memory of the event. The stress response begins with the release of corticotropin-releasing factor, which helps activate autonomic, immune, and endocrine stress responses. The hormonal sequence eventually leads to the release of epinephrine and glucocorticoids, which subsequently activate the sympathetic system. The amygdala also stimulates the midbrain and brain stem causing many of the physical symptoms associated with anxiety.

PAIN AND ANXIETY RELATIONSHIP

The correlation between anxiety and pain continues to be debated. Intuitively, we know that uncontrolled pain may exacerbate present and future states of anxiety. Yet, the causal relationship between anxiety and increased pain is less clear. Indeed, many clinicians view increased pain in anxious patients to be a subjective increase in perceived pain versus nocioception, discounting patient discomfort as either psychosomatic or psychiatric. Often, higher than normal levels of anxiety may be overlooked by medical staff in the preoperative area.

To gain insight into the relationship between anxiety and pain, Kain and colleagues[10] conducted a study to determine if postoperative pain could be predicted based on preoperative anxiety. Their research examined women undergoing abdominal hysterectomy and included evaluations on patients' state and trait anxiety, coping mechanisms, and level of stress. Patients completed the State-Trait Anxiety Inventory preoperatively and both the McGill Pain Questionnaire and the Visual Analogue Scale (VAS) postoperatively. Their results showed positive correlations between the level of anxiety and postoperative pain. Based on their findings, Kain and colleagues[10] suggested using postoperative anxiety-reducing strategies as an adjunct to postoperative analgesics. In a subsequent study, Kain and colleagues[11] examined patients who underwent similar surgical procedures. The patients were divided into 2 groups: one group received an anxiolytic and the other group received a placebo. The research demonstrated that pain was significantly decreased in the anxiolytic group for 1 week postoperatively.

Ploghaus and colleagues[12] measured neural activity in subjects who were given visual cues before receiving thermal stimuli. Patients were given time to associate high-intensity cues with high thermal activity and low-intensity cues with low thermal activity. Subsequently, high-intensity cues were given with low thermal stimulation. The results demonstrated higher anxiety, stronger pain, and hippocampal involvement with preliminary evidence of neural representation of pain and anxiety. Ploghaus and colleagues[12] surmise that hippocampal involvement from increased anxiety results in pain intensity amplification.

However, not all studies support a closed relationship between anxiety and pain. In a subsequent study, Kain and colleagues[13] examined 70 women who received abdominal hysterectomies. Two groups were formed: one group was given an anxiolytic and the other was given a placebo. The results showed no statistical correlation between reduced anxiety and postoperative pain beyond the pharmacologic effect of benzodiazepines combined with anesthesia. These conclusions contradicted Kain and colleagues' previous studies.[13] The investigators noted that previous results correlating reduced anxiety to decreased postoperative pain were for minor surgical procedures and may not be applicable to patients with major surgery.

Large prospective, double-blinded, randomized studies would be helpful to determine if a physiologic causality exists between anxiety and increased pain. Nonetheless, psychiatric and psychosomatic manifestation of increased pain from heightened anxiety is well established.[14] Many health care providers intuitively understand this correlation between psychological and physical health. This understanding coupled with humanitarian motivation should influence our treatment of anxiety from a holistic approach to address the emotional needs of our patients.

MORTALITY AND MORBIDITY OF IMPROPER PAIN AND ANXIETY CONTROL

Improper anxiety and pain management can influence morbidity and mortality for many patients. A heightened level of anxiety or uncontrolled postoperative pain can intensify the sympathetic reaction, which in turn affects almost every organ system in the body.

Cardiovascular effects include hypertension, tachycardia, and increased vascular resistance. Increased myocardial oxygen demand may precipitate ischemia. In cases of ventricular dysfunction, increased workload may lead to reduced cardiac output. The respiratory system responds to increased oxygen demand and CO_2 production by increasing minute ventilation and volume. The neuroendocrine response leads to release of additional adrenocorticotropic hormone, which stimulates the release of glucocorticoids. Cortisol release leads to compromised immune function and the suppression of the reticuloendothelial system, predisposing the patient to postsurgical infections. The gastrointestinal system exhibits decreased motility with an accompanying increase in gastric secretions. Risks are increased for gastric ulcer and aspiration pneumonia. Activation of the sympathetic nervous system leads to hypercoagulation, secondary to decreased fibrinolysis, with increased risk for venous thromboembolism. Activation of the endocrine system results in hyperglycemia, protein catabolism, and sodium retention. Excessive glucose predisposes diabetic patients to poor wound healing, and intracellular fluid retention may exacerbate conditions such as congestive heart failure.

Effective management of pain and anxiety can decrease the incidence of many common postoperative complications. A decreased incidence of these complications reduces recovery time and postoperative pain.[15] However, excessive postoperative pain relief (as in the case of opioid overdose) may result in complications of respiratory and cardiovascular depression, renal failure, and addiction. Careful management of each patient's analgesic regimen should take into consideration pain tolerance and social, physical, medical, and psychiatric history.

CURRENT TRENDS IN PAIN MANAGEMENT

Recent advancements in pain and anxiety management pertains more to current trends and methodology of drug usage versus new pharmaceutical developments. General classes of pain and anxiety management include nonsteroidal anti-inflammatory drugs (NSAIDs), acetaminophen, opioids, benzodiazepines, selective serotonin reuptake inhibitors (SSRIs), tricyclic antidepressants (TCAs), and monoamine oxidase inhibitors (MAOIs). Although most of these drugs have existed for decades, research about their clinical effects, pharmacokinetics, and adverse reactions continues to develop in the current literature.

Tapentadol

Tapentadol is a centrally acting analgesic approved for use in 2008 for moderate to severe pain. It acts through a dual-mode application of activating μ-opioid receptor and inhibits norepinephrine reuptake.[16] Tapentadol is a new molecular entity that has both opioid and nonopioid activity in a single compound.

Side effects include nausea, dizziness, constipation, and central nervous system sedation, which are common to opioid pain medications. Clinical trials demonstrate tapentadol to have equianalgesic effect with a lower incidence of side effects compared with oxycodone and morphine. Studies comparing tapentadol with morphine and NSAIDs found tapentadol to cause less nausea and dizziness than morphine.[17]

Being new to the market, the abuse potential of tapentadol has not been fully discovered. Preliminary data suggest that tapentadol has a relatively limited potential for dependency compared with other strong opioid medications. Nonetheless, tapentadol is currently a class II scheduled drug.

Tramadol

Tramadol (Ultram) is a weak μ-opioid receptor agonist that causes the release serotonin, and inhibits the reuptake of norepinephrine.[18,19] It is used in treatment of moderate to severe pain and chronic pain such as trigeminal neuralgia.

Common side effects include nausea, vomiting, sweating, and constipation. Respiratory depression, common for most opioids, is not clinically significant in normal doses. When taken in combination with other SSRIs or MAOIs, there is an increased risk of serotonin toxicity, which can be fatal.[18,19]

In 2009, the Food and Drug Administration issued a Warning Letter to Ultram's manufacturer, Johnson & Johnson (Titusville, NJ, USA), alleging that the Web site commissioned by the manufacturer had "overstated the efficacy" of the drug, and "minimized the serious risks."[20] In the most recent *Physicians Desk Reference*, new warnings from the manufacturer place greater emphasis on tramadol's addictive nature and risk of respiratory depression, and includes a new list of side effects.

Propofol

Since its inception in 1986, propofol has been the intravenous (IV) anesthetic agent of choice for inducing general anesthesia and providing sedation whether in the outpatient setting or continuously in the intensive care unit (ICU). It has become popular in many outpatient procedures, either alone or in conjunction with a polymodal sedation regimen. Propofol is considered a sedative hypnotic and is not an analgesic. Many poly-modal sedation regimens supplement with fentanyl for analgesia. It is available in a 1% solution with 10.00% soybean oil, 2.25% glycerol, and 1.20% purified egg phospholipid.

Propofol induces sedation through the potentiation of gamma-aminobutyric acid (GABA). It has rapid onset of about 30 seconds, a rapid rate of distribution half-life of 2 to 4 minutes, and a short elimination half-life of 30 to 60 minutes, but maintains a shorter clinical effect. Rapid onset, offset, lack of accumulation, and minimal effect on liver and renal function make this drug a popular choice among clinicians. The general anesthetic induction dose in healthy adults is 2.0 to 2.5 mg/kg, less for the geriatric population.[21] IV sedation requires a slow injection of 100 to 150 µg/kg/min (6 to 9 mg/kg/h) for 3 to 5 minutes followed by a maintenance infusion of 25 to 75 µg/kg/min or incremental bolus doses of 10 to 20 mg.[21] Propofol undergoes hepatic conjugation to inactive metabolites that are renally excreted.

Despite the pharmacologic advantages and many uses of propofol therapy, there are adverse side effects with normal usage and/or overdose. Propofol results in cardiovascular depression that may lead to hypotension, bradycardia, and reduced intracranial pressure. Hyperlipidemia, associated with pancreatitis, respiratory depression, pain with injection, and allergic complications, has also been associated with usage, particularly in the ICU setting.[22] Transient apnea with respiratory depression, particularly with polymodal sedation, as well as mild myoclonic movements and dystonia, have been observed. In the critical care setting, prolonged use of propofol has been associated with propofol infusion syndrome.[22] Clinical features include rhabdomyolysis, cardiac failure, and renal failure. Use of propofol is limited to clinicians trained in advanced airway management.

Remifentanil

Use of narcotic sedation has also changed in the past decade. Remifentanil is a potent ultrashort-acting synthetic opioid derivative. Used as an adjunct in general anesthesia, it has also become popular in outpatient office procedures. It is 100% more potent than fentanyl, and 200 times more potent than morphine.[23] The utility of remifentanil versus alternative opioids resides in its rapid onset and offset. The initial distribution half-life is 1 minute and its effective biologic half-life of is 3 to 10 minutes.[23] This termination time is similar regardless of the duration of infusion. Metabolism occurs by plasma esterases and is unaffected by the renal or hepatic impairment. Remifentanil is a specific mu receptor agonist, resulting in analgesia and sedation. Like other opioids, side effects include reduction in sympathetic tone, respiratory depression, cardiovascular depression, muscle rigidity, nausea, constipation, and urinary retention.[23]

When used in a polymodal sedation regimen, remifentanil allows for rapid postoperative recovery time. Used synergistically, this analgesic allows for the use of high-dose opioid with reduced dose-sedative hypnotics. Rapid distribution and elimination of remifentanil allows it to be used as the rate-limiting drug in initiation and termination of synergistic polymodal sedation. With careful monitoring, adverse events of anesthetic, respiratory, and cardiovascular complication are reduced.

Triazolam

Recent developments regarding triazolam (Halcion) called into question the safety of this common-day anxiolytic. Triazolam is a benzodiazepine derivative used as a sedative in treatment of short-term anxiolysis or insomnia. It has amnesic, sedative, anxiolytic, and anticonvulsant properties. Rapid onset and short half-life (approximately 2 to 4 hours) are the main benefits when compared with other anxiolytics. Mechanism of action is the potentiation of GABA and it is hepatically metabolized. Side effects of using triazolam include anterograde amnesia, addiction, rebound insomnia, rebound anxiety, amnesia, confusion, and disinhibition, with residual lasting up to 24 hours depending on dose. Although frequently used for periods of short anxiolysis in the United States, it has been withdrawn in several countries owing to adverse psychological events. Clinical trials by UpJohn (Kalamazoo, MI, USA) demonstrated an unfavorable risk with about 10% of patients dropping out of one study versus 1.9% of trial subjects taking flurazepam.[24] In other studies, patients on a 3-week course of triazolam became markedly anxious after discontinuation.[25] Its continued use in the United States is under controversy.

Anticonvulsants with Analgesic Properties

Development continues in the medical management of trigeminal neuralgia. Low-dose anticonvulsants have been well established in the treatment of chronic neuropathic pain. Carbamazepine and phenytoin are used to inhibit excessive release of glutamate, thus disrupting the development of central sensitization and decreasing the incidence hyperalgesia and allodynia. Recently studies now add the anticonvulsant gabapentin in the treatment of chronic pain. Cheshire,[26] in a retrospective study, examined the effects of gabapentin on 92 subjects with about two-thirds showing reduction in facial pain at 8 months. Two recent randomized controlled studies found pain reduction in the treatment of diabetic neuropathy and postherpetic neuralgia.[27] In comparison with other anticonvulsants, gabapentin has few interactions with other drugs and fewer side effects.

Current Trends in Pain Management Delivery Systems

In the mid 1990s, a transdermal application of fentanyl was made available to provide continuous opioid administration. Its application is largely in patients with chronic pain or those who cannot take medications orally. Transdermal opioids are contraindicated for use in acute postoperative pain, because of the risk of respiratory depression. They have a slow onset of action, which makes them difficult to titrate. A minimum of 30 days of oral opioid use is required before initiation of transdermal fentanyl.

First developed in 1950, patient-controlled analgesia (PCA) continues to be an effective technique in providing postoperative analgesia. This technique allows the patient to control the amount of analgesia at programmed intervals with set lockout and baseline dosages. PCA provides the advantage of relieving pain at onset and minimizing central sensitization. Recent advances in this field include use of a fentanyl iontophoretic transdermal system, which delivers set doses of fentanyl by iontophoresis through electronic transport. The system uses a low current to move fentanyl stored in a hydrogel reservoir toward the skin. Fentanyl then diffuses into the local circulation and is transported to the central nervous system. The transdermal patch is approximately 10 × 6 cm and is worn on the patient's upper arm. This new system allows for PCA without IV access, bypasses pump failure from traditional IV PCA regimens, and eliminates active metabolites from morphine PCA. Studies have shown fentanyl PCA transdermal systems to be equivalent to IV PCA.[28]

Current Trends in Surgical Modalities

Continued development in imaging has also renewed the application of older technologies. Gamma knife radiosurgery was developed in the 1960s but had limited application because of poor imaging modalities. The gamma knife is a device that focuses the intersection of 201 beams of gamma rays from a cobalt-60 energy source to perform radiosurgery. The evolution of high-resolution computed tomography and magnetic resonance imaging scans coupled with computer technology has allowed for precise targeting of the gamma radiosurgery with improved outcomes in the treatment of trigeminal neuralgia.

Studies from the University of Pittsburgh demonstrated that gamma knife radiosurgery resulted in an 82.3% success rate in the reduction or resolution of trigeminal pain.[29] Possible complications include facial numbness and relapse of pain, which developed in 6% of patients. Unlike traditional surgery, gamma radiosurgery avoids complications of infection, cerebrospinal fluid leak, hematoma formation, facial paralysis, and other nerve injury.[29]

CURRENT ADVANCES IN ANXIETY MANAGEMENT

Advances in management of anxiety have continued to focus on the development of holistic and behavioral therapies. Coping mechanisms and strategies involving imagery, massage, breathing techniques, music intervention, and other relaxation techniques have been used successfully for decades.

One such therapy modality is the ADVANCE protocol used in the preoperative setting for children. The ADVANCE (anxiety reduction, distraction, video modeling and education, adding parents, no excessive reassurance, coaching, and exposure/ shaping) program focuses on family-centered preparation involving both the parent and child. This multimodal program provides procedural information, training in coping mechanisms, and an exposure plan for both parents and children. Studies demonstrated that families participating in the program had lower preoperative anxiety with decreased incidence of emergence delirium, less need for analgesics, and reduced time to discharge.[30]

Music therapy is becoming a popular modality in the treatment of preoperative and postoperative anxiety. Studies from St Mary's Hospital, Milwaukee, Wisconsin, investigated the role of music therapy in the postoperative setting for ambulatory patients.[31] Patients were assigned to a music therapy group along with the preoperative instructions or a control group where they received preoperative instruction alone. Heart rate, blood pressure, and respiratory rates were measured to assess anxiety. Results demonstrated that the patients exposed to music had reduced levels of stress, as indicated by vital signs.[31]

Miluk-Kolasa and colleagues[32] demonstrated that music therapy reduced stress by sampling the cortisol level in saliva in presurgical patients. All subjects were given presurgical instructions, but only half received 1 hour of music therapy shortly after. Results showed markedly higher salivary cortical level in the non-music group,[32] emphasizing again the positive effect of music therapy on stress and anxiety levels.

Imagery is another holistic device used to alleviate anxiety and stress. Patients are guided through their imagination toward a relaxed, focused state. The theory behind guided imagery is based on the concept that the body and mind are connected.

Patients are then instructed to use their senses to help create a mental picture of a safe or relaxing environment. Preliminary data show some promise to these techniques, but more research in clearly needed.[33]

SUMMARY

In light of preoperative and postoperative mortality and morbidity, continued advancement in pain and anxiety management would benefit millions. Although significant strides have been made in the past few decades, it is imperative that research and development continue. The basis of any doctor-patient relationship begins with trust. It is important to remember that among the chief complaints is usually pain accompanied by a dose of anxiety. To ignore these concerns would subvert this trust and ultimately render any subsequent treatment void from lack of patient compliance. Hopefully, with future developments we will be able to treat those patients who were in past generations "beyond treatment."

REFERENCES

1. Meldrum ML. A capsule history of pain management. JAMA 2003;290:2470–5.
2. Pernick MS. A calculus of suffering: pain, professionalism, and anesthesia in nineteenth-century America. New York: Columbia University Press; 1985.
3. Milgrom P, Weinstein P, Getz T. Treating fearful dental patients: a patient management handbook. 2nd edition. Seattle (WA): University of Washington; 1995.
4. Gatchel RJ, Ingersoll BD, Bowman L, et al. The prevalence of dental fear and avoidance: a recent survey study. J Am Dent Assoc 1983;4:609–10.
5. American pain society: press room, media backgrounder. Available at: www.ampainsoc.org. Accessed July 13, 2010.
6. Merskey H, Bogduk N. Part III: pain terms, a current list with definitions and notes on usage classification of chronic pain. IASP Task Force on Taxonomy. 2nd edition. Seattle (WA): IASP Press; 1994. p. 209–14.
7. Loeser JD, Treede RD. The Kyoto protocol of IASP basic pain terminology. Pain 2008;137(3):473–7.
8. Morgan GE, Mikhail MS, Murray MJ. Clinical anesthesiology. 4th edition. New York (NY): McGraw-Hill Medical; 2005.
9. Definition of anxiety. Available at: http://www.thefreedictionary.com/anxiety+control. Accessed September 9, 2010.
10. Kain ZN, Sevarino F, Alexander GM, et al. Preoperative anxiety and postoperative pain in women undergoing hysterectomy. A repeated-measures design. J Psychosom Res 2000;49:417–22.
11. Kain ZN, Sevarino F, Pincus S, et al. Attenuation of the preoperative stress response with midazolam: effects on postoperative outcomes. Anesthesiology 2000;93:141–7.
12. Ploghaus A, Narain C, Beckmann CF, et al. Exacerbation of pain by anxiety is associated with activity in a hippocampal network. J Neurosci 2001;21(24):9896–903.
13. Kain ZN, Sevarino FB, Rinder C, et al. Preoperative anxiolysis and postoperative recovery in women undergoing abdominal hysterectomy. Anesthesiology 2001;94:415–22.
14. Cooper IS, Braceland F. The psychosomatic aspects of pain. Med Clin North Am 1950;34:981.
15. Seeling W, Rockemann M. Influence of postoperative pain on morbidity and mortality. Schmerz 1993;7(2):85–96.

16. Tzschentke TM, Christoph T, Kögel B, et al. A novel μ-opioid receptor agonist/ norepinephrine reuptake inhibitor with broad-spectrum analgesic properties. J Pharmacol Exp Ther 2007;323(1):265–76.

17. Two new analgesics may help patients after bunionectomy. J Anaesthesiol Clin Pharmacol September 26, 2006. Available at: http://www.joacp.org/index.php?option=com_content&task=view&id=48&Itemid=58. Accessed September 20, 2007.

18. Tramadol drug information, professional. Available at: http://www.drugs.com/tramadol.html. Accessed September 9, 2010.

19. Dayer P, Desmeules J, Collart L. Pharmacology of tramadol. Drugs 1997;53(Suppl 2): 18–24.

20. Warning letter, Department of Health and Human Services. Available at: http://74.125.93.132/search?q=cache%253Aplw2Pm_16SMJ%253Awww.fda.gov%252Fdownloads%252FDrugs%252FguidanceComplianceRegulatoryinformation%252FEnforcementActivitiesbyFDA%252FWarningLettersandNoticeofViolationLettersto PharmaceuticalCompanies%252FUCM153130.pdf+ultram+abuse+fda&;hl=en. Accessed September 9, 2010.

21. Diprivan indications and dosage. Available at: http://www.rxlist.com/diprivan-drug.htm. Accessed July 14, 2010.

22. Propofol drug information, professional. Available at: http://www.drugs.com/MMX/Propofol.html. Accessed July 14, 2010.

23. Remifentanil drug information, professional. Available at: www.rxlist.com/ultiva-drug.htm. Accessed July 14, 2010.

24. Adam K, Oswald J. Triazolam. Unpublished manufacturer's research unfavourable. BMJ 1993;306(6890):1475–6.

25. Bramness JG, Olsen H. Adverse effects of zopiclone. Tidsskr Nor Laegeforen 1998;118(13):2029–32 [in Norwegian].

26. Cheshire WP Jr. Defining the role for gabapentin in the treatment of trigeminal neuralgia: a retrospective study. J Pain 2002;3(2):137–42.

27. Backonja M, Hes MS, LaMoreaux LK, et al. US Gabapentin Study Group 210. Gabapentin (GBP, Neurontin) reduces pain in diabetics with painful peripheral neuropathy: results of a double-blind, placebo-controlled clinical trial (945–210). Proceedings of the 16th annual meeting of the American Pain Society. New Orleans (LA), October 23–6, 1997.

28. Viscusi ER, Reynolds L, Chung F, et al. Patient-controlled transdermal fentanyl hydrochloride vs intravenous morphine pump for postoperative pain: a randomized controlled trial. JAMA 2004;291(11):1333–41.

29. University of Pittsburgh, Department of Neurological Surgery. Center for Image-Guided Neurosurgery: trigeminal neuralgia treatment. Available at: http://www.neurosurgery.pitt.edu/imageguided/trigeminal_neuralgia.html. Accessed September 20, 2010.

30. Kain ZN, Caldwell-Andrews AA, Mayes LC, et al. Family-centered preparation for surgery improves perioperative outcomes in children: a randomized controlled trial. Anesthesiology 2007;106:65–74.

31. Augustine P, Hains AA. Effect of music on ambulatory surgery patients' postoperative anxiety. AORN 1996;63:4750.

32. Miluk-Kolasa B, Obminski Z, Stupnicki R, et al. Effects of music treatment on salivary cortisol in patients exposed to pre-surgical stress. Exp Clin Endocrinol 1994; 102(2):118–20.

33. Ackerman CJ, Turkoski B. Using guided imagery to reduce pain and anxiety. Home Healthc Nurse 2000;18(8):524–30.

Advances in Dental Materials

Ram M. Vaderhobli, DDS, MS

KEYWORDS

• Dental materials • Pit and fissure sealants • Glass ionomers
• Composites

The use of materials to rehabilitate tooth structures is constantly changing to the benefit of the patient and clinician. Over the past decade, newer material processing techniques and technologies have significantly improved the dependability and predictability of dental material for clinicians. The greatest obstacle, however, is in choosing the right combination for continued success. Finding predictable approaches for successful restorative procedures has been the goal of clinical and material scientists. Any dental material used in the oral cavity must satisfy some basic perquisites: they must be similar to tooth structures in their physical and mechanical properties, resist masticatory forces, and possess an appearance similar to natural dentin and enamel. Restorative materials used in the oral environment must fulfill form, function, esthetics, and biocompatibility. The ideal material, however, does not exist because many do not fulfill all prerequisites. Fortunately, recent advances in material science, which are described in this article, have closed the gap significantly. This article provides a broad perspective on the advances in functionality of various classes of dental restorative materials, namely pit and fissure sealants, glass ionomers, and dental composites.

PIT AND FISSURE SEALANTS

Several improvements have been made in the materials that are used as sealants. Fluoride-containing sealants were introduced to dentistry with an expected benefit from their anticariogenic properties. This sealant consists of dimethacrylate monomers with sodium fluoride and poly (methyl methacrylate-co-methacryloyl) fluoride.[1] However, compared with the glass ionomers, these resin sealants have less total availability and release of fluoride to induce anticariogenic effects.[2] The addition of fluoride did not alter the retention properties of the sealants, causing manufacturers to develop techniques of incorporating fluoride ions onto the resin chemistry. Clinical data proving the anticaries advantage of these fluoride-containing sealants are still lacking.

The author has nothing to disclose.

Department of Preventive and Restorative Dentistry, University of California San Francisco, Box 0758, 707 Parnassus Avenue, San Francisco, CA 94143-0758, USA

E-mail address: ram.vaderhobli@ucsf.edu

Dent Clin N Am 55 (2011) 619–625
doi:10.1016/j.cden.2011.02.015
0011-8532/11/$ – see front matter © 2011 Elsevier Inc. All rights reserved.

In effort to improve the longevity of these sealants, researchers and clinicians suggest incorporating a bonding agent layer between the sealants and the saliva-contaminated enamel. This technique shows promise, with better retention of these sealants and reduced microleakage in both in vitro and in vivo studies.[3] The addition of a bonding agent decreases the risk for failure by 47% for occlusal sealants and 65% for buccal/lingual sealants.[4] One potential explanation could be attributed to the flexibility features offered by the newer generations of bonding agents, especially when they were analyzed in class v restorations.[5] The combined primer, adhesive, and resin complex layer resulted in a stronger long-term bond.

Subsequently, with the development of the self-etching adhesive resin, clinicians began to evaluate the efficacy of using a self-etching adhesive before sealant placement. This step minimized treatment time and potential errors in technique, and had better patient compliance. One self-etching adhesive clinically tested for 2 years was the Prompt L-Pop (3M ESPE, St Paul, MN, USA). The 2-year data show comparable sealant retention against normal etch and seal methods.[6] Glass ionomers are also being used as a surface protectant because they can flow more readily into pits and fissures, as shown by their clinical effectiveness.[7] The explanation could be attributed to the fact that fluoride content in glass ionomers is higher than in the tooth. When used as sealants, the ion exchange process causes fluoride ions to diffuse from the cement onto the tooth, transforming some of the hydroxyapatite into fluorohydroxyapatite, and making it more caries-resistant.[8]

Official American Dental Association (ADA) guidelines recommend the use of glass ionomer sealers only on partially erupted teeth or deciduous teeth, and the use of resins on permanent teeth. The latest glass ionomer, Ketac Nano (3M ESPE Dental Products, St Paul, MN, USA), is nano-filled and could change the guidelines if clinical trials on wear rates are favorable. Currently, strong support in the literature favors bonding dental sealants or the use of glass ionomers as a pit and fissure sealant on surfaces determined to be at high risk for caries. The drawback, however, is the lack of long-term clinical longevity data.[9]

GLASS IONOMER MATERIALS

The use-based classification for glass ionomer materials includes crown cementation, restorations, liners and bases, fissure sealants, orthodontic cements, and buildups in non–stress-bearing situations. ADA classification for glass ionomers include type 1, which are cements, and type 2, which are filling materials (class 2, 3, 5).

Glass ionomers have been one of the most widely researched dental materials since their introduction in the 1970s. They have a coefficient of thermal expansion similar to dentin and can be bulk-filled and finished faster than a composite. The newer generations of glass ionomer materials are faster setting and no longer sensitive to hydration or desiccation during setting. They are used more regularly as intermediate restorations, adhesive cavity liners (sandwich technique), and atraumatic restorative material. However, their use in load-bearing situations is still unreliable.

One main advantage of glass ionomer materials is their chemical bonding ability to tooth structure, making them more resistant to leaks. Compared with resin system bonding, glass ionomer bonding is more degeneration-resistant and does not breakup, unlike the hydrolytic degradation of the hybrid layer of the resin system.[10] Literature from laboratory studies supports the application of these adhesive materials to perform therapeutic actions on demineralized tissues because of the potential for bother uptake of fluoride ions and release and recharge by fluoride-containing toothpastes. However, clinical trials supporting this work are still uncertain.[11–13]

The most recently accepted uses of glass ionomers have been as a liner and base under deep composite restorations, which has been referred to as the *sandwich technique,* Deep cervical lesions and proximal boxes of class II cavities whose gingival floor is on root surfaces are areas where there is increased diameter of dentinal tubules that will affect the bond strength because of increased chances of hydrolytic degradation. Because of their chemical bonding capabilities, glass ionomer adhere to these surface better then dental adhesive-bonding agents. Based on evidence-based dentistry protocols, the recommendation is to treat the surfaces with a polyacrylic acid conditioner, which is rinsed before glass ionomers are applied. This weak acid modifies the smear layer by leaving the smear plugs behind, improving the seal and eliminating postoperative sensitivity. A new self-conditioner for resin-modified glass ionomers, recently developed by Fuji (GC America, IL, USA), does not require rinsing before applying the glass ionomer material.[14] Both Fuji II and Fuji IX (GC America, IL, USA) have unique automix dispensing capsules, simplifying placement of these materials. Resin-modified ionomers, such as Fuji II LC, are routinely used as liners at 1 mm or less, and a material such as Fuji IX or Riva (SDI, Bensenville, IL, USA) is preferred for larger areas of dentin replacement.

Based on abundant evidence, conventional and metal-modified glass ionomers are not recommended in class 2 restorations in both primary and permanent molars.[15–17] To compensate for this, resin-modified glass ionomer cements were developed to produce better mechanical properties than the conventional ones. The resin hydrox-yethyl methacrylate (HEMA) or bis-glycerol methacrylate was added to the liquid. The resin modification of these cements allowed the base curing reaction to be supplemented by a light or chemical curing process, allowing for a command set. The obvious advantages were better fracture toughness, increased tensile strength, and a decrease in desiccation and hydration problems.[18] The limiting factors were the setting shrinkage, which was found to be greater than with conventional cements, and the limited depth of cure with more opaque lining cements.[19] The mean age of these failed glass ionomer restorations at replacement in permanent teeth in general practice was found to be 5.5 years for patients older than 30 years.[20] Secondary caries, bulk fracture (1.4%–14%), and marginal fracture (from poor anatomic form) constituted the main reasons for failure.[21,22]

In developing countries, highly viscous glass ionomer materials have became popular in atraumatic restorative treatment techniques for class 1 restorations in posterior teeth. In class 2 restorations, these high viscous glass ionomers are still considered satisfactory after 3 years of clinical service, despite large percentages of failed restorations.[23,24] However, a recently concluded retrospective study showed that the failure of class 2 restorations with these materials rose to 60% at 72 months. It was hypothesized that caries-like loss of material was seen on radiographs and that the presence of proximal contacts promoted disintegration of these materials.[25]

In effort to provide easier manipulation and reduced variability of the physical properties, dental material companies have introduced a paste/paste glass ionomer dispensing system. Examples include the Ketac Nano (3M ESPE Dental Products, St Paul, MN, USA) light-curing glass ionomer, which is the first paste/paste resin-modified glass ionomer developed with nanotechnology. The nano fillers are blended with fluoroaluminosilicate technology. Laboratory studies support these nano-ionomers, but clinical data will prove their ultimate efficacy.[26]

Vanish XT (3M ESPE Dental Products, St Paul, MN, USA) is a newly developed resin-modified glass ionomer material that releases fluoride, calcium, and phosphate. It is currently used as a site-specific, light-cured durable coating that provides an immediate layer of protection to relieve dentinal hypersensitivity through occluding the dentinal tubules.

The newer generations of glass-ionomers are anticipated to be amino acid–modified and non–HEMA-containing glass ionomers materials, because they are being researched extensively to reduce deficiencies of the present generation of glass ionomers, especially in terms of their strength. The technique of ultrasound application to improve the mechanical properties during hardening of the glass ionomer cement seems promising and intriguing.[27]

DENTAL COMPOSITES

High polymerization shrinkage, increased marginal leakage with frequent secondary caries, and postoperative sensitivity have been concerns with dental composites. When adhesively bonding restorations, one should keep in mind the C-factor, or the cavity configuration factor. The C-factor is the ratio of the bonded surface area to the unbonded surface area.[28] The higher the C-factor, the greater are the shrinkage stresses on curing. In a class 1 cavity, the C-factor is five (high) and unfavorable, resulting in more shrinkage of the adhesively bonded restoration. One recommended clinical technique to counteract this high polymerization shrinkage is the use of an appropriate layering technique and incremental curing of composites.[29] Theoretically, these problems arise because of shrinkage in composites, which is unavoidable, and range in incidence from 2% to 5%.

These problems occur because when a viscous composite is placed inside the cavity walls and light-cured, it transforms to a viscoelastic and then to an elastic or a cured state. Stress is always initiated and builds up during the viscoelastic state, and is relieved as the material flows to its cured state. However, once the composite gets cured, flow no longer occurs and the stresses that are built up must be relieved. The stresses are relieved as shrinkage stresses, which are transmitted to the surrounding rigid confounding walls of the cavity preparation.[30] If a sterile gap-free hybrid layer is absent, the shrinkage stress forces will exceed the bond strength of the tooth restoration interface, resulting in loss of adhesion and leading to gap formation, marginal leakage, secondary caries, and postoperative sensitivity.

These problems were the inherent limitations of the hybrid and microfill composites, and required dentists to layer both the hybrid and microfill composites to compensate for these inequities, requiring more technical control in creating predictable restorations. Innovation in dental composite manufacturing technology focuses on improving these limitations, particularly to maximize aesthetic potential while simultaneously maintaining the mechanical properties to withstand masticatory forces. Advancements in composite manufacturing technology have included the filers in terms of particle size, particle shape, filler type, and changing the type of monomer.

With the increasing use of nanotechnology in material science, dental material companies have focused on developing nanocomposites with excellent polish retention (typical of a microfill) and mechanical properties ideal for high stress-bearing situations (typical of a hybrid). The use of synthetic chemical processes allowed nanofillers to be produced on a molecular scale (3M ESPE Dental Products, St Paul, MN, USA), ranging from 0.1 to 100 nm. The wavelength of light is known to range from 0.4 to 0.8 μm, and when these fillers are shrunk to a fraction of the visible light, then detection of the particles becomes impossible because they cannot scatter that particular light and become well concealed, replicating optical properties of the natural tooth.[31] Because the filler particles are dramatically smaller in size, they can be packed in high concentrations, imparting excellent mechanical strengths.

Furthermore, because the fillers are in the nano scale, the composites have excellent adhesion to the nanoscopic (1–10 nm) tooth structures, resulting in excellent adhesion and stabilization on the dental joint. Because of these obvious reasons, clinicians are able to construct more predictable conservative tooth preparation designs.[32]

Innovation in monomer technology from DuPont resulted in the development of Kalore (GC America, IL, USA), a new universal composite resin. Researchers at DuPont were able to create a stiff monomer core with flexible arms that resulted in putty-like properties, allowing the composite to be spread easily and sculpted without slumping. The removal of the shorter-chain methacrylate matrix (commonly seen in regular composites) by this new monomer resulted in a universal composite with less shrinkage and less polymerization shrinkage stress.[33] This composite is offered in universal, translucent, and opaque shades, allowing clinicians to layer the resin the way a dental laboratory technician would layer porcelain to create life-like restorations.

Flowable composites are becoming more popular with clinicians worldwide. They are less rigid because of reduced filler content, which imparts favorable modulus of elasticity and results in less polymerization stresses. Furthermore, because of their favorable handling properties, they are used as the first layer of composite resin after the adhesive is placed to ensure precise wetting of the adhesive surface and to act as a stress-absorbing layer before a more rigid composite is placed.[34] Other applications of flowable composites include pit and fissure sealing, orthodontic bracket bonding, and restoration of small-sized class 1 cavities. Newer generations of flowable composites have been developed within the past year using the self-etch adhesive concept of bonding resins (seventh generation). This newer flowable composite (Vertise Flow, Kerr Corp, Orange, CA, USA) combines the adhesive properties of a bonding agent and a flowable composite to simplify direct restoration placement, making it the first self-adhering composite material on the market. Older systems of flowable composite resins relied on the combined use of a dental bonding system to adhesively bond to tooth structure. With the development of all-in-one adhesive systems, the adhesion process is simplified based on the self-etch method and combines etching, priming, and bonding into a single application step.[35]

However, even though the single-step adhesive systems seem attractive, they are still being researched extensively for the long-term durability of their bond. Nevertheless, the self-adhering composite resins eliminate the need for a separate bonding application step and represent what dental material scientists believe to be the eighth generation of dental adhesive systems. This generation of composite resins bond to tooth structure through micromechanical and chemical bonding via the phosphate functional group of the glycerophosphoric acid dimethacrylate monomer and calcium ions of the tooth. Currently, they are being used clinically in small class 1 stand-alone cavities and require a brushing motion of 15 to 20 seconds with 0.5 mm of the material and light curing for 20 seconds. As for any new material, clinical studies are required to prove their strengths. A 6-month clinical trial on 40 subjects exhibited satisfactory clinical performance with no reported postoperative sensitivity.[36] However, long-term clinical studies are required to substantiate their preliminary promising characteristics.

SUMMARY

The goal of dental material research is to augment the practice of dentistry. Use of technology such as nano technology has improved the mechanical characteristics of materials for clinical use and will definitively prolong their clinical life. According to the BCC Research report, *The Dental Market: Techniques, Equipment & Materials*,[37] the United States dental market is projected to grow to almost $10 billion by 2013, with the professional equipment and supplies expected to grow at a compound annual growth (CAG) of 5.8% to reach $4.2 billion in 2013. Changes in monomer technology will result in the next generation of restorative materials having physical, optical, and mechanical properties similar to natural tooth structures. Clinicians have wide array of materials to choose from to achieve their restorative goals, and therefore must know the bonding quality of the material to tooth structures. Bonding to etched enamel is more predictable, but in many clinical situations, because of the lack of enamel, one must know how to choose the best material to provide the best clinical results for patients.

REFERENCES

1. Tanaka M, Matsunaga K, Kadoma Y, et al. Use of fluoride-containing sealant on proximal surfaces. J Med Dent Sci 2000;47(1):49–54.
2. Garcia-Godoy F, Abarzua I, De Goes MF, et al. Fluoride release from fissure sealants. J Clin Pediatr Dent 1997;22(1):45.
3. Hebling J, Feigal R. Use of one-bottle adhesive as an intermediate bonding layer to reduce sealant microleakage on saliva-contaminated enamel. Am J Dent 2000; 13(4):187.
4. Feigal RJ, Musherurue P, Gillespie B, et al. Improved sealant retention with bonding agents: a clinical study of two-bottle and single-bottle systems. J Dent Res 2000;79(11):1850–6.
5. Kemp-Scholte C, Davidson C. Complete marginal seal of Class V resin composite restorations effected by increased flexibility. J Dent Res 1990;69(6):1240.
6. Feigal R, Quelhas I. Clinical trial of a self-etching adhesive for sealant application: success at 24 months with Prompt L-Pop. Am J Dent 2003;16(4):249.
7. Da Covey W, L Hopper. 2004. Penetration of various pit and fissure sealants into occlusal grooves [abstract 3471]. J Dent Res 83(A):Sequence #359.
8. Forss H, Seppä L. Prevention of enamel demineralization adjacent to glass ionomer filling materials. Eur J Oral Sci 2007;98(2):173–8.
9. Feigal R, Donly K. The use of pit and fissure sealants. Pediatr Dent 2006;28(2): 143–50.
10. Pashley D, Tay F, Yiu C, et al. Collagen degradation by host-derived enzymes during aging. J Dent Res 2004;83(3):216.
11. Kielbassa A, Schulte-Monting J, Garcia Godoy F, et al. Initial in situ secondary caries formation: effect of various fluoride-containing restorative materials. Oper Dent 2003;28(6):765.
12. Gao W, Smales R, Gale MS, et al. Fluoride release/uptake from newer glass-ionomer cements used with the ART approach. Am J Dent 2000;13(4):201.
13. Papagiannoulis L, Kakaboura A, Eliades G, et al. In vivo vs in vitro anticariogenic behavior of glass-ionomer and resin composite restorative materials. Dent Mater 2002;18(8):561.
14. Bishara S, Ostby A, Lafoon J, et al. A self-conditioner for resin-modified glass ionomers in bonding orthodontic brackets. Angle Orthod 2007;77(4):711–5.
15. Hübel S, Mejare I. Conventional versus resin-modified glass-ionomer cement for Class II restorations in primary molars. A 3-year clinical study. Int J Paediatr Dent 2003;13(1):2–8.
16. Naasan M, Watson T. Conventional glass ionomers as posterior restorations. A status report for the American Journal of Dentistry. Am J Dent 1998;11(1):36.
17. Qvist V, Laurberg L, Poulsen A, et al. Eight-year study on conventional glass ionomer and amalgam restorations in primary teeth. Acta Odontol Scand 2004; 62(1):37–45.

18. Davidson C. Advances in glass-ionomer cements. J Appl Oral Sci 2006;14:3–9.
19. Attin T, Buchalla W, Keilbassa AM, et al. Curing shrinkage and volumetric changes of resin-modified glass ionomer restorative materials. Dent Mater 1995;11(5–6):359–62.
20. Mjör I, Dahl J, Moorhead JE, et al. Age of restorations at replacement in permanent teeth in general dental practice. Acta Odontol Scand 2000;58(3):97–101.
21. Hickel R, Manhart J. Longevity of restorations in posterior teeth and reasons for failure. J Adhes Dent 2001;3:45–64.
22. Mjör I, Moorhead J, Dahl JE, et al. Reasons for replacement of restorations in permanent teeth in general dental practice. Int Dent J 2000;50(6):361.
23. Burke F, Wilson N. Glass-ionomer restorations in stress-bearing and difficult-to-access cavities. In: Davidson CL, Mjör IA, editors. Advances in glass-ionomer cements. Chicago (IL): Quintessence Publishing Co; 1999. p. 253–8.
24. Taifour D, Frencken J, Beiruti N, et al. Effectiveness of glass-ionomer (ART) and amalgam restorations in the deciduous dentition: results after 3 years. Caries Res 2000;36(6):437–44.
25. Scholtanus J, Huysmans M. Clinical failure of class-II restorations of a highly viscous glass-ionomer material over a 6-year period: a retrospective study. J Dent 2007;35(2):156–62.
26. Uysal T, Yagci A, Uysal B, et al. Are nano-composites and nano-ionomers suitable for orthodontic bracket bonding? Eur J Orthod 2010;32(1):78–82.
27. Kleverlaan C, van Duinen R, Feilzer AJ, et al. Mechanical properties of glass ionomer cements affected by curing methods. Dent Mater 2004;20(1):45–50.
28. Feilzer A, De Gee A, Davidson CL, et al. Setting stress in composite resin in relation to configuration of the restoration. J Dent Res 1987;66(11):1636.
29. Ferracane J. Developing a more complete understanding of stresses produced in dental composites during polymerization. Dent Mater 2005;21(1):36–42.
30. Feilzer A, Dooren L, dee Gee AJ, et al. Influence of light intensity on polymerization shrinkage and integrity of restoration-cavity interface. Eur J Oral Sci 1995; 103(5):322–6.
31. Mitra S, Wu D, Holmes BN, et al. An application of nanotechnology in advanced dental materials. J Am Dent Assoc 2003;134(10):1382.
32. Terry D, Leinfelder K, Blatz MB, et al. Achieving excellence using an advanced biomaterial: part 2. Dent Today 2009;28(11):69.
33. Lowe R. Combining technologies to improve aesthetics. Dent Today 2010;29(4): 118, 120–3.
34. Unterbrink G, Liebenberg W. Flowable resin composites as "filled adhesives": literature review and clinical recommendations. Quintessence Int 1999;30(4):249.
35. De Munck J, Van Landuyt K, Peuman M, et al. A critical review of the durability of adhesion to tooth tissue: methods and results. J Dent Res 2005;84(2):118.
36. Vichi A, Goracci C, Ferrari M. Clinical study of the self-adhering flowable composite resin Vertise Flow in Class I restorations: six-month follow-up. International Dentistry-Australasian Edition 2010;5(2):14–24.
37. BCC Research Web site. The dental market: techniques, equipment & materials. Available at: http://www.bccresearch.com/report/HLC028C.html. Accessed March 4, 2011.

Technological Updates in Dental Photography

Josh Shagam, BS[a],*, Alan Kleiman, DMD[b,c,d]

KEYWORDS

- Digital photography • Image workflow • Imaging equipment
- Digital storage • Dental photography

The purpose of this article is to highlight the changes and developments related to digital photography specifically, within the context of dentistry. As with all technology, each year brings updates and improvements to the newest software and hardware available. Software that streamlines digital workflow management, increasingly inexpensive storage media, and better camera sensors have all pushed the use of dental photography forward in the past 5 years. In the following sections, the intention is to provide a brief overview of the overarching elements of the medium as it pertains to dental photography.

One of the most comprehensive and informative resources pertaining to traditional external photography for dental applications is Dr Wolfgang Bengel's[1] *Mastering Digital Dental Photography*. Due to the inherently evolving nature of technology, some new elements not covered in that publication are highlighted here. Software in particular has adopted a very consistent, albeit rapid, development cycle whereby new editions supplant earlier ones every 12 to 18 months. Owning the newest piece of software or hardware is far from necessary, but an overall understanding of the developments in the medium is a powerful way to best use it as a tool.

FILE FORMATS

Today, the majority of "prosumer" (professional consumer) and professional digital single-lens reflex (DSLR) cameras have the ability to record captured images in a type of file known as "raw"—though the actual file extensions and compatibility of

a Department of Biomedical Photographic Communications, Rochester Institute of Technology, Rochester NY 14623, USA
b Department of Oral & Maxillofacial Surgery, New Jersey Dental School, University of Medicine and Dentistry of New Jersey, 110 Bergen Street, Newark, NJ 07103-2400, USA
c Department of Community Health, New Jersey Dental School, University of Medicine and Dentistry of New Jersey, 110 Bergen Street, Newark, NJ 07103-2400, USA
d Private Practice, 21 East Main Street, Moorestown, NJ 08057-3309, USA
* Corresponding author.
E-mail address: josh.shagam@gmail.com

Dent Clin N Am 55 (2011) 627–633
doi:10.1016/j.cden.2011.02.016
0011-8532/11/$ – see front matter © 2011 Elsevier Inc. All rights reserved.

dental.theclinics.com

these is not completely standardized or universal. The raw format essentially holds on to all of the recorded data at the time of capture without making postprocessing decisions that irreversibly alter the interpretation of this data. This information can be adjusted after it is uploaded to computer, maintaining the flexibility to always go back to the original, unaltered image file. Analogous to the latent image recorded on film, the image data must be processed to create a useable photograph. The Joint Photographic Experts Group (JPEG) format is perhaps the most widely used file format for general sharing of digital photos and is used by point-and-shoot cameras; JPEG images are actually a compressed form of the original data that a camera sensor is capable of capturing. This compression trades some data for more manageable file sizes. When elements of a photograph are critical to keep accurate and repeat editing is a concern (saving a JPEG repeatedly will compound data compression and enhance noise), the photographer should shoot in the raw format.

There is no single raw format, however. Different camera manufacturers—namely, Nikon and Canon—develop their own file language that requires their own code to decipher them. Raw editing software is capable of handling more than one type of raw file, but it must be updated with multiple file types (there are over 100 different raw formats).[2] The proprietary nature of these formats is a subject of concern for some photographers, raising the question of the lifespan of digital photographs over that of physical film. Since raw files are proprietary by nature, much of the data interpretation and usability is controlled by the manufacturers and software developers. If a format ceases to be supported by the software, the user is left with files that cannot be opened.

In an effort to address this concern, Adobe Systems Incorporated introduced a new type of raw file in 2004: the Digital Negative (DNG), with the goal of establishing a "legacy" format that will remain compatible for years to come and to establish a future-proof solution for archiving digital photographic files. As Adobe's press release of the time stated, "current raw formats are unsuitable for archiving because they are generally undocumented and tied to specific camera models, introducing the risk that the format will not be supported over time."[3] The format is naturally supported by Adobe's own product line (Bridge, Photoshop, Photoshop Elements, Lightroom), but is also supported by GIMP, Corel Paint Shop Pro X, and Apple's Aperture 3.[4,5] The debate continues on whether the DNG format is a suitable legacy format.

If long-term storage and organization of dental photographic files is an important element to the photographer's workflow and archiving needs, the DNG format is worth exploring in depth. A small number of cameras are able to output directly to DNG, including some Leica, Samsung, and Hasselblad models; any common raw format such at NEF (Nikon) or CR2 (Canon) can be converted after the fact using software such as Adobe Camera raw or Adobe's DNG Converter.[6] The DNG files retain raw functionality and in some cases can prove to be more compatible with other software.

DIGITAL CAMERAS AND EQUIPMENT

Digital cameras are constantly evolving with more megapixels, better low-light performance, and dozens of other features to stand out among the numerous options available to the professional and the consumer alike. One issue that has plagued DSLR cameras is dust accumulating on the Charge-Coupled Device (CCD) sensor. This occurs because of the interchangeable-lens capability of the DSLR, something that a photographer will make use of when switching between a "normal" lens (18 mm–50 mm) to a macro lens for close-up work. As a point of reference, in 2005, one of the only cameras designed to address this issue in its hardware was the Olympus E-1.[7] This camera featured a vibrating sensor that knocked any resting dust particles off the CCD. Since then, many camera models have adopted similar technologies. The Canon 5D Mark II, for example, uses ultra-sonic vibrations each time the camera is turned on and off to ensure that new dust particles do not hinder photographs taken after switching lenses. This camera also features a 21.1 megapixel sensor, which may be more pixel resolution than is necessary for screen display or small prints.[8] This is a key aspect to consider when upgrading camera bodies; the upgrade should be justified in terms of other factors and not simply megapixels because this alone does not offer a benefit to workflow or output potential in the context of a dental practice, especially when considering the additional storage space needed to the accommodate larger files sizes that a larger sensor produces.

For general dental photography, the combination of a macro lens and ring flash is a highly capable imaging system. The Canon MR-14EX Macro Ring Lite[9] is Canon's own flash unit that has been around for a number of years, while Nikon users have the R1 Wireless Close-Up Speedlight System.[10] Though they have somewhat different form factors, they have the flexibility of controlling lighting ratios and firing one or both sides for more directional or even light, respectively. A second option for Nikon cameras is the Canfield Twinflash,[11] a third-party flash unit that has the option of attaching a flip-down set of polarizing filters to eliminate reflections from wet surfaces.

For the advanced user with a strong grasp on raw processing, including a calibrated reference such as a color checker in photographs for postprocessing color accuracy is a great idea. Many portable products have emerged recently for the "on-the-go" photographer that double as useful macro photography color checkers. These products include the X-Rite ColorChecker Passport[12] and the Macbeth ColorChecker Mini.[13] By including these small cards in dental photographs, the "eyedropper" or comparable tool in Photoshop, Lightroom, or other similar software can establish an accurate white point. This means that sensitive colors such as the shades of teeth can be consistently processed over multiple images and thus over time.

ARCHIVING AND BACKUPS

As cameras continue to increase in megapixel counts and subsequently produce larger files, it is necessary to have a file storage and backup system capable of handling the large volume of data. Personal storage via internal hard drives, external drives, and network-attached solutions offer ease of access, transfer speed, and security. Redundant Array of Independent Disks (RAID) configurations offer increased reliability by providing redundancy in the event of hardware failure, thus limiting loss of data.

Storing digital images also necessitates removable media for off-site storage in case the primary means of storage fails or becomes damaged. The most common approaches have traditionally included burning CDs and DVDs, and investing in additional portable hard drives. DVDs remain an inexpensive option and hard drives consistently grow in size while dropping in price. This characteristic of digital storage is reciprocated by cameras that create increasingly larger file sizes and software; inviting the creation of even larger edited documents (ie, Photoshop Document [PSD] files, composite images). Nevertheless, for smaller-scale photo archiving, DVDs are a readily available option. The use of Blu-ray discs, which expand the typical DVDs' 4.7 gigabyte (GB) limits to 25 GB (single layer, dual-layer can hold 50 GB). Disc drives capable of reading and burning Blu-ray discs, however, are not yet commonplace.

A storage and backup solution that is gaining momentum is the use of the "cloud." Cloud computing is an Internet-centric method of access that puts resources such as software and storage "away" from the user's computer, instead locating them in a virtual space that links to physical storage in another location. Having cloud storage means that there is no need to burn discs or purchase additional hard drives to backup image files—automated backups can be set up that make copies of files that are transferred over the Internet. Services such as Carbonite[14] and Dropbox[15] allow for such off-site storage; Dropbox has the additional functionality of being able to synchronize files and data across different machines that can access the cloud information collaboratively. This can make home-to-office file management easy and secure.

Google Docs is another viable method of sharing and collaborating information. Although it has a stronger emphasis on nonvisual data such as text documents and spreadsheets, archived files such as images can be uploaded to Google's servers where other users can be given access with password protection to view and edit them. Amazon Web Services[16] also offers highly scalable, reliable, and low-latency cloud storage infrastructure on a pay-for-what-you-need basis while addressing the limitations.

Limitations of cloud storage are access to the Internet, connection speed, cost, support, reliability, security or privacy, ownership of data, and retrieval of data in the event of the service provider going out of business. For security, encryption of data during transmission is recommended. Encrypted storage provides an additional layer of security, but may hamper indexing of data at the storage site for easy retrieval. Comparing monthly costs and services that fit the needs of the individual will determine which service offers the best fit for off-site file backup and storage.

EDITING AND WORKFLOW

Adobe Photoshop continues to be the industry standard for image editing. However, a notable shift has come to the available software and workflow methods when handling digital files. In February of 2007,[17] Adobe announced a new program called Photoshop Lightroom (often referred to more simply as Lightroom) designed for the professional photographer to combine some of the features of both Adobe Bridge and Photoshop into an interface that made global adjustments and workflow more streamlined. As with other Adobe products, Lightroom has seen multiple revisions with Lightroom 3 launched in mid-2010.[18]

Adobe Lightroom is a versatile solution for dental photography because it helps simplify the potentially complex workflow of downloading, editing, and archiving photographs. If complex image manipulation is needed such as mocking up treatment outcomes, Photoshop remains the most powerful tool. However, if the needs of the photographer fall more in line with overall adjustments such as exposure, contrast, and color temperature, Lightroom provides these controls while making file management a less difficult task. It also allows adjustments to be made to entire set of images at once, making uniform editing easy. The user interface is broken up into distinct workflow steps: namely, "Library" (organizing and viewing files), "Develop" (adjusting exposure, contrast, etc), "Slideshow" (useful for showing patients directly from the computer monitor), "Print" (discussed below), and "Web" (for Web site publishing) (**Fig. 1**).

When importing images, Lightroom provides the ability to embed metadata in each file as well as batch file renaming. This means that images could be tagged by patient name, treatment, or any other relevant category. At any point following file importation, image files can be sorted and organized by a given metadata tag,

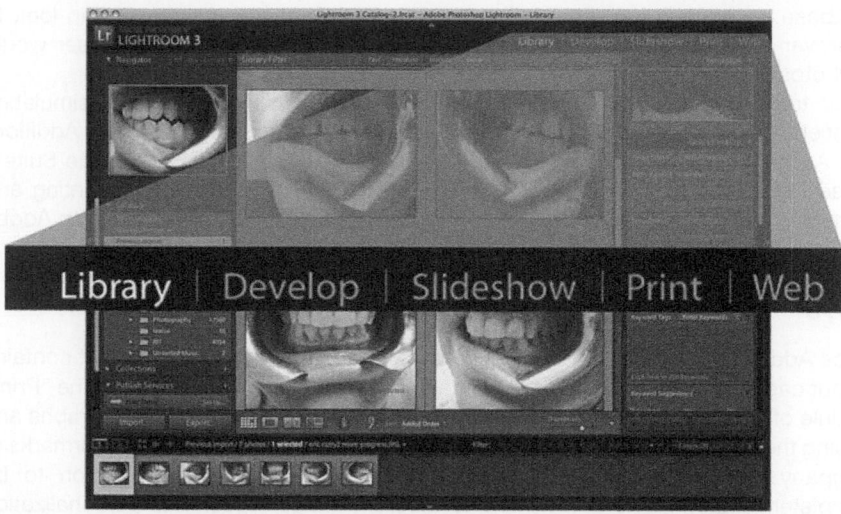

Fig. 1. The Adobe Lightroom 3 interface with workflow modules for organizing, editing, and outputting digital images. (*Courtesy of* Edward Shagam, DDS PA, Medford, NJ.)

including the information recorded by the camera at the time of capture (ie, date, aperture setting, white balance). Such highly configurable file organization is conducive to efficient workflow—with the ability to reorganize and search through archives on demand without setting up a complex image retrieval system or external

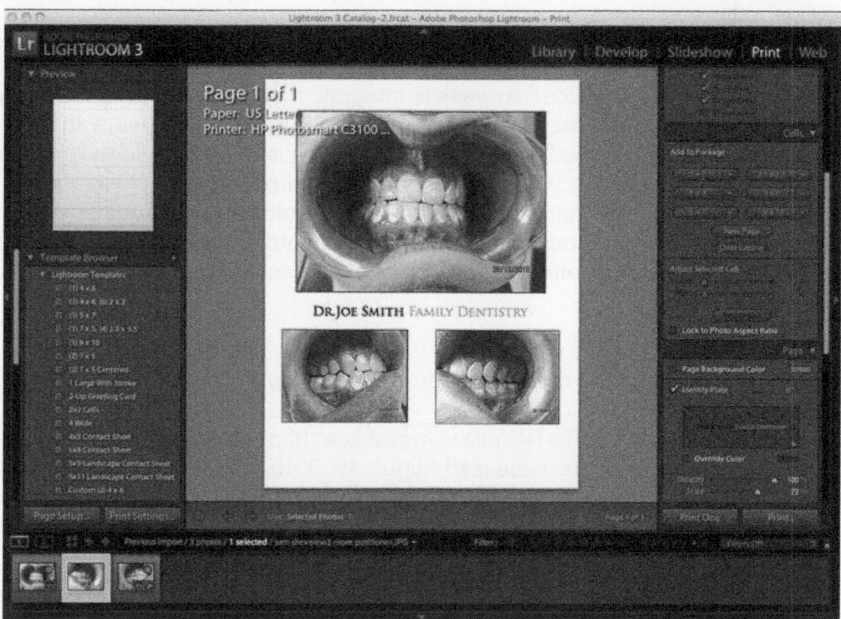

Fig. 2. An example of a custom print template for dental images including a custom logo. (*Courtesy of* Edward Shagam, DDS PA, Medford, NJ.)

database. Lightroom functions more like a catalog in the sense that it can look to wherever the files are stored without opening and editing them as the user would in Photoshop.

For tasks that require more retouching and reconstructing such as simulating a patient's smile after treatment, Adobe Photoshop is the ideal tool to use. Additionally, Adobe introduced a version of its Photoshop line starting with Creative Suite 4 called Photoshop CS4 Extended that includes a number of tools for counting and measurement for the scientific and medical community. The latest release from Adobe is Photoshop CS5, released in April of 2010.[19]

OUTPUT

Since Adobe Lightroom is designed as a workflow tool from start to finish, it contains output capabilities that are useful for patient presentations and education. The "Print" module of Lightroom has straightforward options for taking a set of photographs and placing them proof-style on a page to be printed with options to include watermarks or company logos (**Fig. 2**). Many preset templates allow this presentation to be completely customizable and flexible to different image types. This personalization makes the output product uniquely part of the doctor's approach to patient care. By easily rendering printouts with in-progress or before-and-after photographs, patient consultations can be extremely informative and personal, even providing the option to have them walk out of the office with a visual reminder of the work.

The ability to print photographs using templates is not entirely new to digital photography. However, the development of Adobe Lightroom has made the workflow to create such presentation tools a practical and easy option for getting the most out of digital photography in dentistry. Using the "Slideshow" module, additionally, offers the ability to show the patient the images on the monitor during consultations.

SUMMARY

Digital photography continues to evolve and offer new and exciting utility for dental imaging applications. A practice may seek to integrate these tools and workflow solutions to take advantage of the latest technology. However, as is always the case, having the "latest and greatest" hardware and software is not critical to have a functional dental imaging system that serves a valuable purpose in documentation and illustration. No single combination of equipment and software will produce the best imaging system; the desired personal application of photography to a dental practice necessitates a unique, cost-effective, and comfortable solution.

REFERENCES

1. Bengel W. Mastering digital dental photography. Chicago: Quintessence Publishing; 2006.
2. Reichmann M, Specht J. The RAW flaw. Available at: http://www.luminous-landscape.com/essays/raw-flaw.shtml. Accessed August 15, 2010.
3. Adobe unifies raw photo formats with introduction of digital negative specification. Available at: http://www.adobe.com/aboutadobe/pressroom/pressreleases/200409/092704DNG.html. Accessed August 15, 2010.
4. DNG hardware and software support. Available at: https://www.adobe.com/ap/products/dng/supporters.html. Accessed August 15, 2010.
5. Wide support for RAW formats from leading cameras. Available at: http://www.apple.com/aperture/specs/raw.html. Accessed August 15, 2010.

6. Digital negative (DNG). Available at: http://www.adobe.com/products/dng/supporters.html. Accessed August 15, 2010.
7. Olympus America web site. Available at: http://www.olympusamerica.com/cpg_section/cpg_archived_product_details.asp?fl=2&id=919. Accessed August 15, 2010.
8. EOS 5D mark II. Available at: http://www.usa.canon.com/cusa/consumer/products/cameras/slr_cameras/eos_5d_mark_ii. Accessed August 15, 2010.
9. Macro ring lite MR-14EX. Available at: http://www.usa.canon.com/cusa/consumer/products/cameras/speedlite_flash_lineup/macro_ring_lite_mr_14ex. Accessed August 15, 2010.
10. R1 wireless close-up speedlight system. Available at: http://www.nikonusa.com/Find-Your-Nikon/Product/Flashes/4804/R1-Wireless-Close-Up-Speedlight-System.html. Accessed August 15, 2010.
11. Canfield twinflash & filters. Available at: http://canfieldsci.com/imaging_systems/photography_equipment/Canfield_Twinflash_&_Filters.html. Accessed August 15, 2010.
12. ColorChecker passport. Available at: http://www.xrite.com/product_overview.aspx?ID=1257. Accessed August 15, 2010.
13. ColorChecker mini. Available at: http://www.xrite.com/product_overview.aspx?ID=824. Accessed August 15, 2010.
14. Carbonite web site. Available at: http://www.carbonite.com/. Accessed August 15, 2010.
15. Dropbox web site. Available at: http://www.dropbox.com/. Accessed August 15, 2010.
16. Amazon web services web site. Available at: http://aws.amazon.com. Accessed August 15, 2010.
17. Schewe J. Announcing adobe Lightroom. Available at: http://photoshopnews.com/2006/01/09/announcing-adobe-lightroom/. Accessed August 15, 2010.
18. Adobe photoshop Lightroom 3 now available. Available at: http://www.adobe.com/aboutadobe/pressroom/pressreleases/201006/060810AdobeLightroom3.html. Accessed August 15, 2010.
19. Adobe creative suite 5. Available at: http://www.adobe.com/products/creativesuite/. Accessed August 15, 2010.

Technological Advances in Minimally Invasive TMJ Surgery

Joshua Wolf, DDS[a],*, Adam Weiss, DDS[a], Harry Dym, DDS[a,b]

KEYWORDS

- TMJ surgery • Arthrocentesis • Arthroscopy
- Temporomandibular joint

The technological advances in temporomandibular arthroscopy and arthrocentesis have given oral surgeons a treatment for patients who have not responded to conservative and pharmacologic treatment without the surgical risks and long-term recovery of open joint surgery.

The development of a less-invasive surgical treatment of temporomandibular joint (TMJ) pathology began in 1975 when Ohnishi first used an arthoscope to enter and study the TMJ.[1] The major surgical procedures that would follow to be used with the arthroscope were diagnostic, by attaching the arthroscope to a screen to visualize the joint and the lysis and lavage of the joint (**Fig. 1**). This procedure most commonly involves the placement of two arthroscopic portals, one of which is for the arthroscope and the other for a blunt probe. As the joint is observed and the adhesions are encountered, the probe can be used in a sweeping fashion to break up the adhesion. The use of the probe along with the hydraulic distention of the joint allow for stretching of the joint space. Images of preparation for and performing the procedure can be seen in **Fig. 2**. When the adhesions are broken down and the joint space distended, the joint movement improves and range of motion increases. Drugs, such as corticosteroids and sodium hyaluronate, have also been injected following the joint to reduce inflammation and improve lubrication, respectively. By 1991, Nitzan and colleagues showed that performing lavage of the TMJ without the scope, a procedure called arthrocentesis, gave similar results in the reduction of pain with success rates in up to 91% of patients.[2] Arthrocentesis involves placement of two cannulas into the superior joint for hydraulic distension and joint lavage. The initial application of the procedure was

[a] Department of Oral and Maxillofacial Surgery, The Brooklyn Hospital Center, 121 Dekalb Avenue, Brooklyn, NY 11201, USA
[b] Department of Dentistry, The Brooklyn Hospital Center, 121 Dekalb Avenue, Brooklyn, NY 11201, USA
* Corresponding author.
E-mail address: wolfjoshuac@gmail.com

Dent Clin N Am 55 (2011) 635–640
doi:10.1016/j.cden.2011.03.001
0011-8532/11/$ – see front matter © 2011 Elsevier Inc. All rights reserved.

dental.theclinics.com

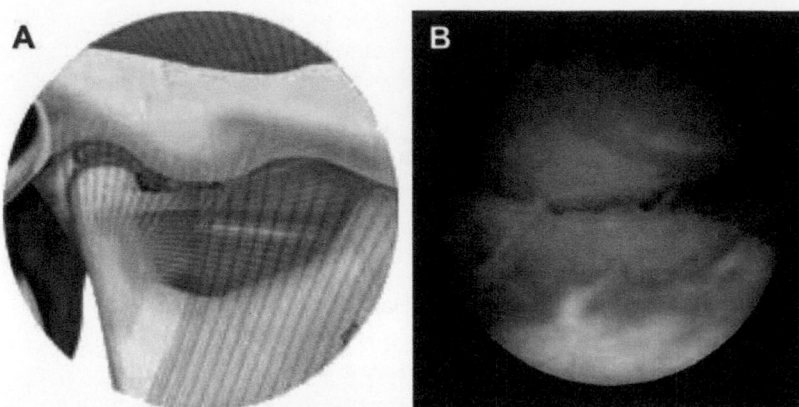

Fig. 1. (A) Drawing of the TMJ. The articular disc positioned between the mandibular condyle and articular fossa and eminence divide the joint into upper and lower compartments. (B) Arthroscopic view of upper compartment using the Onpoint 1.2 mm Scope System.

for the treatment of internal derangement of the TMJ. Later stages in this disorder can eventually lead to anterior disc displacement without reduction, also called closed lock because of the limited mobility of the jaw. This disorder is often accompanied by pain but the exact mechanism seems multifaceted. With the procedure's success in reducing pain and increasing mobility, arthrocentesis was expanded for treatment in other joint disorders. Recent comparisons between arthroscopy and arthrocentesis have shown both procedures to be successful (82% to 75%, respectively) with no significant difference in their success rates. Some investigators have argued that patients with chronic long-standing closed lock are more resistant to arthrocentesis and require TMJ arthroscopic lysis and lavage.[3]

There have been many theories as to the etiology of TMJ dysfunction and of how it results in pain. The focus of TMJ research at one time was on the shape and anatomic position of the deranged disc but the focus has changed to the biochemical

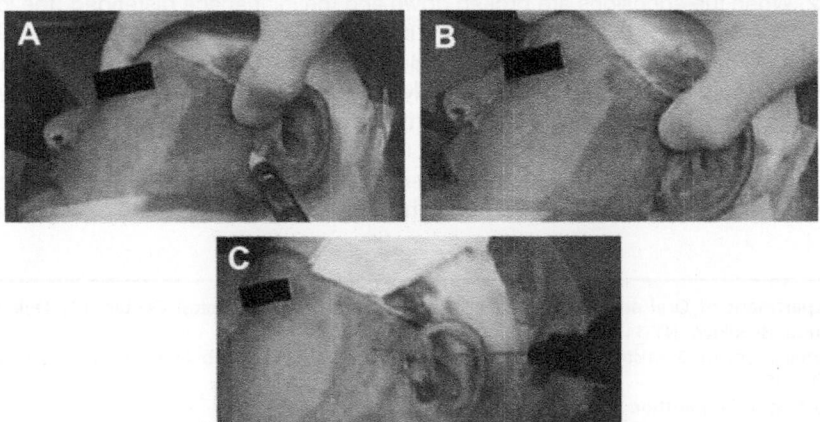

Fig. 2. (A) Patient is properly draped and local anesthetic is given into planned puncture point. (B) The upper joint compartment is entered and joint is insufflated with lactated Ringer solution. (C) Scope is placed into the cannula to perform arthroscopy.

environment and inflammatory mediators related to the pathologic joint. One theory for the success of arthrocentesis comes from the active elimination of the altered synovial fluid, which, together with physiotherapy, produces improved joint function with a diminished pain sensation.[4] Despite many studies showing that disc position and perforations do not improve with arthrocentesis, many patients have experienced improved TMJ function with less pain from this procedure.[5]

Before arthroscopic surgery or arthrocentesis is performed, conservative management must be attempted to see if symptoms can be relieved with out surgery. Literature has shown that nonsurgical management, which includes physical therapy, behavioral changes, and pharmaceuticals for internal derangement, can improve a patient's symptoms without the need for surgical treatment from 74% to 85% of the time.[6,7] Those who do not respond to conservative treatment may still benefit from arthrocentesis and/or arthroscopic lysis and lavage. Kim and colleagues[8] conducted a study investigating closed lock patients who had not shown response to the conservative treatment for more than 3 months. TMJ lysis and lavage were performed using an ultrathin arthroscopy, and positive outcomes were found in 80% of patients.

The other major indications for arthrocentesis are[9]

1. Acute and chronic limitation of opening because of anteriorly displaced disc without reduction
2. Chronic pain with good range of motion and anterior disc displacement with reduction
3. Degenerative osteoarthritis
4. A condition of TMJ open lock where the condyle is entrapped anterior to the condyle.

Contraindications to TMJ arthrocentesis are patients who have undergone successful conservative treatment, demonstrate bony or fibrous ankylosis, or have extracapsular sources of pain.

Arthrocentesis of the TMJ may be performed with the patient receiving a local anesthetic, intravenous conscious sedation, or general anesthetic depending on surgeon and patient preference.

As TMJ arthroscopy and arthrocentesis have gained popularity, new techniques, entry portals, and technology have been developed to enhance the classic arthroscopic procedure of the TMJ.

Moses[10] highlighted the general principles that all arthroscopy techniques must include the following:

1. The joint should be fully distended allowing easier trocar puncture and minimizing the risk of iatrogenic intracapsular damage.
2. The skin should be punctured with a sharp trocar.
3. All intracapsular procedures should be done with care to prevent articular surface damage.
4. Attention should be given to preserve as much healthy synovium as possible to enhance its physiologic effects on the joint.
5. The joint space should be kept expanded during instrumentation by a slow infusion irrigation system.

Over the past two decades the popularity of arthroscopy and arthrocentesis has grown because it has been considered a safe and effective procedure for TMJ pain with a low complication rate. Tsuyama and colleagues[11] first reported a 10.3% complication rate after arthroscopic procedures but a larger and more recent study showed a complication of only 1.3%, demonstrating the success of the new techniques and surgeons' increased experience with arthroscopy.[12] The major portion of complications was otologic problems, including blood clots in the external auditory meatus, perforation of the tympanic membrane, partial hearing loss, ear fullness, and vertigo. Other injuries included neurologic injury to fifth and seventh cranial nerves and TMJ injury possibly causing osteoarthritis. Correct portal placement lowers the chances of complications and decreases the chances of limited access within the TMJ during the arthroscopic technique. McCain and de la Rua[13] are given credit for combining anatomic knowledge with a surgical perspective, giving detailed, precise anatomic measurements for portal placement. Due to the anatomic variations from one patient to another, the portals are anatomically measured, then palpated for confirmation before cannulization is started.

Some of the major contributions to TMJ arthroscopy have come from the technological advances in arthroscopes. The improvements in camera and lens technology have advanced the ability to diagnose a wide variety of pathologic conditions within the TMJ. The Onpoint 1.2 mm Scope System is an innovative breakthrough that provides minimally invasive visualization of the joint in the convenience of an office-based setting (**Fig. 3**). The button on the hand piece allows still image and video recording for the visual effect of patient instruction, and visualization and smaller size could prevent complications. The disposable fiberoptic scope tube is approximately the size of an 18-gauge needle and is sterile packaged for single use. The Onpoint system is a single-portal system, thereby requiring only one puncture of the joint, and the new fiberoptic design tolerates more flexion to help avoid tissue trauma.

Advances in TMJ arthroscopy have also benefited from the addition of new laser surgery techniques. Procedures that can be performed with the holmium:YAG laser system include anterior muscle release procedures, lysing fibrous adhesions, treatment of chondromalacia, tissue débridement in symptomatic degenerative joint disease, treatment of synovitis, cauterization of bleeding vessels of hemostasis, discoplasty, removal of bone spurs and osteophytes, and discestomy. The major advantage of performing these procedures arthroscopically as opposed to as an open procedure is that it is minimally invasive and results in less periarticular tissue disruption and better preservation of vascular and lymphatic drainage to the joint.[14] By using the holmium:YAG laser instead of conventional cutting instrument fluid, surgeon precision is increased and diseased tisssue can be removed without mechanical contact, minimizing trauma

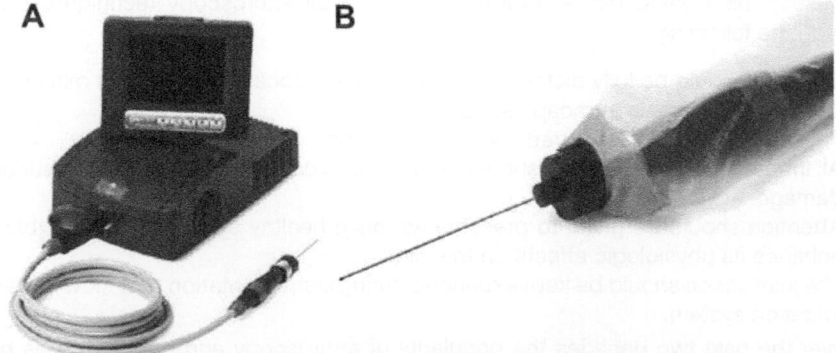

Fig. 3. (*A*) The OnPoint system is a small tube-like camera that projects the image onto a monitor with video and audio capabilities. (*B*) The disposable fiberoptic scope tube is approximately the size of an 18-gauge needle and is sterile packaged for single use.

to the articular cartilage. Arthroscopic laser surgery also produces significantly less tissue damage because the laser has less penetrance into surrounding tissue, allowing a surgeon to cut and ablate tissue while minimizing iatrogenic damage.

Arthrocentesis and arthroscopy have filled a major gap in the armamentarium of oral surgeons by providing a procedure to relieve pain and increase mobility in the joint for patients not responsive to conservative treatment and not having to perform open joint surgery. As the field has evolved, new techniques have made arthroscopy and arthrocentesis more successful, less invasive, and with fewer complications. In a recent study, Israel and colleagues[15] conducted a study analyzing the effects of TMJ arthroscopy early and later in patients' clinical courses. They found that TMJ arthroscopy reliably decreased pain and increased the maximum interincisal opening distance in both the early and late intervention groups. The early intervention group had better surgical outcomes than the late intervention group. They concluded that arthroscopic surgery should be considered earlier in the management of patients with inflammatory/degenerative TMJ disease. Israel and colleagues[15] recommend, "although a defined period of nonsurgical therapy is necessary before consideration for surgical intervention, continued treatment with non-surgical therapy that does not effectively relieve symptoms is not conservative. Arthroscopic surgery should be considered early in the management of patients with inflammatory/degenerative TMJ disease."[15]

REFERENCES

1. Ohnishi M. Arthroscopy of the temporomandibular joint. J Jpn Stomatol 1975; 42:207.
2. Nitzan DW, Dolwick MF, Martinez A. Temporomandibular joint arthrocentecis: a simplified treatment for severe, limited mouth opening. J Oral Maxillofac Surg 1991;49:1163.
3. Emshoff R, Rudisch A. Determining predictor variables for treatment outcomes of arthrocentesis and hydraulic distension of the temporomandibular joint. J Oral Maxillofac Surg 2004;62:816–23.
4. Nitzan DW, Price A. The use of arthrocentecis for the treatment of osteoarthritic temporomandibular joints. J Oral Surg 2001;59:1154.
5. Carvajal WA, Laskin DM. Long-term evaluation of arthrocentesis for the treatment of internal derangements of the temporomandibular joints. J Oral Maxillofac Surg 2000;58(8):852–5 [discussion: 856–7].
6. Green CS, Laskin DM. Long term evaluation of treatment for myofacial pain dysfunction syndrome: a comparative analysis. J Am Dent Assoc 1983;107:235–8.
7. Okeson JP, Hayes DK. Long term results of treatment for temporomandibular disorder: an evaluation by patients. J Am Dent Assoc 1986;12:473–8.
8. Kim YK, Im JH, Chung H, et al. Clinical application of ultrathin arthroscopy in the temporomandibular joint for the treatment of closed lock patients. J Oral Maxillofac Surg 2009;67:1039–45.
9. Ziccardi VB. Arthrocentecis of the temporomandibular joint. In: Fonseca RJ, editor. Oral and maxillofacial surgery. 2nd edition. Philadelphia: WB Saunders Co; 2000. p. 912–8.
10. Moses J. Temporomandibular joint arthrocentesis and arthroscopy: rationale and technique. In: Miloro M, editor. Peterson's principles of oral and maxillofacial surgery, vol. 2. 2nd edition. Hamilton (Ontario): BC Decker; 2004. p. 963–88.
11. Tsuyama M, Kondoh T, Seto K. Complications of temporomandibular joint arthroscopy: a retrospective analytic study of 301 lysis and lavage procedures performed using the triangulation technique. J Oral Maxillofac Surg 2000;58:500.

12. Gonzalez-Garcia R, Rodriguez-Campo FJ. Complications of temporomandibular joint arthroscopy: a retrospective analytic study of 670 arthroscopic procedures. J Oral Surg 2006;64:1591.

13. McCain JP, de la Rua H. Principles and practice of operative arthroscopy of the human temporomandibular joint. Oral Maxillofac Surg Clin North Am 1989;1: 135–52.

14. Mazzonetto R. Long term evaluation of arthroscopic discectomy of the temporo-mandibular joint using the Holmium YAG laser. J Oral Maxillofac Surg 2001;59: 1018–23.

15. Israel HA, Behrman DA, Friedman JM, et al. Rationale for early versus late intervention with arthroscopy for treatment of inflammatory/degenerative temporo-mandibuar joint disorders. J Oral Maxillofac Surg 2010;68:2661–7.

Index

Note: Page numbers of article titles are in **boldface** type.

A

AAPD caries-risk assessment tool, 424
Accupal, for anesthesia delivery, 486–487
Acetic acid, to detect oral lesions, 546
ActCel, 437
Alveolar buccal atrophy, in need of preimplant reconstruction, 454
Anesthesia, 482–483
    local, in dentistry, advances in, **481–499**
        delivery devices for, 485–494
      reversing of, 484–485
Anticonvulsants, with analgesic properties, 615
Antiseptics, dental caries and, 421
Antral communications, oral, polyurethane foam for closure of, 510–511
Anxiety, management of, current advances in, 616–617
    pain and, improper control of, mortality and morbidity of, 612–613
        management of, current treatments and advances in, **609–618**
        physiology of, 611
        relationship of, 611–612
Apexum device, in endodontics, 467–468
Arthrocentesis, of temporomandibular joint, 637–639
Arthroscopic surgery, of temporomandibular joint, 637–639
Articane, 482–483
    and paresthesia, 483
    efficiency of, 482
    in pediatric patients, 482–483
    metabolism of, 483
    safety of, 482
    structure of, 481

B

Bioengineering, in orthodontics, 582–583
Bleaching, dentin hypersensitivity due to, 601
Bone graft materials, bone regenerative properties of, 455
Bone grafting procedures, advanced techniques in, **453–460**
    safety assessments for, 456
    surgical procedure for, 456–457
Bone marrow aspirate concentrate, 459–460
Bone recombinant human bone morphologic protein-2, 454
Bone substitute synopsis, 454
Bone wax, 436–437
Brackets, self-ligating, in orthodontics, 571–573

Dent Clin N Am 55 (2011) 641–648
doi:10.1016/S0011-8532(11)00084-X
0011-8532/11/$ – see front matter © 2011 Elsevier Inc. All rights reserved.

dental.theclinics.com